Alzheimer's & Dementia

for

dummies®

A Wiley Brand

Alzheimer's & Dementia

for **dummies®**
A Wiley Brand

in conjunction with The American Geriatric Society and The Health in Aging Foundation

Alzheimer's & Dementia **For Dummies**®

Published by: **John Wiley & Sons, Inc.,** 111 River Street, Hoboken, NJ 07030-5774, www.wiley.com

Copyright © 2016 by John Wiley & Sons, Inc., Hoboken, New Jersey

Published simultaneously in Canada

No part of this publication may be reproduced, stored in a retrieval system or transmitted in any form or by any means, electronic, mechanical, photocopying, recording, scanning or otherwise, except as permitted under Sections 107 or 108 of the 1976 United States Copyright Act, without the prior written permission of the Publisher. Requests to the Publisher for permission should be addressed to the Permissions Department, John Wiley & Sons, Inc., 111 River Street, Hoboken, NJ 07030, (201) 748-6011, fax (201) 748-6008, or online at http://www.wiley.com/go/permissions.

Trademarks: Wiley, For Dummies, the Dummies Man logo, Dummies.com, Making Everything Easier, and related trade dress are trademarks or registered trademarks of John Wiley & Sons, Inc., and may not be used without written permission. All other trademarks are the property of their respective owners. John Wiley & Sons, Inc., is not associated with any product or vendor mentioned in this book.

For general information on our other products and services, please contact our Customer Care Department within the U.S. at 877-762-2974, outside the U.S. at 317-572-3993, or fax 317-572-4002. For technical support, please visit www.wiley.com/techsupport.

Wiley publishes in a variety of print and electronic formats and by print-on-demand. Some material included with standard print versions of this book may not be included in e-books or in print-on-demand. If this book refers to media such as a CD or DVD that is not included in the version you purchased, you may download this material at http://booksupport.wiley.com. For more information about Wiley products, visit www.wiley.com.

Library of Congress Control Number: 2016930756

ISBN 978-1-119-18773-8 (pbk); ISBN 978-1-119-18777-6 (ebk); ISBN 978-1-119-18776-9 (ebk)

Manufactured in the United States of America

10 9 8 7 6 5 4 3 2 1

Contents at a Glance

Table of Contents

Introduction

Pick up a newspaper or turn on the television or radio, and it won't be long before you come across a reference to Alzheimer's disease (AD) or dementia. Either someone is touting a breakthrough in research, or someone famous has been diagnosed with it, or an expert has decided that some food or other, which people have previously enjoyed without a second thought, is now believed to double our risk of developing the condition.

But its media popularity isn't really that much of a shock, because dementia is on the rise. In fact, scientists estimate that every four seconds someone somewhere in the world is diagnosed with dementia, so the number of cases is rising pretty fast.

Put simply, that increase means that more and more families are dealing with dementia or AD, trying to provide care for a loved one while maintaining some semblance of balance in their own lives. If you have a family member who's been diagnosed with AD or dementia, chances are you've got a lot of questions. *Alzheimer's and Dementia For Dummies* tries to help you find the answers that are right for your particular situation.

The media paints a big, frightening picture of how the increasing number of Americans with dementia will affect the economy, the healthcare industry, lost productivity, and a dozen other markers. However, little of that information is likely to hold much meaning for you as the family member that now must care for a loved one with a memory disorder. You want to know how Alzheimer's or some other form of dementia is going to affect your loved one as time goes on. As a caregiver, you want to know how to provide the best care for the person with dementia while you keep all the other balls in the air (work, spouse, the rest of the family, and other obligations).

About This Book

Dementia and AD are progressive conditions that affect sufferers more as time goes on. At present no cures are available. Although that is tough to swallow, we want to help you realize that you can do many things to improve the quality of life both for your loved one with a memory disorder and yourself, particularly if you're the primary caregiver.

Alzheimer's and Dementia For Dummies takes a realistic look at dementia and AD and offers pertinent, practical advice for dealing with the myriad of concerns and responsibilities that a primary caregiver must assume when managing a patient with a memory disorder. We look at the treatments available, both from mainstream medicine and complementary therapies, and review the evidence of what works and what doesn't. Other sections give tips to caregivers about how to handle difficult symptoms that may occur as the condition progresses. We emphasize the importance of taking care of yourself as the caregiver as you care for your loved one. We provide advice on the financial and legal issues that need to be considered. And we walk you through the details of how to choose the right residential care facility for your loved one should the need arise. Plus much more.

The main information about each topic is contained in the main text of each chapter, but you'll also notice shaded boxes of text in each chapter, called sidebars. These boxes offer interesting asides, designed to complement the rest of the chapter, rather than essential information. So if a sidebar doesn't interest you, just skip it; you'll still be able to understand everything else without it.

Within this book, you may note that some web addresses break across two lines of text. If you're reading this book in print and want to visit one of these web pages, simply type in the address exactly as it's noted in the text, pretending that the line break doesn't exist. If you're reading this as an e-book, you've got it easy: just click or tap the web address to be taken directly to the page.

Foolish Assumptions

As we wrote this book, we kept in mind everyone who has dementia or AD, or who may one day be affected by them. It's for those who are just generally worried about dementia and AD and want to find out more about the conditions and how they develop. If you're currently experiencing symptoms that you think may mean you have a memory disorder and want to know what to do next, you'll find valuable information here. We've also written this book for people who've already been given the diagnosis and need advice about how to get the best care available. People who are looking after people with dementia or AD can also use this book as a resource for being the best caregivers they can be.

But despite the wealth of information, we've designed this book so you don't need to have a degree in medicine or biology to understand the science stuff or be a lawyer to write a watertight will. Everything in this book should make sense to everyone with an interest in dementia and how best to care for the people who develop it.

Icons Used in This Book

As you go through the book, you'll notice that a variety of different icons pop up in the margins. These are designed to identify information that you need to know; information that may be interesting, but that you can live without; and hints about how to understand what you're reading:

TIP

These are handy bits of information that are worth remembering because they will help you deal with problems and perhaps head them off before they arise.

REMEMBER

These are key facts and important words that anyone wanting to get a handle on dementia or AD and what they're all about will want to know.

WARNING

This icon flags potential dangers and pitfalls that can lead to problems when managing dementia or AD.

TECHNICAL STUFF

This icon points out information that's interesting or in-depth but that isn't necessary for you to read.

Beyond the Book

In addition to the material in the print or e-book you're reading right now, this product also comes with some access-anywhere goodies on the web. These resources are crammed with useful summaries about everything you need to know about dementia. Check out the free cheat sheet at www.dummies.com/cheatsheet/alzheimersanddementia for more information about early symptoms of dementia and AD and tips about finding a suitable residential facility when your loved one can no longer be cared for at home.

You'll also find online articles at www.dummies.com/extras/alzheimersanddementia. One gives advice on how to cope with a patient who wanders; another discusses whether you should turn over power of attorney to a lawyer; the third talks about ensuring the patient's spiritual needs are met in her final days; and the last one lists ten points to tell the hospital staff if the person with the memory disorder is hospitalized for more than a few hours.

Where to Go from Here

We didn't design this book to be read from the front cover to the final page in order — although if you want to do that, it takes you on a logical journey from finding the diagnosis to dealing sensitively with end-of-life care. Instead, each chapter is designed to stand alone. You can read the chapters just as easily in a completely random order, according to your area of interest, as in numerical order by chapter.

If you don't know a thing about dementia or AD (or you just can't bring yourself to begin a book in the middle), start from the beginning with Chapter 1. If a loved one has received a diagnosis of dementia or AD and you want to know what treatments and care are available, check out Part 2. If you need advice on caring for someone with dementia or AD, see Part 3. If you're at the end of your rope and need some advice about maintaining your own mental and physical health, flip to Part 4.

Basically, thanks to the organization of all *For Dummies* books, the choice of how you read through this book is completely yours. But, however you decide to set off, we hope you enjoy learning more about this increasingly important subject.

1

Getting Started with Alzheimer's and Dementia

IN THIS PART . . .

Get an overview of dementia and Alzheimer's disease and see how the two are related.

Know what symptoms lead a doctor to consider the diagnosis of a memory disorder.

Discover the causes of dementia, the risk factors for developing it, and ways to possibly protect yourself from getting it.

Look at some other medical conditions whose symptoms, although similar to dementia, can be reversible with appropriate treatment.

Chapter 1

An Overview of Dementia and Alzheimer's Disease

I f you're reading a book about dementia, you first need to understand what the term means. People have a whole lot of different ideas about what sort of condition the word *dementia* suggests. For some, it's the diagnostic label you give to people who keep having "senior moments" and regularly forget names and where they put their eyeglasses. To others, it refers to people who are old and confused and spend all day shouting at the television and letting their friends and neighbors know exactly what they think of them.

Although some of these symptoms clearly can be part of the picture of dementia, neither of the people described actually fit the diagnosis. The first is probably just forgetful but otherwise well, and the second may simply be grumpy and bad-tempered. Dementia has a very clear definition, and the diagnosis should never be made lightly.

This chapter looks in detail at what dementia is and what it certainly is not and serves a jumping-off point for what you can expect to face when your loved one receives a dementia or Alzheimer's disease (AD) diagnosis.

Defining the Relationship between Dementia and Alzheimer's Disease

This section explains what dementia is and isn't and then does the same for Alzheimer's. As you read this text, keep in mind the relationship between dementia and AD. In many cases, what we write about dementia applies to AD, but what we write about AD may not apply to dementia in all of its forms.

Understanding what dementia is

Dementia is a general term for a decline in mental ability (including impaired memory, language, reasoning, judgment, visuospatial skills, and orientation) severe enough to interfere with daily life. Think of dementia as a big general category like the word "building." Just as there are many specific types of buildings (stores, houses, cabins, skyscrapers, factories, and so on), there are many specific forms of dementia. AD is the most common cause of dementia, making up about 60 percent of dementia cases. We discuss other forms of dementia later in this chapter.

Dementia isn't a single entity. Multiple different medical conditions that affect normal brain functioning are causes of dementia.

TECHNICAL STUFF

The World Health Organization (WHO) defines dementia thus:

[A] syndrome — usually of a chronic or progressive nature — in which there is deterioration in cognitive function (i.e. the ability to process thought) beyond what might be expected from normal aging. It affects memory, thinking, orientation, comprehension, calculation, learning capacity, language, and judgment. Consciousness is not affected. The impairment in cognitive function is commonly accompanied, and occasionally preceded, by deterioration in emotional control, social behavior, or motivation.

This definition, however, still contains a fair amount of medical jargon. So we tried to come up with a simpler, but still accurate, version by considering each of the key terms used by the WHO:

>> **Syndrome:** This word describes the symptoms that together are characteristic of a particular medical condition. People with the condition have most of these symptoms but don't have to show all of them to receive the diagnosis. Thus with dementia, one person may have poor memory and language but still have judgment enough to not walk out into a busy road,

whereas another may have problems with both memory and judgment but have no changes in language skills.

>> **Chronic and progressive:** These terms mean that the condition is ongoing long term and gets steadily worse with time. Many people think that the word *chronic* means that something is severe. Although dementia may be severe for some people, it's mild in others; *chronic* here means long-lasting.

>> **Consciousness:** Used in relation to dementia, this word takes on both of its meanings. People with dementia are both awake (as opposed to unconscious) and mentally aware of their surroundings, although what's going on around them is confusing to them.

REMEMBER

A number of diseases of the brain that lead to a collection of progressively worsening symptoms affecting a person's thought processes, mood, and behavior can cause dementia; eventually, the person loses the ability to carry out the basic tasks of daily living.

In the "Realizing that Dementia Doesn't Just Mean Alzheimer's" section later in this chapter, we explain the four main types of dementia to help you understand the bigger picture of memory disorders.

Grasping what dementia is not

In the past, dementia has been referred to as "senility" or "senile dementia." This terminology reflects the previously common but incorrect belief that serious mental decline is a normal part of aging. Many myths and misunderstandings circulate about dementia. And to get a grasp of what dementia actually is, it's important to have a clear idea about what it certainly isn't. So here's a selection of some of the most common misconceptions to help sort fact from fiction:

>> **All old people get dementia.** Although the chances of developing dementia do increase as people get older, it's not a normal part of the aging process. In the United States, 1 in 9 people older than 65 and 1 in 3 older than 85 suffer from it.

>> **Dementia is the same as Alzheimer's disease.** Alzheimer's disease is just one of a number of brain diseases that lead to dementia.

>> **Memory loss equals dementia.** Dementia does affect memory, but for someone to be diagnosed with the condition, he needs to show many other more complex symptoms rather than simply poor memory alone.

>> **Everyone with dementia becomes aggressive.** Even though some people with dementia can become agitated, aggression isn't a universal feature of dementia and is usually triggered by the way someone is treated or communicated with rather than being a symptom of the dementia alone.

>> **A diagnosis of dementia means a person's life is over.** Despite the fact that the condition is chronic and progressive, many medical, social, and psychological treatments and strategies are available to help make life as fulfilling as possible for someone with dementia, for many years.

>> **Everyone with dementia ends up in a nursing home.** Although one-third of people with dementia do eventually need this level of intense care in the later stages of their condition, many people are able to access enough help and support to stay in their own homes.

>> **My aunt has dementia, so I'm going to get it too.** Some forms of dementia do have a genetic component and may run in families, but these are in the minority. For most people, it doesn't follow that because a relative has dementia, they'll get it too. And contrary to what one patient thought, you can't catch it from your aunt either.

Understanding what Alzheimer's disease is

As previously stated, AD is a form of dementia. Although all AD patients have dementia, not all dementia patients have AD. The Alzheimer's Association defines Alzheimer's disease as "an irreversible, progressive brain disease that slowly destroys memory and thinking skills, eventually even the ability to carry out the simplest tasks." AD is a fatal disease, ending inevitably in death.

Alzheimer's disease was named after a German physician, Alois Alzheimer, who first identified the condition in 1906 when he performed an autopsy on the brain of a woman who'd been suffering severe memory loss and confusion for years. He observed microscopic amyloid plaques and neurofibrillary tangles in the woman's brain tissue under a microscope. He then correctly hypothesized that these abnormal deposits were responsible for the patient's loss of memory and other cognitive problems. To this day, AD can only be diagnosed with 100 percent accuracy through an autopsy that reveals the presence of the characteristic plaques and tangles in the brain. However, a comprehensive examination and good work-up do provide a reliable diagnosis with greater than 90 percent accuracy.

Abnormal deposits of specific proteins inside the brain disrupt normal brain function and cause the cognitive and functional problems typically associated with AD. Eventually, as these deposits spread throughout the brain, brain tissue starts dying, which leads to further cognitive impairment. The resulting brain shrinkage can be seen in CT scans and MRI scans. Current research is focused on trying to determine what causes these deposits and is looking for ways to prevent or reverse them before they cause permanent brain damage.

Seeing what AD is not

The preceding section talks about what AD is. Now allow us to go over what it isn't. AD is *not*

>> Curable

>> Contagious

>> A natural part of the aging process

>> Something you get from using deodorant or cooking in aluminum pans

>> Inevitable if you live long enough

Although certain familial forms of AD do run in families, these forms are extremely rare, accounting for less than 5 percent of all cases. So just because your mother or your brother got AD doesn't automatically mean that you're going to get it as well.

No test can predict whether you'll get AD unless you have the very rare inherited form of AD. A blood test exists that can tell you whether you have a certain form of a cholesterol-carrying protein associated with a higher incidence of AD, but that's all that it can tell you. The test can't tell you whether you'll actually develop the condition because at least 50 percent of the people who have the risk factor never get AD.

For ethical reasons, healthcare professionals advise against taking this blood test or undergoing other genetic testing because they want to spare their patients unnecessary worry about something that'll probably never happen even if the tests do come out positive. They also recommend against testing because if a person does find that he has inherited the gene or the risk factor, this information may negatively impact the person's ability to get long-term care coverage and lead to increased cost for health insurance.

Looking at the Link between Age and Dementia

A clear correlation exists between increasing age and the chances of developing dementia. In fact, less than 1 percent of people are diagnosed under the age of 65. Table 1-1 breaks down these figures.

The obvious question is whether dementia will become more common as people live longer. Thanks to advances in science, medicine, and technology, as a species we're living increasingly longer. Life expectancy until 30,000 years ago is believed to have been less than 30 years, and right up until the 1800s it was common for adults to die by the age of 40. Now the average man in the United States can expect to live for 76.4 years, whereas a woman can make it to the ripe old age of 81.2.

TABLE 1-1   **Dementia Diagnosis by Age**

Age	Number diagnosed
Younger than 65	1 in 1,500
65–70	1 in 100
71–79	1 in 20
80–89	1 in 4
90+	1 in 3

REMEMBER

These figures represent an average, and life expectancy across the United States varies depending on levels of poverty and other factors. To the same extent, life expectancy in some countries is much lower than in the United States; in the African nation of Chad, for example, it's only 49.5 years.

Over the next few decades these figures are expected to rise along with the proportion of older people in the population as a whole. According to government figures, currently 44 million people in the United States are older than 65 years of age. By 2030, it's estimated that 25 million more elderly people will be residing in the United States, rising to around 79 million by 2050.

A boy born in the United States in 2030 will have a good chance of living until he's 85, and a girl to 90. Given the rising chance of developing dementia with age, it's feared that cases will become far more common as a result of this boom in life expectancy.

Realizing that Dementia Doesn't Just Mean Alzheimer's

One of the most common misconceptions about dementia is that it means AD. Alzheimer's disease certainly does mean dementia, but numerous other causes of dementia also exist.

Also consider mild cognitive impairment, which isn't yet dementia but not part of the normal aging process either. For 40 percent of those patients who show signs of mild cognitive impairment, dementia is unfortunately their next step, but for the remainder, their symptoms will either not develop further, or may even be reversible if they are due to depression or the effects of an acute infection.

Considering the big four types of dementia

On safari in Africa, the guides bust a gut to make sure you get the best chance of glimpsing the so-called "big five": lions, African elephants, Cape buffalo, leopards, and rhinoceros. Dementia can be broken down into the "big four," Alzheimer's disease, vascular dementia, Lewy body disease, and frontotemporal dementia. Here is a quick field guide to each.

Alzheimer's disease

Alzheimer's disease is the most common cause of dementia worldwide. In the United States, it's the cause of dementia in 62 to 80 percent of cases, accounting for the symptoms of more than 5.3 million people in 2015. According to the Alzheimer's Association, one in nine Americans older than age 65 have Alzheimer's disease. Alzheimer's disease is the sixth leading cause of death in the United States and the fifth leading cause of death in Americans age 65 and older. Refer to the earlier section, "Understanding what Alzheimer's disease is" for more information about this form of dementia.

Vascular dementia

After AD, vascular dementia is the next most common cause of dementia, affecting more than half a million people — roughly 10 percent of the total cases of dementia in the United States. It was previously known as *multi-infarct* or *post-stroke dementia*. It occurs because decreased blood flow from blood vessel blockage or bleeding from infarcts (strokes) in the brain, which limits oxygen supply to brain cells.

Vascular dementia symptoms are similar to those seen in AD, but depend on which parts of the brain the reduced blood flow affects — what parts of the brain have experienced oxygen deprivation from strokes and how many brain cells have been affected. A person who has experienced strokes may also suffer additional weakness or even paralysis of limbs and speech difficulties.

Circulation problems become more common as we get older and can affect people who already have AD. As a result, at least 10 percent of people have *mixed dementia*; that is, they have Alzheimer's disease alongside vascular dementia, and a mix of symptoms of both.

Lewy body disease

A much rarer diagnosis, Lewy body disease makes up less than 4 percent of the number of dementia cases. Lewy bodies are protein deposits that damage brain cells. They're also found in the brains of people with Parkinson's disease, and as a result an overlap exists in the symptoms of people with these two conditions.

The symptoms of Lewy body dementia are also similar to those of Alzheimer's, but in addition these sufferers also develop muscle stiffness, tremors, and shakiness in their limbs, and slower movement. They also frequently experience visual hallucinations, commonly seeing animals or people around them that aren't really there.

Frontotemporal dementia

Frontotemporal dementia is the least common of the "big four," affecting about 50,000 people in the United States and representing less than 2 percent of total dementia cases. It's also the most likely of the four types of dementia to be diagnosed in people under the age of 65.

This type of dementia is named because of the areas of the brain that it affects most: the frontal and temporal lobes. These areas of the brain are involved in memory and personality. Thus frontotemporal dementia shares many of the features of AD, but has additional symptoms, including strange or sexually disinhibited behavior, lack of empathy, poor personal hygiene, apathy and loss of motivation, increased appetite for sweet or fatty foods, and repetitive and compulsive speech and actions.

Mild cognitive impairment: Dementia lite?

Dementia clearly isn't simply a memory problem, because it affects other thought processes along with mood and the ability to carry out all sorts of everyday tasks. Mild cognitive impairment involves more than the limitations that occur as a result of a normally aging brain, but not enough to constitute dementia. Long-term studies suggest that 10 to 20 percent of people age 65 and older may have mild cognitive impairment.

Like dementia, mild cognitive impairment can affect a variety of normal thought processes including memory, planning, and judgment, but it doesn't impact mood or a person's ability to perform day-to-day functions. And, although it can be a sign of future dementia (most likely AD) for some people, around 60 percent of people who develop mild cognitive impairment don't get any worse and some even get better.

The normally aging brain

It's no secret that as people get older, bits start to wear out and don't work quite as well as they once did. Joints become creakier, backs ache, eyesight isn't quite as clear, hair falls out or goes gray, once excitable parts of the body barely raise a smile, and memory isn't necessarily as sharp as it used to be.

TECHNICAL STUFF

Failing memory was once thought to result simply from a progressive loss of brain cells as people get older, but that's no longer believed to be the case. Research now suggests that unless people have a disease that wipes out their brain cells, they die with the same number as they had when they were born. And although human brains do shrink in overall size — by about 10 percent during adulthood — that loss of volume isn't the culprit behind memory problems.

A combination of factors actually conspires to create the infamous "senior moments." These include a decreased effectiveness of communication between nerve cells that whizz information around the brain, increase of inflammation in brain tissue in response to infection and disease reduction in blood supply, and damage caused by exposure to free radical molecules such as oxygen throughout life.

All these factors make up the recipe for the wear-and-tear type changes seen in the aging brain. Reflexes become slower, and it may take longer to finish a crossword puzzle. It's normal, although by no means universal, for people to experience these changes. Some people don't have even this level of deterioration and are as sharp as tacks well into their 90s (and even beyond).

The abnormally aging brain

In a person with mild cognitive impairment (MCI), the symptoms are more significant than those just described for normal aging. It's not uncommon for people to notice the following:

>> Forgetfulness

>> Difficulty following conversations

>> Declining ability to make sensible decisions

>> Getting lost easily

>> Poor concentration and attention span

Those people with MCI that do progress to dementia generally follow the progression charted by the Global Deterioration Scale (GDS) developed by Dr. Barry Reisberg in 1982. This score has seven stages:

>> **Stage 1:** No problems identified by doctors or the patient.

- **>> Stage 2:** The patient recognizes that he has a problem, perhaps with remembering names, but he scores normally on diagnostic tests.

- **>> Stage 3:** Subtle problems carrying out thought processes start to affect work and social activities. Tests may begin to pick up problems (this is mild cognitive impairment).

- **>> Stage 4:** Clear-cut difficulties develop in terms of memory and carrying out tasks such as dealing with finances or traveling. Denial is common. Early dementia has set in.

- **>> Stage 5:** The person needs some assistance but is still quite capable of washing, dressing, eating, going to the bathroom, and choosing appropriate clothes. Forgetfulness in relation to names and places is becoming more severe.

- **>> Stage 6:** The person is largely unaware of anything that's happened to him in the recent past. He needs help with most of the basic activities of daily living and may need to be looked after in a nursing home. Incontinence is common.

- **>> Stage 7:** By this stage the person is experiencing severe dementia. He's completely dependent on others for everything, often including mobility. Verbal communication skills are extremely restricted.

Recognizing the causes of mild cognitive impairment and taking steps to avoid it

Some cases of MCI are caused by the development of similar protein deposits to those found in AD. This finding isn't surprising, considering that those people with MCI who go on to develop dementia mostly develop AD. Other brain changes noted in MCI include worsening blood supply and shrinkage of the part of the brain called the hippocampus, which is involved with memory.

No specific treatment for MCI exists and, in particular, no evidence suggests that the drugs used to treat Alzheimer's disease are of any use. You can gain some mileage, however, by addressing risk factors for poor circulation by controlling your blood pressure, eating a low-carbohydrate and high-fiber diet, quitting smoking, drinking alcohol within the limits of recommended guidelines, and getting regular exercise.

Increasing evidence suggests that keeping the brain mentally active by doing word and number puzzles, reading and maintaining stimulating hobbies, and social activities can help too. (Consider reading *Staying Sharp For Dummies (John Wiley & Sons, 2016)*, which discusses this evidence in detail.)

Chapter 2

Spotting the Symptoms

As doctors, we love to be able to categorize diseases, and our ability to do our jobs properly depends on it. It's important to know that a certain set of symptoms means a patient simply has a nasty bout of the common cold, whereas another set of symptoms means she's more seriously ill with influenza. Without knowing what someone is up against, we can't advise on treatments or tell her the likely outcome of what she's going through.

In this chapter, we look in some detail at the symptoms that show that someone has dementia, including Alzheimer's disease (AD). And we help you understand when it may be time to see a doctor for a possible diagnosis.

Identifying the Early Warning Signs

Although dementia affects everyone slightly differently, a few common symptoms can alert you to the fact that it may well be on its way. In the early stages, though, it's important not to panic and see dementia lurking behind every forgetful or confused senior moment, because these types of memory lapses are often a normal part of the aging process. And it's important to bear in mind that there's much more to all types of dementia than simply becoming forgetful. These sections explain what dementia is and isn't so you know what to be worried about.

Differentiating between dementia and a few senior moments

Many things can make most people absentminded, from simple tiredness and poor concentration to a period of low mood or actual depression. How many people, busily caught up in an engrossing task or conversation, have forgotten a dental appointment or burned dinner?

Only when these symptoms become a regular feature of your behavior, or that of someone you love, may they be signs of something more serious. And the symptoms only really become significant when they start to interfere with a person's ability to carry out the tasks of everyday life.

Also, it's rare for memory issues alone to be enough to suggest that dementia is manifesting itself. Problems with finding the right words and confusion over using money or how to follow a favorite recipe are also likely to be evident, alongside changes in mood and loss of confidence in social situations.

REMEMBER

Dementia is not just about losing memory. It's also a decline in mental ability severe enough to interfere with daily life.

Knowing what to look out for

Here is a run-down of the top ten most important early symptoms to look out for, as voted for by pretty much every dementia charity website or research article you're likely to come across.

REMEMBER

As this list demonstrates, the symptoms of dementia are certainly more varied than simply being a bit forgetful. To be diagnosed, someone must show at least two, if not more, of these ten warning signs, which can themselves sometimes be fairly subtle to start with.

As the disease progresses, the symptoms become more obvious, because they become more permanent. Theses ten symptoms become part of a person's usual day-to-day life and behavior, and there's little doubt that the person has developed dementia.

In the rest of this chapter, we look in more detail at the symptoms, which can become more severe as time goes on. We split them into symptoms affecting thought processes, mood, and the way people function, for ease of explanation, but often a great deal of overlap exists between groups.

For now, we focus on some of the more general symptoms of dementia. People with different types of dementia can develop other symptoms that are particular to their specific diagnosis — for example, AD or Lewy body disease. Also bear in mind that some people may be lucky enough to develop few of the symptoms we describe, and that the examples in the following sections are offered as a guide to what may happen and not what always happens to someone with dementia.

Number 1: Memory problems that affect daily life

Forgetting the odd thing every now and again is perfectly normal as you get older; generally, you remember these things later. In dementia, you don't remember things later; those forgotten things are gone. Unfortunately, you need to remember things such as the following to be able to function normally every day:

» Important dates and events

» The route taken on well-traveled journeys

» Where you've left important paperwork

» Names and faces of friends, neighbors, and work colleagues

Number 2: Difficulty with planning and problem solving

Co-author Dr. Atkins's grandmother could cook a turkey with all the trimmings with her eyes closed — until she started to develop dementia. As the disease took hold, her ability to time the cooking of meat and vegetables completely deserted her, and she'd regularly burn some of the vegetables while undercooking the meat. In the end, grandpa had to take over the chef's duties or everyone would regularly go hungry.

As well as having trouble following recipes, people in the early stages of dementia may also

>> Become confused using a debit card, credit card, or checking account

>> Lose track of what their bank statement or credit card statement shows

>> Have difficulty paying bills or filing taxes

>> Become confused while trying to put gas in the car

Number 3: Problems finding the right word

Most people will have had the experience of frantically hunting for the right word when chatting with someone or, worse still, when giving a presentation to a group of colleagues. Eventually, the word comes to mind, the panic's over, and you stop feeling stupid.

In early dementia, many people find that words regularly become elusive, leading to difficulty communicating effectively and to huge amounts of frustration. People with early dementia may also substitute the word they're after for something similar, such as a football becoming a *kick ball,* or a wristwatch becoming a *hand clock.*

People may also have problems following the thread of other people's conversations and may therefore become less inclined to join in and socialize with others to save themselves embarrassment. Socializing can become a particular problem in noisy environments or in situations where other background conversations are going on, because people with dementia find it harder to focus on the conversation that they're supposed to be having.

Number 4: Confusion about time and place

People with early dementia often lose track of time or become muddled about the date. They may also forget where they are or how they got there. As an example, a patient of Dr. Atkins's sat in the waiting room for ages, expecting to be called in for his appointment. Unfortunately, although he did have an appointment at that time, it was across town with his dentist.

Number 5: Poor judgment

Another of the losses that occurs in early dementia is that of good judgment. Normally frugal people may end up spending money on things they don't need and can be a telemarketer's dream customer, signing up for all kinds of special offers.

Judgment about appropriate dress may also suffer, with people heading off to the beach wearing a coat, hat, and scarf or, conversely, going shopping in the pouring rain with only a T-shirt and sandals to protect them from the elements.

Number 6: Visuospatial difficulties

Increasing clumsiness can herald the start of dementia. As people are robbed of their ability to judge widths and distances, falls and breaks are common, as are bumps (or worse) when parking or driving a car.

Number 7: Misplacing things

Although everyone forgets where they've put their keys or cellphone from time to time, you can usually retrace your steps and eventually find them. This ability to retrace steps is lost in dementia. Coupled with an increasing tendency to leave things in the wrong place as well (such as slippers in the refrigerator), important objects go missing more often.

Number 8: Changes in mood

When our children were teenagers, rapid mood swings were an extremely common feature of life in our homes. One minute a decision we'd made meant we were the worst people in the world, and the children felt angry and a bit sorry for themselves; the next (usually when cash had changed hands), we were great people, and they couldn't think of anyone they'd rather have as parents.

As people grow into adulthood, these extremes of mood and temperament thankfully tend to be much less evident. But in the early days of dementia, this type of fluctuating mood can return, with people often rapidly switching between extremes of sadness, fear, and anger. Low moods and depression are also extremely common in dementia. At times it can be hard to work out whether the symptoms of dementia are causing the depression or vice versa.

Number 9: Loss of initiative

Although anyone can become fed up with work, hobbies, and even social obligations, it's often a passing phase after a tough day or a bad night's sleep, and you snap out of it. People with dementia may lose interest in taking part in their usual activities altogether and repeatedly need prompting about what they should be doing or simply to join in with what friends or family are doing.

Number 10: Personality change

A number of different changes are possible here, and not all people who are developing dementia will change in the same way. In fact, often what changes is their normal behavior, so a reserved and quiet person may become flirty and disinhibited, whereas the life and soul of many an extrovert may become withdrawn and reclusive. Common changes include becoming

>> Confused

>> Suspicious

>> Withdrawn

>> Angry

>> Sexually disinhibited

Recognizing Thought-Processing Problems

The *thought-processing* (cognitive) symptoms of dementia are all those of loss. People with dementia will, to one degree or another, lose their memory, their judgment, and quite literally their way. These sections examine these problems a bit more so you can see how dementia may impact someone.

Forgetting things

When my (co-author Dr. Wasserman) uncle Eddie developed AD, he'd pop into my mom's house around the corner four or five times a day to ask her what she was up to. If he got no reply, he'd put a note in her mailbox that simply said, "Fern, where are you?" And all this despite the fact that on his first and no doubt second visit, she'd told him exactly what she was up to that day and where she was going.

In contrast, my aunt, who had vascular dementia, was well aware of everything that was going on each day, but she had an awful memory for names and faces. Not only would she mix me up with my brother, but she'd also often call me Bill, which was her son's name.

And the many aspects of forgetting that can occur in dementia go way beyond these two examples from family history.

REMEMBER

Memory can be affected by dementia in more than one way. People with AD may experience problems learning new material or may forget information that they previously knew or both. Problems learning and retaining new information often precede the loss of already learned information.

The key point regarding memory loss due to AD is that it's not static. As AD progresses, you realize you're not seeing just occasional forgetfulness but a pattern of steadily worsening memory loss.

MEMORY FOR DUMMIES

A fully functional memory is vital for human existence. That's because without some way of remembering what's happened, every waking moment stands alone as a brand-new experience; you have no past and can't plan for the future. Sadly, memory is one of the main casualties of the different dementia processes.

Two main types of memory exist: short-term and long-term memory. You also possess an emotional memory, which is completely preserved in dementia, and which we mention at the end of this sidebar.

- **Short-term memory:** *Short-term memory* is your working memory, which stores information for a short time only (hence its name) before it's either forgotten or transferred to long-term memory for storage, potentially for the rest of your life. Short-term memory, it's believed, allows people to remember lists of only seven to nine items, for around 30 seconds. Repeating these items over and over in your head can help keep them there, but if you're distracted by something else or the 30 seconds run out, the items are gone.

- **Long-term memory:** *Long-term memory* has unlimited capacity, and memories can be stored until your dying day. It has two main forms:

  - **Declarative memory:** This is memory for facts such as bank account or phone numbers, computer passwords, meanings of words, general knowledge, and events in your past.

  - **Procedural memory:** This allows you to remember how to carry out tasks without having to relearn them each time. It's what makes riding a bike easy when you haven't done it for a while. And it's what enables us to know how to hold a knife and fork each time we pick them up, or to brush our teeth using the same technique each day.

The development of a long-term memory in the brain involves three crucial steps. If any of these steps don't work, the memory is effectively lost — and that's what can happen in dementia:

- Encoding (which ensures that all types of sensory input are in a suitable form for storage)

- Storage

- Retrieval

(continued)

(continued)

Encoding can be thought of as the way in which the nervous system labels a fact, emotion, smell, image, or whatever is to be remembered so it can be stored for further use. It's very similar to the way in which librarians assign specific numbers to books depending on their subject matter so someone searching for them among the many bookshelves can easily find them.

Emotional memory

Emotional memory allows you to recall the really important moments in your life, both good and bad. It stores not only the information about what happened, but also an exact memory of how you felt. It means that if you find yourself in a similar situation in future, you'll probably experience those feelings again.

Classic short- and long-term memories are created in a part of the brain called the *hippocampus*, and long-term memories are stored in different parts of the outside of the brain called the *cerebral cortex*. Cells in these areas and those that communicate between them can be damaged in dementia, stopping the encoding, storage, and retrieval processes.

In contrast, emotional memory appears to occupy much more primitive parts of the brain, particularly in the brain stem. These areas aren't affected by dementia, meaning that emotional memory can remain intact.

The implication here is that people with dementia can still be troubled by stored memories of negative events, such as the experience of being beaten by a parent as a child. If, because of dementia, a person believes that a long-dead father is still alive, that person may experience some strong negative emotions. Likewise, an action carried out in the present, such as an injection, that provoked an unhappy response in the past may cause the person with dementia to respond negatively to it. These emotional memories are thought to lead to some of the disturbed and aggressive behavior seen in people with dementia.

With more advanced AD, your loved one may have trouble recalling familiar people and places as well as forming new memories; recent events seem to drift away as soon as they're over. For example, a person with dementia may forget that a grandchild visited only two hours before.

Memory for dates and times

The caricature of a person with dementia is someone who can remember every detail of World War II, which she lived through as a child, but can't remember what she had for breakfast today, or even what day it is. And in a sense, this caricature can be accurate. Dementia tends to involve a loss of short-term memory while many aspects of long-term memory are preserved.

Short-term memory is, in effect, working memory, helping you to function day by day by allowing your brain to remember lists, appointments you need to attend, phone numbers, or where you put your door key. *Long-term memory*, on the other hand, stores all sorts of information from the past, mingling sights, sounds, smells, and the dates of events to give you a rich picture of your life going all the way back to childhood.

In dementia, this loss of short-term memory presents all sorts of problems and can lead to difficulties remembering appointments, important messages, and especially the day and date, so that the person becomes completely disorientated.

Memories of people and places

Forgetting other people's names and faces is another common problem associated with dementia. These memories are often stored in long-term memory, but when a person experiences problems retrieving these memories, even family members can feel like strangers. For example, a wife awakened in the night thinks that her husband sleeping next to her really is a stranger and she yells at him to get out of her bed. This effect on memory can be particularly significant in the workplace, leading to the person with dementia forgetting her boss or important clients.

Forgetting places increases the chance that someone with dementia will easily get lost, even in the most familiar surroundings, and find it hard to follow the directions of any new route you try to tell her. A person with dementia may get lost and end up across town when he was trying to drive to the neighborhood grocery store only two blocks away, despite driving there hundreds of times in the past.

CHILDHOOD MEMORIES

I (Dr. Wasserman) vividly remember the first time my grandfather took me to a baseball game on July 4, 1967. Not simply because my home team, the Dodgers, beat our archrivals, the Giants, 4-2, but because my long-term memory has stored the associated smell of cigar smoke that in those days wafted around the grounds, the sounds of the chanting supporters, and the emotional feeling of an 8-year-old doing something grown up with his grandpa. To this day, every time I get a whiff of cigar smoke, I'm transported back to that day, sitting in the bleachers at Dodger Stadium watching Drysdale overpower the Giants.

Memories of self

When short-term memory malfunctions, it's believed to result in people with dementia losing their sense of self. This mostly affects the present self, and such people may have an intact sense of who they were when they were younger, thanks to their long-term memory.

People with dementia who constantly follow their partners or caregivers around and keep repeating the same questions may be seeking reassurance and protection from that person to make up for this loss of their own sense of self.

Problems with language (aphasia)

Although memory loss is a key symptom that doctors look for when trying to assess the presence of AD, language impairment, which is also called aphasia, is another symptom that may be present.

Many people develop language problems early in the course of AD. You may notice someone who used to be an avid talker now has trouble finding the right word to express himself. Or you may notice hesitations in his speech that weren't there before or find yourself filling in words for him or anticipating or interpreting his speech. A person with AD may say a similar but incorrect word or give a description of what he's trying to say but never recall the word he wanted to use. Unlike the memory problems that are present in all AD patients, difficulty with speech doesn't affect every AD patient.

REMEMBER

As AD progresses, problems with language tend to become more noticeable. Your loved one may have trouble putting together a coherent sentence or start speaking in a nonsensical or fanciful language that is hard to understand. Patients who are particularly sensitive to their language difficulties may withdraw socially, become more passive in social situations, and rely on you because they're frustrated with their inability to express themselves. They may also withdraw because they fear embarrassment or that someone will find out they have a problem comprehending or following conversation.

As language skills deteriorate, so do reading comprehension and the ability to understand what others are saying. Some families find it helpful to label everyday objects to assist their loved one in maintaining some feeling of control over their environment; other families find that signs or labels do no good because their loved one can't understand them.

Getting lost and wandering

When someone's memory for places has ceased to function as it used to, it's very common for her to get lost, even when traveling on extremely familiar routes. In addition, people with dementia tend to wander, which adds to the likelihood that they'll get lost.

REMEMBER

Wandering is rarely an aimless activity and would actually be better described as walking without purpose. It's not often obvious to caregivers why people with dementia sometimes wander, but some suggested reasons include the following:

>> **Continuing with a habit:** People who enjoy walking as either their main means of transport or as a hobby are very likely to continue doing it.

>> **Relieving boredom:** People with dementia often don't have a lot to do, especially as the condition progresses and they withdraw from work and socializing. Going for a walk relieves this boredom and provides a sense of purpose.

>> **Using up energy:** People who were normally quite active and enjoyed exercise may feel restless if they're unable to continue to go out. Going for a walk is a very simple solution.

>> **Being confused:** People with dementia may have an idea they have to be somewhere to do something, but as soon as they've headed off, they become lost and keep wandering, trying to identify familiar landmarks. Sometimes, when confused about time, people with dementia get up in the night thinking it's morning, get dressed, and go out.

>> **Relieving pain:** People with arthritis stiffen up if they're inactive for long periods, which makes their joints extremely painful. Going for a walk loosens things up and temporarily relieves this pain.

>> **Searching:** The person with dementia may be looking for a particular place or person. It may be a former home or the house she grew up in. She may be searching for old friends, family members, or even long-dead parents.

Progressive lack of judgment

Sensible decision making is key to so many areas of adult life, particularly when it comes to dealing with money, health, and the assessment of a multitude of potential risks. Once again, dementia can rob people of this ability, creating potential physical and financial dangers.

Dealing with money

This potential danger can range from people with dementia simply forgetting how to use an ATM to writing checks or running up credit card bills for all sorts of charitable causes that they wouldn't normally support or services they don't need and will never use.

WARNING

We know lots of stories about people who've lost the ability to maintain a balance in their checking account or pay credit card bills on time, and who've been sold unnecessary insurance policies over the phone. In one case, this lack of financial judgment cost the person's employer thousands of dollars.

Awareness of danger

Poor judgment in relation to danger can not only have personal ramifications but also put others at risk. In particular, people with dementia

>> Have difficulty evaluating the relative risk of situations they find themselves in

>> Lose the ability to determine the relative importance of things

>> Misjudge environmental conditions and go out unprepared

>> Find it hard to think through the logical outcomes of their decisions

>> Misjudge the intentions of others

>> Overestimate their capabilities

WARNING

Put all these elements together and dementia puts people at significant risk of being manipulated or taken advantage of by others, getting robbed or mugged, being a liability behind the wheel of a car or on a bicycle or motorcycle, jaywalking (one patient was picked up by the police as she wandered along a major street in her nightgown), and developing hypothermia as a result of going out in unsuitable clothing and then getting lost.

Observing Emotional Changes

Emotions comprise the next big category of mental functions affected by dementia. In fact, for some people with dementia, the term *emotional rollercoaster* isn't an exaggeration. For families and caregivers, the emotional changes wrought by dementia can be a huge challenge. The following sections address some of these emotional changes.

Maintaining a sense of humor can really help a family make it through the challenges of caring for an AD patient. If you respond to a difficult situation with humor instead of anger, you're gaining two benefits: first, your humor can help defuse your loved one's anger or aggression, and second, your humor helps you avoid becoming overly stressed.

Aggression and agitation

One of the biggest myths about dementia is that everyone who develops it will become angry and aggressive. Although it can happen to some people (some studies suggest a range of 30 to 50 percent), it's by no means a universal problem and, like anger in other aspects of life, it rarely happens for no reason.

Types of aggression

The aggression expressed by a person with dementia can be both verbal and physical:

>> **Verbal:** Shouting, swearing, screaming, threatening, and refusing to comply with a request

>> **Physical:** Hitting, kicking, slapping, biting, scratching, pulling hair, and making offensive hand gestures (although these can simply be forms of nonverbal gesturing with no offense intended)

This behavior can occur in people who were quite aggressive and confrontational before they developed dementia, but can also arise in people who normally wouldn't hurt a fly. The aggression may just be a phase that the person is going through and may settle down with time and appropriate support. And the outbursts may have more to do with the way they are being handled or spoken to, rather than with an intrinsic change in their personality.

Reasons behind aggression

A host of physical, psychological, and social causes can trigger aggressive behavior that if adjusted can sometimes alleviate this symptom:

>> **Physical:** Physical aggression can be a direct result of changes in the brain caused by the dementia, or side effects from some of the medication prescribed to treat it. Paranoia, delusions, and hallucinations can also prompt protectively aggressive reactions.

- *Paranoia* is an unfounded or exaggerated distrust or irrational suspiciousness of others.

- *Delusion* is an irrational and unshakeable belief in something untrue despite obvious proof to the contrary.

- *Hallucination* is a sensory experience in which a person can see hear, smell, taste, or feel something that isn't there.

Equally, however, aggression can be caused by things that would annoy anyone but that generate a more extreme reaction as a result of the disinhibition that can occur due to changes in the brain. These other triggers include noisy surroundings, pain, hunger, thirst, and the person simply not getting along with someone.

>> **Psychological:** A sense of fear and uncertainty is common in dementia because of the memory and other cognitive problems that it can cause. Feeling frightened and unsure can make people overprotective of themselves, which can lead to anger. Misinterpretation of caregivers' actions is another common cause of anger. Frustration with their loss of ability to carry out some tasks can also make people irritable, as can, conversely, people being too helpful and not letting patients with dementia do things for themselves.

>> **Social:** Loneliness, boredom, personality clashes with others, and even the well-meaning but poorly performed actions of caregivers can trigger anger and aggression. If someone poked a sponge on a stick at you while you were in the shower, you'd certainly get agitated!

Social problems

As AD progresses, your loved one may develop social problems. He may become so disoriented and disconnected from his normal routine that withdrawing just seems easier. He also may withdraw because of an increased awareness of his problems. This self-imposed isolation is a common behavior in AD patients.

AD patients may become embarrassed because they can't keep up with their personal hygiene or laundry. Poor personal care may result in social isolation, particularly if the person with AD is living alone. If a family member asks her about her hygiene or whether she has been eating regularly, she may become argumentative, combative, or simply withdraw into silence.

Alzheimer's daycare facilities can help families meet their loved one's social needs by providing structured activities with other AD patients in a controlled, secure environment. Many patients respond favorably to this sort of planned activity. (For more benefits of adult daycare, see Chapter 14.)

Sexual disinhibition

Sexuality is a normal part of life whether you're young or old, have dementia, or don't. People with dementia, however, lose control of the social mechanisms that keep their romantic desires in check at inappropriate moments.

This inability to control sexual impulses can manifest itself very mildly — for example, some people are simply more flirtatious or overly familiar with others — but in extreme cases can involve exhibitionism and making unwanted sexual advances. This behavior is more common in men with dementia than in women and can involve the following, in descending order of frequency:

>> Making inappropriate comments

>> Touching

>> Fondling

>> Undressing in public

>> Making sexual advances

>> Masturbating in public

The top two on this list are the most common and probably least offensive; the bottom three happen in up to 10 percent of people with dementia, most commonly as their condition progresses.

Paranoia

People with dementia can develop unfounded fears of being persecuted and can become unnecessarily suspicious of the actions and motives of other people. This paranoia can stem directly from damage to the brain by the process of dementia itself or as a byproduct of the confusion that dementia causes. In the latter case, the confusion causes people to misinterpret the actions of others, which they then misconstrue as either negative or outright persecutory. An example here is a husband living in a nursing home believing his wife has maliciously abandoned him because he can't remember her daily visits or recognize the photographs of her in his room.

TIP

If Alzheimer's patients become suspicious to the point of delusion, their suspicions may involve one or more of these common themes:

>> They believe a stranger is living in the house and going through their things (known as the *Phantom Boarder syndrome*).

>> They believe someone is stealing their personal belongings.

>> They believe someone is stealing their money, although they may have actually given it away or misplaced it.

>> They believe their spouse is having an affair.

Without careful management, this paranoia can provoke unnecessary anxiety, distress, and agitation, leading perhaps to more disruptive and aggressive behavior. Caregivers can also help reduce it by making sure they aren't communicating with the person in oppressive ways or repeatedly reprimanding her.

Mood swings

Variations in mood are a normal part of life for everyone. On a basic level, you often feel differently on a Monday morning at the start of a long workweek than you do on a Friday, just four mornings later, with the weekend in sight. Your mood goes up before a party, before a hot date, or after receiving good news, but can swing the other way after learning of a death, when you've been dumped by the hot date, or when you experience financial worries.

What's different in dementia is that these mood swings can occur rapidly and without the obvious triggers just mentioned. One minute someone may be sitting calmly chatting away to you, and literally the next minute she's pacing the room or crying. The tiniest things can also cause major reactions with mountains frequently being made out of molehills. This symptom is particularly noticeable if the person concerned has always been calm and collected.

Noting Functional Problems

Alongside the memory problems and emotional changes that happen to someone with dementia, getting in a pickle carrying out practical tasks is the other noticeable development that goes hand-in-hand with the other problems to lead to a diagnosis.

Of course, some people can make even the simplest practical tasks — from changing a light bulb to hanging a picture — seem extraordinarily difficult. But in a person with dementia, a combination of changes in the brain can make struggling with many of life's little tasks that the following sections discuss the rule rather than the exception.

Which shoe on which foot?

As a young man, co-author Dr. Atkins's uncle was an engineer in the army. In later life he taught often extremely intricate engineering skills to young recruits in the Royal Electrical and Mechanical Engineers (the UK equivalent of the Army Corps of Engineers). Unfortunately, as an elderly man he developed dementia and became incapable of dressing himself without ending up with something inside out or the buttons fastened incorrectly, and even his shoes on the wrong feet.

As a former military man, he certainly knew how to dress, and when Dr. Atkins was a young man at school, his uncle taught him how to shine his shoes until he could see his reflection in their toecaps. But these changes in his attire weren't due to sloppiness because he was running late or had dressed in the dark, which explains most of Dr. Atkins's wardrobe malfunctions. This uncle got it wrong every time, in different ways, and when his shoes looked scuffed and unpolished, Dr. Atkins and his family knew that something was seriously wrong.

This sort of confusion is extremely common in dementia and is associated with a slowing down of the whole dressing process, because each stage needs to be focused on and is invariably carried out incorrectly. Clothes that were always spotless may start to appear dirty or un-ironed, and the person's appearance may well show a lack of the effort previously put into maintaining it.

REMEMBER

This is an example of a problem with what is called executive function: putting plans into action. The more steps involved, the more difficult they are to perform. Executive functions include planning, organizing, sequencing, and abstracting abilities. Any loss in executive functions impacts a patient's ability to make decisions, make and follow plans, establish goals, control impulses, think abstractly, and reason and solve problems.

Kitchen nightmares

Although most people are able to go through the process of preparing a familiar meal without much effort, and can certainly follow a recipe fairly easily, people with dementia start to find this a struggle and would soon have Gordon Ramsay yelling expletives at them if they were cooking in one of his kitchens.

One function of long-term memory is to help you remember how to carry out various common practical procedures so you can do them on autopilot rather than think each stage through every time. The retrieval of these memories can be impaired in dementia, making the process of changing a light bulb, riding a bike, or whipping up a plate of ham and eggs more difficult.

Short-term memory problems and difficulties with timing also mean that food can often be burned, undercooked, or left cold in the oven long enough to grow a layer of mold on top. People with dementia may have stacks of spoiled rotten food in their refrigerator due to their inability to properly perform food preparation as well as their forgetting to eat the prepared food family members so graciously bring to them.

Housework becoming a chore

Now, we know that not everyone is fastidious when it comes to housework and tidiness. We've visited enough homes as geriatricians to know that not everyone's floor is clean enough to eat off. (In fact, we've had to sit on our doctor's bags on more than one occasion, because the patient's sofa was teeming with wildlife.)

But a change in the way a formerly independent person keeps her home can be another indicator of dementia when coupled with any of the other changes we describe in this chapter. The person may forget to do housework or simply become distracted halfway through, but a dirty home may also be the result of the loss of initiative that features in the top ten early warning signs earlier in this chapter. The houses of the chronically untidy can, of course, simply just become even worse. Dr. Atkins remembers visiting an old man who was sitting in his armchair surrounded by piles of dirty, moldy plates and old newspapers, with a bucket in the middle of the room that served as a toilet.

WARNING

Hoarding is another common behavior in dementia patients. Especially if the individual developing dementia has always been a bit of a pack rat, such behavior as collecting things can go to the extreme of hoarding. Newspapers can become stacked everywhere in the living room, mail (including unpaid bills) can be piled on the counters, trash can accumulate in the kitchen, and plastic grocery bags can fill closets. Medications may become stockpiled because the patient forgets why he is taking them or doesn't remember how much to take. Sometimes this behavior comes from the person with dementia being confused at how to handle a situation, like his inability to pay bills so they stack up unpaid. Other times items are hoarded because the person with dementia fears his memories will be lost without tangible evidence of the past. As brain function decreases and confusion increases, hoarding can become a safety hazard with junk piles throughout the house that are a tripping as well as a significant fire hazard.

Picking Up on Physical Symptoms

Unlike memory problems, which are noticeable almost from the onset of AD, with few exceptions early-stage patients display almost no significant physical disabilities. However, some patients do experience the following physical symptoms.

Identifying extrapyramidal signs

As the disease advances, some patients may display what is known as *extrapyramidal* signs including tremors, rigidity, and slowness of movement. This kind of physical symptom may also indicate the development of another condition or a problem with medications interacting.

More commonly, patients who exhibit extrapyramidal signs early in the disease are at risk for developing non-Alzheimer's dementia, such as that caused by a vascular accident like a stroke. Parkinson's disease or some antipsychotic drugs like haloperidol (Haldol) may cause the symptoms.

If your loved one has an odd shuffling gait or swings his legs in wide circles from the hip as he walks, have him evaluated immediately. These extrapyramidal symptoms may respond well to treatment if caught early enough.

TECHNICAL STUFF

If you're thinking that extrapyramidal means outside the pyramid, you're almost right. Many of the nerves that control movement and sensation run through a part of the brain stem called the *medulla,* which is shaped somewhat like a pyramid. The nerves running from the medulla to the spinal cord are called the *pyramidal tract,* and they control all voluntary muscle movement like walking or raising your hand. Nerves outside of this main bundle are called extrapyramidal and run from a group of brain structures called the *basal ganglia.* The extrapyramidal nervous system controls involuntary motor movement like posture, balance adjustments, and non-intentional gross motor movements that are part of a more complex act like walking. Damage to the extrapyramidal nerve system can result in a disruption or impairment of motor ability.

Patients with more advanced AD may display extrapyramidal signs; it depends on how the AD progresses in each case. If the neurofibrillary tangles and amyloid plaques that are characteristic of AD (see more about this in Chapter 3) invade the basal ganglia, extrapyramidal symptoms follow because the functioning of this part of the brain is disrupted. Remember that if extrapyramidal symptoms occur, these degenerative changes are more likely to happen in the later stages of the disease.

Restlessness

Another significant physical symptom that develops as AD progresses is restlessness. The patient can't seem to sit still for a moment and is constantly pacing around with no real purpose in mind.

Restlessness may also manifest as sleep disruption, occurring in as many as 45 percent of all AD cases. Some patients withdraw and sleep almost all the time, while others barely sleep at all. Many families report that their AD patient roams around all night long, making it impossible for other family members to sleep soundly. Sometimes families have to install special locks high up on doors to the outside to avoid the nighttime wanderer from getting outside and roaming in the night. In some cases, the patient may experience a reversal of their nights and days, sleeping all day and staying awake and active all night. Such day-night reversal can be very burdensome for family caregivers. In addition to physical aggression and incontinence, families cite sleep disturbances as a major reason why they decide to put their loved one in a residential care facility.

Other physical symptoms

The following physical symptoms may also be present in an AD patient, but they generally don't appear until the disease profoundly affects the patient:

>> Impaired motor ability: Even though muscle function remains intact, the nerve signals that initiate voluntary movement may degrade as AD progresses into the sections of the brain that control these movements. When this happens, your loved one may move more slowly or with a marked degree of uncertainty.

>> Difficulty walking.

>> Problems with pacing.

>> Trouble maintaining balance, resulting in falls.

These kinds of physical symptoms generally don't appear until later in the course of AD. If they appear early on, you may be looking at something else altogether, such as Parkinson's disease, stroke, or Normal Pressure Hydrocephalus (NPH), all of which produce gait disturbances right from the onset of the problem. See Chapter 4 for a complete discussion of conditions that may mimic the symptoms of AD.

Figuring Out Whether Your Loved One Needs an Assessment

So how do you decide whether you need to take your loved one to a doctor for assessment? Any ongoing memory loss requires professional evaluation. Remember that doctors are looking for memory loss and at least one other cognitive deficit or problem in day-to-day functioning in order to make a diagnosis of dementia. Dementia may be the cause if memory loss is accompanied by

>> Difficulty speaking or comprehending information

>> Confusion

>> Disorientation (for example, confusing the days of the week or problems estimating or telling time)

>> Problems recognizing or identifying objects

>> Difficulty with finding words

>> Problems with motor skills

>> Personality changes (such as sudden irritability)

>> Agitation (such as restlessness, pacing, unprovoked verbal or physical aggression)

>> Problems recognizing similarities or differences between ideas and concepts

>> Problems planning, reasoning, judging, and other kinds of higher-level thinking

>> Any significant change in day-to-day functioning that contradicts your loved one's normal conduct

If you suspect dementia or AD, start keeping a record of any symptoms and behavioral changes that you notice in your loved one. Gathering this information gives your doctor a leg up as she starts the diagnostic process. (See Chapters 5 and 6 for more about getting a diagnosis.)

One of the biggest problems healthcare professionals face when diagnosing dementia is that other conditions mimic many of its most common symptoms. That's why it's important for you to present the big picture to your doctor; looking at a patient's entire range of emotional and behavioral difficulties along with problems in their cognitive skills helps doctors make a better diagnosis. Any bit of information that you don't include in your comments to your loved one's doctor may be the missing key that prevents an accurate diagnosis or a diagnosis at all.

For example, if you forget to mention that your loved one has a low thyroid condition but refuses to take the prescribed thyroid supplement medication, or if you don't know whether she's taking it, then your doctor may believe that some of the symptoms caused by the thyroid condition are an early manifestation of AD. Such medical history is essential to assist the doctor in making a proper assessment of a potentially reversible and treatable problem that may mimic dementia. That's why it's so important to maintain complete healthcare records and to make sure you share *all* the information you have with your doctor, even if it doesn't seem important.

REMEMBER

Giving the doctor an accurate list of all medications (both prescription and over-the-counter) as well as all vitamins and herbal supplements that your loved one is taking is critical. Explaining to the doctor exactly how your loved one uses these medications (especially if different from how they were prescribed) is also important, which may range from non-use to underuse or overuse compared to the instructions on the bottle. This is one time that the truth of what is really being done becomes paramount to communicate to the doctor. Such honesty can prevent incorrect medical decisions by letting the doctor know what is really happening.

You may be thinking that seems like an awful lot of work, and you'd be right. Some concentrated effort is required to gather all the information your doctor may need to make an accurate diagnosis of your loved one's condition. Write things down as you notice them. The most important thing is to record events as they happen, noting the time of day and whatever incident may have preceded the behavior you're noting. In time, you may see emerging patterns of behavior that may help both you and the doctor to address recurring problems.

The idea is to give your doctor as much information as you can about your loved one's symptoms and behavior. Only an experienced healthcare professional can determine whether a particular fact truly raises a red flag of concern or is simply a red herring that can lead in the wrong direction if it's given too much importance. If your doctor isn't familiar with dementia, seek a second opinion.

Chapter 3

Considering Causes and Risk Factors

You probably know that an ounce of prevention is better than a pound of cure. And with dementia, for which no cure exists and the symptoms are so devastatingly awful, surely anything is worth trying to prevent the disease. Unfortunately, no one single thing that you can do or not do prevents dementia. The situation isn't as simple as it is with prevention of some other conditions.

Doctors can't put their fingers on a single trigger for dementia, which perhaps isn't surprising given that it manifests itself in many different ways. Thankfully, however, some scientific evidence suggests that changing diet and lifestyle — keeping mentally and physically active — can help you avoid developing dementia.

This chapter looks at the different risk factors, from genes to environmental pollutants, from lack of exercise to a pack-a-day smoking habit. First, though, it offers a quick overview of how your brain and memory work normally when they're not affected by disease. Understanding a normal brain function better can help you to have a better understanding of what goes wrong in dementia. Secondly, we focus on ways you can help yourself to reduce your risk for dementia.

Taking a Quick Look Under the Hood

Computers are now ubiquitous. Pretty much everyone, regardless of their age — from nursery school children to silver surfers — has at least one electronic gadget. Cellphones, tablets, laptops, and gaming consoles are so common that everyone's familiar with machines containing microchips that are so clever they seem to think for themselves. Maybe one day they will.

Thus looking inside the skull at the human brain (or at least a picture of it) and discovering that it contains no shiny components or intricate circuitry can be a shock. Unlike other organs in the body, the brain doesn't look like what it does. The heart, for example, is unmistakably a pump; the long, tubular guts are clearly designed to have something passing through them; and the lungs, with their tiny airspaces, are obviously used for breathing. Thankfully, the strange, waxy-looking organ inside your head is a lot cleverer than it looks. In fact, it's the cleverest and most complex object in the whole of the known universe.

Think of what your brain does when you sit down at your computer to type a letter. It's seriously multitasking! Your brain controls your hands as they tap on the keyboard; your eyes are sending it images of the words as they form on the screen; you can hear music from your iPod. As well as processing all that information, your brain is also thinking of the next words to write, composing sentences with them and planning the paragraphs that they'll eventually construct. And all the while your brain is controlling your breathing, heart rate, balance, and everything else needed to keep you alive and conscious, while simultaneously storing and recalling memories. And it does all this, and so much more, 24 hours a day, seven days a week for many years without breaking a sweat.

These sections take a closer look at the ins and outs of the brain and the different functions that the brain does, how it remembers things, and what happens to the brain during dementia.

Considering normal brain structure and function

This is obviously an ambitious heading for a small section in a book, because you could fill whole libraries with books on which bits of the brain are where, the routes through which they communicate with each other, and the chemical processes involved, and still not have all the answers. The pathways controlling muscle movement are complicated enough, let alone the ones scientists think determine personality and stimulate feelings such as love.

But you have to start somewhere, so here's a rough outline of the brain's anatomy and the method by which messages whizz around it, allowing you to do all the clever physical things you can do as well as the more complicated emotional and philosophical stuff.

Understanding the anatomy (what goes where)

The brain consists of a large blob called the cerebrum, sitting on top of a stalk that joins to the spinal cord, with a bump hanging off the back called the cerebellum, as shown in Figure 3-1.

An adult brain weighs around 3.3 pounds and has the consistency of tofu. It's made up of around 86 billion nerve cells, called *neurons*, arranged into two halves, called *hemispheres*, which are each divided further into four lobes: *frontal*, *parietal*, *temporal*, and *occipital*.

Neurons are the main components inside the brain. They're a bit like insulated wires carrying electrical signals around the brain to communicate between its different regions. Nerves (see Figure 3-2) pass these signals between each other at gaps called synapses (Figure 3-3). Here, the signal from one cell causes the release of chemicals across the synapse, which then attach to receptors on the next neuron, triggering a further electrical signal in the next cell, and so on; Figure 3-4 illustrates this process. Of these chemicals, called *neurotransmitters*, dopamine, glutamate, and acetylcholine have the most relevance to dementia.

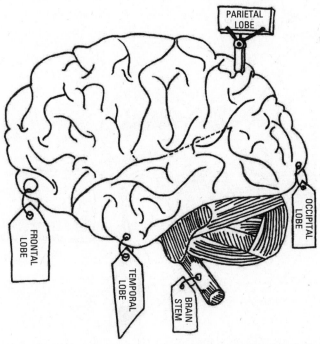

FIGURE 3-1:
The human brain.

Illustration by Sam Atkins

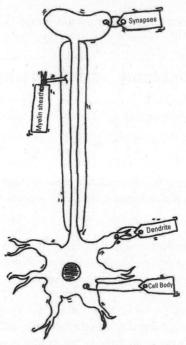

FIGURE 3-2:
A nerve cell.

Illustration by Sam Atkins

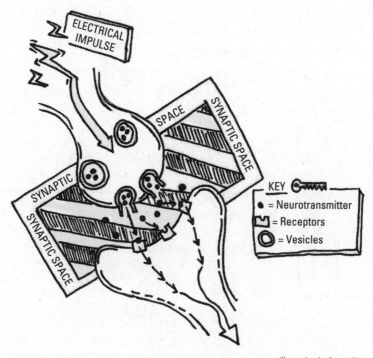

FIGURE 3-3:
A synapse.

Illustration by Sam Atkins

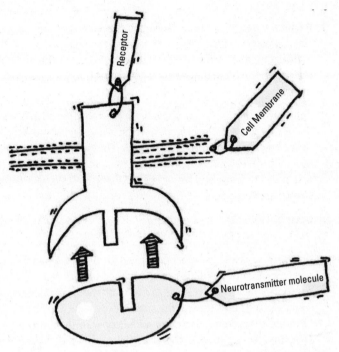

FIGURE 3-4:
A transmitter "plugging" into a receptor.

Illustration by Sam Atkins

Fathoming functions (which bit does what)

In order to get a handle on what goes wrong in the brain in dementia, a basic knowledge of which parts of the brain are responsible for doing what is helpful. Here's a quick rundown:

>> **Cerebral hemispheres:** The two cerebral hemispheres make up the majority of the structure of the brain. The right and left hemispheres are mirror images of one another. They're separated by a deep groove called the *longitudinal fissure.* The surface of the hemispheres, called the *cortex,* looks gray from the outside, hence the colloquial term for the brain: *gray matter.*

>> **Frontal lobe:** Not surprisingly, given its name, this lobe is situated at the front of each hemisphere. This area is far more developed in humans than it is in other species. It's where the higher intellectual functions are carried out, such as planning and mental reasoning. This part of the brain has allowed humans to evolve to the point of not only controlling their environment on earth, but also sending rockets to the moon and beyond. The frontal lobe is also involved in speech and movement and is the main center for emotions.

>> **Parietal lobe:** This area is involved in movement and also houses the primary sensory cortex, which allows you to analyze and make sense of all the information that comes in from your sense organs. The parietal lobe is also the part of the brain that lets you know which way up you are in relation to the floor.

>> **Temporal lobe:** This area of the brain is often affected in dementia. Given that it contains the *hippocampus,* which is involved in memory, it's not difficult to see how memory problems are a significant feature of dementia. The temporal lobe also contains the *primary auditory cortex,* which deals with sound and hearing, and *Wernicke's area,* which allows you to understand speech and language.

>> **Occipital lobe:** This part of the brain is involved in vision, allowing you to see shapes and colors.

>> **Brain stem:** This is the most primitive part of the human brain and is found in one form or another in the brains of other, far less evolved creatures through-out the animal kingdom. It sits underneath the cerebral hemispheres and communicates directly with the spinal cord below it. It controls all the basic functions that you need to carry out unconsciously to stay alive, like breathing and a regular heartbeat. If this area of the brain is damaged, the game is over.

>> **Cerebellum:** The cerebellum may look like a piece of cauliflower glued onto the back of the brain, but don't let looks deceive you. It's vital for balance, posture, and coordination; when the cerebellum is prevented from doing its work properly, most commonly after a boozy night out, these functions just don't work.

>> **Cerebrospinal fluid (CSF):** CSF circulates around the outside of the spinal cord and around and through the brain. It's the liquid that doctors are trying to extract when they do a lumbar puncture. CSF has two main jobs:

- Removing the waste products made during metabolism by brain cells

- Acting as a cushion, especially just under the skull, to protect the brain and spinal cord from damage during trauma (for example, after head injuries and car accidents)

>> **Ventricles:** These are spaces within brain tissue through which CSF circulates. They're situated symmetrically in both hemispheres and enlarge in certain types of dementia as the brain cells around them shrink or die off.

>> **Cortex:** The cortex is the outer most layer of the brain. Depending on the lobe involved, the cortex has different functions, such as memory, thought, language, and consciousness — all the things, in fact, that make you human.

Understanding how memory works

Again we're trying to simplify a subject that could fill a library and that's actually still somewhat mysterious despite the research techniques available to 21st-century science. That said, understanding a few of the basics helps you to make sense of what goes wrong in dementia.

REMEMBER

Memory is obviously vital to normal functioning, hence the disability that results when it starts to fail. Without memory, you can't learn from or make links to the past, and so can't plan for the future. You can also get lost, not only geographically but also emotionally, while carrying out tasks and even in the middle of conversations. Lack of memory prevents you from being able to follow instructions and even to recognize those you love.

Humans have two main types of memory: short term and long term.

Short-term memory

Sometimes called *working memory*, *short-term memory* allows you to remember things like telephone numbers or drink orders at the bar. It has limited storage capacity and empties quickly so new items can be remembered.

People are thought to be able to retain lists of up to nine items for around 30 seconds in short-term memory before they're lost (unless those people repeat the items over and over again to try to hold on to them for longer). Retaining memories longer requires that they be transferred into long-term memory. Then the memories can stay for the rest of your life, and storage is seemingly limitless.

Long-term memory

In long-term memory, people lay down their memories for keeps. Examples include the address of your first home, the name of your elementary school teacher, the Super Bowl final score in 1968 (New York Jets 16, Baltimore Colts 7, in case you're interested), the recipe for Grandpa's dill pickles, or Pythagoras's theorem. Memories aren't stored in one particular part of the brain but involve the interaction and cooperation of a few different regions.

Long-term memory can be subdivided further into two main types:

>> **Declarative memory:** This type is general information knowledge that includes sights, sounds, and smells from the past, phone numbers, general knowledge, meanings of words, and memories of events that have happened to you.

>> **Procedural memory:** This is the memory needed for performing tasks requiring certain procedures and sequences such as riding a bike, tying shoelaces, and driving a car.

Memory processing

For memory to work, each of the following three stages has to happen:

1. Encoding (your ability to take in information)
2. Storage
3. Retrieval

A failure of all or any of these individual processes can cause memory impairment. Thus, for example, encoding and storage may be fine, but with no capacity for retrieval you won't recall what you've stored. Likewise, encoded information won't be retrieved if it wasn't stored.

Realizing what goes wrong in dementia

Dementia interferes with the functioning of brain cells, which stops them communicating between each other and therefore carrying out their normal processes. The process of dementia inflicts two major types of damage on nerve cells, which then produce symptoms:

>> The cells can be killed off or rendered largely inactive because they receive insufficient oxygen in the bloodstream, as in vascular dementia.

>> Protein deposits, such as plaques and tangles in Alzheimer's disease (AD) and Lewy bodies in Lewy body dementia, form within and mess up the internal workings of the cells.

Obviously, this view is simplistic. However, it does give you an idea of what can go wrong in an individual brain cell, although, of course these changes have to occur in many cells to impair how the whole brain works. This loss of function coupled with a reduction in levels of some of the neurotransmitters that let cells "talk" to each other can cause large parts of a person's central nervous system to fail.

Not only is the type of damage important in generating symptoms in the different dementias, but also where this damage occurs in the brain is also crucial in bringing about the changes observed in people with dementia. Each type of dementia has specific features, as well as more generalizable symptoms:

>> **Frontotemporal dementia:** The changes are mainly in the two frontotemporal lobes, which are involved in both higher intellectual functions and memory processes. This damage then leads to the typical symptoms of dementia — from difficulty with planning and motivation to changes in personality and behavior.

>> **Alzheimer's disease:** The main area affected is the hippocampus, which is involved in converting short-term memories into long-term memories, hence the initial classic symptom whereby the person has difficulty remembering what's just happened. Memories already stored long term can, however, sometimes still be recalled.

>> **Lewy body disease:** The damage is largely inflicted throughout the cortex, where Lewy bodies can form in all the different lobes. Lewy bodies also crop up in the brain stem. Because the cortex is involved in both sensory and motor functions, people with Lewy body disease can develop hallucinations and difficulties with movement, leading to its particular cluster of symptoms.

>> **Vascular dementia:** The areas that can be damaged are even more widespread still, given that blockages to blood supply (strokes) or reductions in blood flow can happen pretty much anywhere. Thus if the hippocampus is damaged, memory is affected. If the frontal lobes are involved, issues with planning and personality develop. If the motor control center in the parietal lobe is damaged, then movement can be impaired, resulting in paralysis.

WARNING

Because the brain is so complex, the symptoms of the different types of dementia aren't quite as well demarcated as this. In the brain, many different areas can be involved in certain processes, especially memory. Damage to connecting cells between lobes can result in difficulties of a mixed picture, not just the loss of a specific cognitive function.

Taking age into account

If you had a dollar for every senior who has said, "I'm just getting old," you'd have more money than Warren Buffet and would currently be sitting on a sun-drenched beach on an island in the Caribbean. Although dementia isn't a part of normal aging, human brains and bodies do undergo changes as a person grows older. You may need bifocals in order to read a book and your eyes may develop cataracts. Your ability to hear high-pitched tones tends to fade. Your hair turns gray (or white) and may desert you all together if you're a man. Your skin gets thinner, making bruises show up more easily and for longer. Reaction time increases. You may start to tell the same stories over and over again. And most frustrating, you may forget what you went into the bedroom to get or where you laid down the car keys. *But*, contrary to popular belief, not everyone develops dementia.

Although dementia does become a more common occurrence with advancing years, dementia isn't limited to the aging generation. Some younger people can fall victim to it too. Although the Alzheimer's Association (www.alz.org) estimates that 1 in 14 people older than the age of 65 will develop dementia, its statistics also show that 200,000 of the 5.3 million people with dementia in the United States are younger than 65. And given that the Alzheimer's Association also estimates that less than 50 percent of people with dementia in the United States have actually been diagnosed, this number is likely to rise as pick-up rates improve.

In younger people the cause of dementia can be any one of the following: AD, vascular dementia, Lewy body disease, or frontotemporal dementia. As a person's age at time of diagnosis goes up, there's distribution changes. Over the age of 75 most people diagnosed with dementia are diagnosed with AD or vascular dementia with some cases of mixed dementia thrown in too.

Understanding the Role of Genes and Family History

Unfortunately, many medical conditions run in families and are thus passed on from one generation to the next simply by the act of reproduction rather than being picked up from elsewhere or developed because of bad habits. Common examples are color-blindness and, more rarely, Huntington's disease.

Many more conditions don't develop automatically but are more likely to develop in someone given the right (or wrong in this case) conditions as a result of genetic predisposition. A mental health problem such as schizophrenia, which may only develop if someone experiences particularly difficult life events, is one such example.

The following sections examine more closely genetics and answers whether dementia runs in families or not.

Explaining what genes are and how they work

Each person has between 20,000 and 25,000 genes in her body. *Genes* are found within each of your cells; you can think of them as the blueprint of how people are put together. Thus you have genes that dictate your hair color, the shape of your nose, ears, and feet, how tall you become, whether you have a hairy chest and, of course, whether you're male or female. These genes are bundled up on your *chromosomes.* Everyone has 23 pairs of chromosomes, making 46 in total; half come from your mother, and half from your father.

Your genes, and therefore your chromosomes, are made of a chemical called deoxyribonucleic acid, or DNA for short. DNA is itself made up of four different types of protein molecule:

>> Adenine (A)

>> Cytosine (C)

>> Guanine (G)

>> Thymine (T)

DNA comes as long strands of these proteins that provide the code for hair color and other inherited traits, depending on their order. For example, a gene (which in reality would be much, much longer) with the order AGTACCCTTACGACT would code for one characteristic, while CCCGTTATATGCTA would code for another. The process is obviously much more complicated than that, but hopefully this example gives you the idea. Figure 3-5 illustrates how DNA forms genes and then chromosomes.

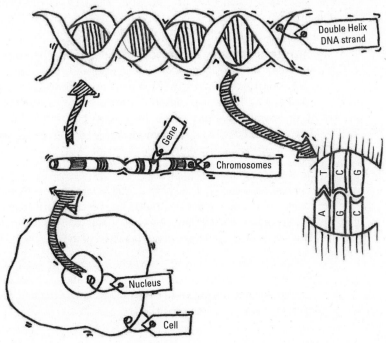

FIGURE 3-5: How DNA forms genes and then chromosomes.

Illustration by Sam Atkins

In an ideal world, your DNA would be perfect and your genes and chromosomes would give you only healthy characteristics, movie-star good looks, and the gift of eternal life. However, disease is rife, most people don't look in the mirror and see Angelina Jolie or Brad Pitt looking back, and everyone dies one day, some people sooner than others. Actually, during the process of evolution, these genetic abnormalities have worked to the advantage of the species, making some people stronger, brighter, or better looking than others, and thus enabling the human race to advance. Unfortunately, the other side of that coin is that the genes that disadvantage people can also be passed on to the next generation and cause disease.

The fact that half of your genes come from one parent and half from the other does provide the opportunity for "bad" genes to die out through dilution over many generations. But some bad traits are persistently inherited down the line. Those families suffer from conditions that run in the family generation after generation.

Identifying whether dementia runs in families

Relatives of people with dementia frequently ask if they will develop dementia as well. Unfortunately, no easy answer exists, and even the experts aren't clear about the genetics of each type of dementia. The case is different for each sort of dementia:

>> **Alzheimer's disease:** The situation depends on whether someone has early or late-onset Alzheimer's. A very rare type of early-onset AD exists that definitely runs in families, with some members developing symptoms as young as 30. This type is caused by a mutation in the gene that makes amyloid protein, which is responsible for the plaques and tangles that form in sufferers' brain cells. People in these families are advised to see their doctor to arrange genetic testing.

In the case of late-onset dementia, you may possibly but by no means definitely develop AD if you have a relative with the condition. The gene responsible is *apolipoprotein E* (APOE for short), which is found on chromosome number 19. This gene has four variants, and the likelihood of the disease being passed on depends on which of these variants a person has.

>> **Vascular dementia:** No proven genetic risk exists for most cases of vascular dementia, although its associated risk factors, such as heart disease, diabetes, and strokes can run in families. The only exception to this is CADASIL, which is a rare genetic form of the condition.

>> **Frontotemporal dementia:** In contrast to vascular dementia, a risk of frontotemporal dementia runs in families. Researchers have identified genes for two different abnormal proteins that could be responsible for this. It's believed that around 40 percent of people with frontotemporal dementia have a family history with it.

TIP

If you have a close relative with frontotemporal dementia, seek genetic counseling via your primary care physician.

>> **Lewy body dementia:** No clear answer can be given to the question of whether a genetic component exists in the development of this form of dementia. Some overlap in genetic mutations with those who have AD and Parkinson's disease is thought to be evident, but no one can yet say for certain.

Dementia doesn't discriminate. It affects people from all ethnic backgrounds. In the United States the numbers of people from certain ethnic groups do appear low, but that may be the result of other factors, including

>> Access to diagnostic services

>> Poor experiences when seeking help from primary care physicians

>> Cultural understanding of the condition

>> Stigma attached to being given the diagnosis

We hope that this situation will change so all people with dementia can be identified and then can receive the treatment and care they need regardless of their ethnic background.

Taking a Long, Hard Look at the Risk Factors for Dementia

Everyone loves a conspiracy theory. If you believed all the newspaper headlines about the risks various pollutants, drugs, cosmetics, and foods pose to your health and very survival, you'd never venture outside the front door. But the impact of these risks — and particularly whether dementia can be triggered by factors in your everyday environment — remains an open question.

THE INFAMOUS CASE OF ALUMINUM

In 1965 some very creative, not to mention cruel, scientists carried out an experiment whereby they injected rabbits' brains with aluminum. At post-mortem, the animal-friendly scientists found that the rabbits had developed the textbook neurofibrillary protein tangles that are found in the brains of people with AD. And so began the story linking the third-most common chemical element on the planet with the most common form of dementia.

Since then all sorts of scares have suggested that even using aluminum saucepans or deodorants containing the stuff will lead to dementia. After years of research, this link hasn't been proved, and currently aluminum is viewed as safe. Just don't inject it directly into your brain!

We've scoured the Internet and the research journals to make sure we're not missing anything, but we think we can safely say that although you should always be careful about what you swallow and breathe in, no clear evidence suggests that environmental factors are involved in developing dementia. Air pollution may apparently predispose older people to cognitive decline, but no link has yet been made to a progression to dementia. In fact, in our career, we're used to seeing people with AD who are otherwise quite healthy. If some kind of environmental toxin caused the disease, one would expect all sorts of other health issues to come along for the ride.

Lifestyle

Here, at last, we discuss some factors with actual proven risk for dementia. These are factors you can do something about from a prevention point of view. No one lives a completely healthy lifestyle all the time. We may run marathons and take part in 100-mile bike rides, but we still enjoy a pizza and a beer.

However, these factors won't surprise anyone. Doctors and nurses drone on about these issues every time someone has an appointment. The government has agencies that warn against them, and the walls of every health center and clinic in the country are decorated with posters that promote a healthy lifestyle that includes

>> Don't use illicit drugs

>> Keep caffeinated beverages use to a moderation

>> Drink alcohol responsibly, if at all

>> Don't smoke

>> Eat more fruit and fiber

>> Eat fewer burgers and other fast food

>> Exercise more

Drugs and alcohol

Flippancy aside, illicit drugs are bad. People who have a serious drug habit don't emerge unscathed. Evidence supporting a link between street drugs and full-on dementia is flimsy at best; however, cannabis, heroin, ecstasy, amphetamines, and cocaine are known to cause cognitive impairment.

Alcohol can cause its own form of dementia, Korsakoff's syndrome. Try to stick to current recommended daily intakes: two drinks per day for a man and one for a woman. If you're gulping down more than that a day, you need to have a chat with your doctor about getting help to reduce your intake. Not only does alcohol increase your risk of developing dementia, but it also rots pretty much every organ in the body.

Smoking

If we could sum up our advice on smoking in one word, it would be *don't*. This includes smoking (and tobacco use) in all its forms: cigarettes, cigars, pipes, e-cigarettes, snuff, and chewing tobacco. Smoking is the biggest risk factor for every form of premature death known to medical science, from cancer of every organ in your body (no exaggeration) to heart attack and stroke. The smoking habit also doubles your risk of dementia, especially AD and vascular dementia, by damaging brain cells and blood vessels.

Thankfully, lots of things are available to help you stop, such as nicotine-replacement therapies, pills, patches, and hypnosis. You can obtain pills and patches from your doctor. Your doctor can also point you in the direction of a support group if you think you'll struggle with quitting alone.

REMEMBER

If you want to avoid dementia and don't have a strong family history of the disease, quitting cigarettes will do you far more good than chucking out your aluminum saucepans.

Diet

People who are obese are four times more likely to develop dementia than those who aren't overweight. People who eat high carbohydrate diets are in general more at risk of damaging their blood vessels and thus reducing the blood supply to the brain, making them more at risk of dementia. According to the Alzheimer's Foundation of America (www.alzprevention.org), you should avoid red meats, saturated fats, trans-fats, salt, added sugars, fried foods, and processed foods for brain health.

A diet relatively low in carbohydrates and high in fiber is best. Eliminating sugars (simple carbohydrates) and unhealthy fats is probably the best approach. Eating five portions of fruit and vegetables per day is strongly recommended. Doing so reduces the risk of clogging up your arteries, and these foods are also rich in anti-oxidants, which protect brain cells from damage.

The only supplements that seem to be of potential benefit are methyl cobalamin, vitamin D3, fish oil, and coenzyme Q10. There is also some evidence that it is beneficial to fast for a minimum of 12 hours between dinner and breakfast, and for a minimum of three hours between dinner and bedtime. (Refer to Chapter 9 for more information about these supplements.)

Exercise

Not only does exercising regularly fend off heart disease, but it can also protect against Alzheimer's and vascular dementia. Fortunately, this doesn't mean you have to rush out and join a gym, deck yourself out in exercise garb, or sign up to run the Boston Marathon. Obviously, you can if you like, but five half-hour sessions of brisk walking every week will do you just as much good.

TIP

To build exercise into your daily activities, park farther away from your workplace, take the stairs rather than the elevator, or walk the dog every day.

Swimming, cycling, aerobics, and many other forms of exercise can help, but it's most important to add in a bit more sweat to your normal daily routine.

Mental health

So-called brain-training exercises are big business. You can buy brain-training apps for your phone or tablet and programs for every kind of games console. But these specific programs aren't the answer.

In fact, increasing evidence supports that keeping your brain active by learning new skills, trying out different hobbies, and doing crosswords, Sudoku, and other puzzles do far more good. Check out the book *Staying Sharp For Dummies* (John Wiley & Sons, 2016) for more information. Socializing with others can also protect your brain from cognitive decline — so join a bridge club, take up salsa dancing, or set up a book club.

There is some evidence that meditating twice a day and participating in yoga to reduce stress can be helpful. Getting seven to eight hours of sleep per night is more beneficial than just four or five.

Examining risk factors specific to Alzheimer's disease

Advancing age increases the likelihood of developing AD, but other risk factors may play a contributing role in the development of the disease as well. Just remember that risk factors don't cause the disease — they just give you a better idea of what your odds are of developing a given condition. A few of the better-recognized risk factors for AD are a family history of the disease, presence of the E4 variant gene, and high blood pressure and high cholesterol.

Family history

Families that have two generations or more of close relatives (a parent or sibling) who developed early onset AD (ages 65 or under) may have Familial Alzheimer's Disease (FAD). Families that have a history of AD have a greater chance of developing FAD than people who have no family history of the condition. The good news is that FAD accounts for only 1 to 5 percent of all AD cases.

E4 variant

People who have at least one E4 variant gene are twice as likely to develop late-onset AD than people who don't have this gene variant. People who have the E4 variant gene and high blood pressure have a five times greater chance of developing the condition; if they also have high cholesterol, their risk is eight times greater. Remember, though, that just having the E4 variant gene doesn't automatically mean that you'll get AD. Having the gene is simply one of the risk factors. The use of genetic testing to determine the presence of the E4 variant in unimpaired individuals isn't recommended.

High blood pressure, high cholesterol, and diabetes

Researchers are starting to explore the possibility that many of the well-established risk factors for cardiovascular disease, including high cholesterol, high blood pressure, and diabetes may also be risk factors for AD. A large study conducted by researchers in Finland showed a strong link between elevated cholesterol and high blood pressure and the eventual development of AD — all the more reason to keep these two conditions under control.

Considering Some Theories on the Causes of Alzheimer's Disease

When it comes to pinpointing the causes of AD, the jury is still out. Researchers believe several factors may contribute to someone developing the condition. A lot of work still needs to be done before any definitive answers about the causes of AD are known.

Researchers have identified age as the most important risk factor for developing AD. But this isn't to imply that dementia is an inevitable consequence of aging; people who manage their risk factors and are proactive about their health have a statistically significant improvement in their odds of staying both mentally and physically healthy as they grow older.

According to the Alzheimer's Disease Education and Referral Center, for every five years past the age of 65, the number of people with AD doubles.

Researchers are examining a plethora of ideas in their attempts to isolate the cause of AD. The most current thinking is that AD has no single cause, but rather a cascade of events that may be triggered by one precipitating event, like an infection or an injury. The following sections consider a few of these theories.

Aging theories

Aging increases the risk for developing AD, but scientists are only now beginning to theorize why this may be so. A body of evidence has accumulated over the past 25 years that *free radicals* (highly reactive molecules produced as a byproduct of metabolism) cause damage to cells throughout the body. Some speculate that this kind of age-related change in brain tissue may be responsible for triggering the onset of AD.

Another theory involves something called messenger RNA. *Messenger RNA* is a class of ribonucleic acid that serves as a template for protein synthesis. As people age, mutations in their messenger RNA lead to mistakes in the amino acid sequences of the proteins they manufacture. Those damaged proteins (amyloid precursor protein and ubiquitin-B) are found in the brains of AD patients along with their corresponding mutated messenger RNA; however, these substances aren't found in the brains of people who don't have AD. Researchers haven't determined if this buildup of protein that can damage other molecules in cell membranes is a cause or a consequence of AD.

Unfortunately, that's as far as research has currently gone. The proteins have been identified, and it's certain that they appear in the brains of all AD patients. But what causes these proteins to form isn't known. What is known is that the chances of getting abnormal protein deposits in the brain increase dramatically with age.

Genetic theories

Scientists have done a lot of work in recent years with genes, trying to determine if and how genes may increase the risk for, modify the course of, or influence the onset of AD. People who have a family member with AD can take heart in this research. Although several genes have been identified as having something to do with the development of AD, only three (amyloid precursor protein, presenilin 1, and presenilin 2) have been linked to the early onset form of AD, called *autosomal dominant inheritance.* This is the same as the Familial Alzheimer's Disease (FAD) that we discuss earlier. Most people with this inherited form of AD first develop symptoms between the ages of 40 to 60.

A2M gene

The A2M gene, or the alpha 2-macroglobulin, has been identified as a sort of trash collector in the brain. The A2M's job is to pick up potentially toxic peptides, such as the amyloid precursor protein, and carry them out of the brain to an area of the body where they're degraded and excreted. Researchers now believe that when the A2M gene undergoes mutation, it no longer performs its trash collecting chores as effectively, allowing dangerous deposits of amyloid protein to build up in the brain, perhaps leading to the onset of AD.

Research is underway to find out whether there is a familial component to this mutation or whether the mutation is something that happens randomly throughout the population. Remember that gene mutation is the least common pathological cause of AD.

E4 variant

The E4 variant of the APOE gene has been associated with an increased risk of developing AD. But the presence of the E4 variant isn't predictive of AD; it's simply another risk factor for developing the condition. Forty to 50 percent of patients with AD have the E4 variant, but half of the people who have E4 never develop AD; so some additional factor must trigger AD.

Long before any clinical symptoms appear, some people with the E4 variant show declines in visual attention that may be suggestive of the eventual onset of AD. This discovery excited researchers because it was the first time they were able to use genes to identify subtle cognitive changes in an at-risk segment of the population that wasn't yet showing any signs of the disease.

Microbial theory

Some researchers are looking into whether a viral or bacterial infection may trigger the onset of AD. The microbial theory has gained credibility in recent years because of similar studies that have proven a hitherto little-known bacteria (*Helicobacter pylori*) is responsible for many ulcers, and bacterial or viral inflammations are now suspected as causative factors in heart attacks.

Researchers are studying several pathogens (organisms that cause disease). *Chlamydia pneumoniae,* a common bacterium that causes pneumonia or bronchitis and is easily spread by coughing or sneezing, has recently been identified as an underlying causative factor in hardening of the arteries. Researchers have proposed that the same organism may also play a role in the development of such diverse conditions as asthma, arthritis, and even AD. It's interesting to note that as people age, the prevalence of *Chlamydia pneumoniae* infection increases.

Nutritional theory

A growing body of evidence suggests that people who follow a diet high in essential fatty acids, low in saturated fats and trans fatty acids, and rich in naturally occurring antioxidants like vitamins E and C, may have a lower risk of developing AD. Numerous studies have shown that people who had high dietary consumption of vitamin E had a 67 percent lower risk of developing AD than people who consumed very little vitamin E. Interestingly, the effect was seen only in vitamin E consumed in the diet and couldn't be duplicated with vitamin E supplements.

Another study showed that people who ate primarily fresh fruits and vegetables along with lean fish and poultry had a lower risk of developing AD than people who ate high-fat, high-sugar diets.

Although much more research is needed, the findings certainly are thought provoking and reason enough for people interested in maintaining long-term health to take a hard look at their diet and make changes to benefit their overall wellbeing.

Cardiovascular risk

Some researchers speculate that cardiovascular disease may increase the risk of developing AD. High levels of the amino acid homocysteine increase the risk for cardiovascular disease by increasing inflammation in the heart and arteries. Several studies are underway to determine whether high levels of homocysteine may also increase the risk of developing AD and whether statin drugs (used to lower cholesterol in cardiovascular patients) may also reduce the incidence of AD in at-risk patients.

Head trauma theory

A number of studies have found a link between traumatic brain injuries that resulted in a loss of consciousness with an increased incidence of AD. The link is particularly significant in people who have not only suffered a serious head injury at some point during their lives but who also have the E4 variant of the APOE gene.

Early life education and stimulation theory

Some studies show the more years of education someone has, the less likely he or she is to develop AD. The theory is that the additional years of study force the brain to develop denser networks of synapses, making the brain less susceptible to AD because it has, to use a sports term, a "deeper bench" or cognitive reserve of brain cells to draw upon to compensate for any damage caused by early AD.

Immune system theory

Dr. Zhi-Qi Xiong and Dr. James McNamara of Duke University published a study in the journal *Neuron* outlining their theory that AD is an autoimmune response to some outside provocation that causes the body to attack itself. They postulate that such a response may follow a seizure, traumatic brain injury, or stroke. Although other doctors disagree with their findings, their theory represents another intriguing idea about the underlying cause of AD.

Environmental triggers

Some of the most interesting AD research is being conducted by scientists looking for a link between environment and the onset of AD. Preliminary studies suggest that people with a large number of siblings have a higher risk of developing the disease, while people who were raised in the suburbs have a lower risk. Researchers theorize that some unknown environmental or socioeconomic factor that directly impacts brain growth and development in young children may translate to a higher risk of developing AD later in life.

COUNTING THE COST: ALZHEIMER'S DISEASE STATISTICS AND PREVALENCE

Although AD isn't our most deadly disease (heart disease claims that dubious distinction), it is one of our more expensive ones, mainly because people live with it for so long and require so much supervision and care. AD puts a huge drain on our healthcare resources, and the problem is only getting bigger. In 1900, only 3 million Americans were ages 65 and older; currently, the United States has approximately 34 million senior citizens who make up 13 percent of the population.

By 2040, the year when the last of the baby boomers hits age 65, the number of new cases of AD is expected to more than double, from an average of 377,000 new cases a year now to more than 959,000 new cases annually by 2040. By the year 2050, experts estimate that about 50 million older Americans will comprise 18 percent of the population, with approximately 16 million cases of AD, more than three times the current 5 million cases.

Take a look at these interesting statistics regarding AD:

- Average age at onset: 72.8 years

- Average length of time between onset of symptoms and diagnosis: 2.8 years

- Average length of survival following diagnosis at age 65: 8.3 years

- Average length of survival following diagnosis at age 90: 3.4 years

- Number of deaths from AD in 2013: 84,767

- Alzheimer's rank among causes of death in U.S.: 6

- Alzheimer's relative cost: third most expensive disease

- Average cost of AD to the U.S. economy annually: $100 billion

- Annual cost of lost productivity due to work disruptions related to caregiving: $26 billion

- Annual cost of caregiver absenteeism to businesses: $7.89 billion

- Average annual cost of caregiving per family: $27,200

- Average lifetime caregiving cost per AD patient: $174,000

- Average length of nursing home stay for AD patients: 2.5 years

- Average cost of nursing home care for AD patients: $139,000

- In 2014, family and friends of AD and other dementia patients provided an estimated 17.9 billion hours of unpaid care, values at $217.7 billion.

Chapter 4

Distinguishing Dementia and Alzheimer's Disease from Other Medical Conditions

After you've been told that your loved one has dementia, you may assume that means she is suffering from Alzheimer's disease (AD). But, the diagnosis isn't that simple. The doctor still has some detective work to do to distinguish which type of dementia is involved. Although AD is the most common form of dementia, making up 60 percent of all dementia cases, there are multiple types of dementia and many medical conditions that may look like dementia but aren't.

Although all Alzheimer's patients have dementia, not all dementia patients have AD. Because some dementias are at least partially reversible and respond very well to treatment, it's important to identify the type of dementia involved. That's why a diagnosis of just dementia isn't sufficient. Proper treatment varies widely depending on the root cause of the symptoms and so depends entirely on accurately identifying what type of dementia is present.

The *differential diagnosis* of dementia includes the multiple explanations that doctors must consider when trying to discover the true cause of symptoms. This chapter introduces you to the many other conditions that must be ruled out before a diagnosis of dementia or AD can be made.

Making Sure That You Have a Reliable Diagnosis

We can't overemphasize the importance of making sure you have an accurate diagnosis of your loved one's condition (for more about getting a diagnosis, see Chapter 5). Assuming that your loved one is suffering from AD won't help if a reversible condition like severe vitamin B12 deficiency that can be identified with a simple blood test actually caused his memory loss and cognitive impairment. Such a vitamin deficiency can be treated with vitamin B12 tablets or injections. The best Alzheimer's treatments in the world will have no effect in someone with vitamin B12 deficiency because this cause of cognitive impairment demands vitamin replacement. In addition, depression and delirium must be ruled out as the cause of your loved one's symptoms before diagnosing dementia, especially because these are usually treatable conditions as well.

You may be asking, "Well, heck, I'm not a doctor. How am I supposed to know if my mom or dad has Alzheimer's, another form of dementia, or something else entirely?"

REMEMBER

Dementia is a clinical state characterized by loss of function in multiple areas. Its most common symptom is memory impairment, accompanied by problems in at least one other area — language, personality, the ability to perceive objects, and *executive functioning* (the ability to plan and carry out complex actions). Not only does a person with dementia need to exhibit these symptoms, but they must also be severe enough to interfere with that person's function in daily life. There are approximately 50 different types of dementia. Depending on which study you believe, 3 to 15 percent of all dementias are potentially reversible. However, AD is an irreversible progressive type of dementia.

No one expects you to know what is the specific root cause of your loved one's symptoms, but you *do* know your loved one. Therefore, you do have the best chance to observe him and keep a record of the symptoms and behavior you observe that caused you to take him to the doctor in the first place. If you keep a good record of your loved one's symptoms, you can play a huge role in helping the doctor find the correct diagnosis. For instance, symptoms of memory loss alone may tell your doctor one thing, but memory loss accompanied by lethargy may lead her to check for substance abuse, medication side effects, or urinary infection. The clues you provide in the initial interview with the doctor are incredibly valuable in helping to determine which tests should be ordered and which aren't needed. (Refer to Chapter 5 for ways to help your loved one's doctor with medical records and familial history.)

THE DIAGNOSIS IS IN THE DETAILS

Giving your doctor accurate information may save you and your loved one years of suffering. For example, if your loved one is suffering from NPH, or *normal pressure hydrocephalus,* its accompanying dementia, incontinence, and gait disturbances may make your loved one look as though he's in the late stages of AD. This condition frequently goes undiagnosed, which is tragic, because proper treatment can sometimes alleviate the symptoms and restore sufferers to normal or near-normal functioning, depending on how advanced it is at the time of diagnosis.

The key here is timing. People in the early stages of Alzheimer's do *not* suffer from gait disturbances; this symptom, if it occurs at all, shows up much later in the disease process after Alzheimer's has attacked the part of the brain that disrupts the gait. NPH sufferers show gait disturbances right from the onset of their disease. Giving your doctor an accurate timetable can help turn her thoughts in the direction of NPH if she knows that the gait disturbances started at the same time as the dementia symptoms.

Admittedly, NPH is a dramatic example, and the outlook for recovery is much rosier than the outlook for most other dementias. But you definitely want to rule out this condition before assuming that your loved one has AD. If your physician has reason to suspect NPH, then she can confirm the diagnosis with CT or MRI brain scans that show the fluid collection in the brain. To treat NPH, a shunt is placed to drain the excess brain fluid, which can help restore the NPH patient to near-normal functioning.

That's why doctors are so careful and deliberate to order appropriate tests when they're trying to establish a diagnosis of AD. Think how tragic it would be if an NPH sufferer was misdiagnosed with AD, when a simple surgical procedure could relieve the NPH and restore a greatly improved quality of life to the patient.

According to the Alzheimer's Association, AD is the most common type of dementia, accounting for about 60 percent of all dementias, with *vascular dementia* (caused by problems with the brain's blood supply) responsible for another 10 percent. The remaining 30 percent of cases consist of both the less common dementias and mixed dementia or combined causes. So even if your loved one acts like he has AD, don't go jumping to conclusions until you get the test results and a good diagnosis.

Considering Copycat Conditions

A whole host of medical conditions can trigger symptoms that are similar to dementia but don't fit the full diagnostic criteria for it. These conditions often cause mental confusion and can stop people functioning normally in daily life, but they're largely reversible with correct treatment and thus, thankfully, aren't progressive in the same way as dementia is.

REMEMBER

Accurately identifying the underlying cause of confusion to determine the proper course of treatment is vitally important. With proper diagnosis and treatment, some people who are severely impaired can be restored to health. Even if the prospect for your loved one doesn't turn out to be so rosy, proper treatment can still alleviate many troubling symptoms and preserve a better quality of life.

When people visit their doctor with symptoms that could mean dementia is setting in, they have several lab tests run on blood and urine samples. Such tests are performed to rule out any reversible causes — most frequently, conditions that either affect the brain and nervous system or result from imbalances in various blood chemistry or hormones. Acute infections can also trigger confusional states, and long-term alcohol abuse can lead to problems with memory (alongside its more commonly seen propensity to render people confused and disoriented).

Neurological causes

Some of the most well-known medical conditions affecting the brain and nerves have symptoms that can mimic dementia features alongside their own, more specific features. So doctors may want to rule out some of these diseases before coming to a final diagnosis:

>> **Parkinson's disease:** This condition has a genuine overlap with dementia, because people with Parkinson's disease have a higher-than-average risk of also developing dementia. In fact, Parkinson's disease-related dementia accounts for 2 percent of all cases.

The symptoms of Parkinson's disease-related dementia are very similar to those of Lewy body disease, and researchers think a link may exist between the two. Thus, alongside problems with cognitive function and movement, people also experience significant visual hallucinations, mood swings, and irritability. Unfortunately, medication to help treat the movement difficulties found in Parkinson's disease, such as tremor and stiffness of muscles, may make the symptoms of this dementia worse.

>> **Subdural hematomas:** A *subdural hematoma* (SDH) is a large blood collection that occurs underneath the *dura mater,* or the tough, fibrous, protective covering of the brain, but is external to the brain itself. Because your skull doesn't have a square centimeter of extra space inside it, the pressure of an SDH can cause brain swelling, which produces a variety of symptoms including abnormal neurologic findings, intense headaches, nausea, vomiting for the acute variety, and confusion and combativeness for the chronic variety. The symptoms get worse as the clot grows larger. An acute subdural hematoma is a life-threatening condition. The chronic variety is the type that produces symptoms that can be confused with AD.

SDH can be the result of traumatic injury or blunt-force trauma to the head. People who are on aspirin therapy or taking a blood-thinning medication such as Coumadin have a higher risk. Alcoholism also increases the risk.

>> **Brain tumors:** Depending on their size and location within the brain, brain tumors may cause a variety of symptoms, some of which may mimic AD. Although most significantly large brain tumors cause intense headaches, nausea, and vomiting, tumors located in the frontal lobe of the brain cause the type of symptoms that mimic AD, including memory loss, personality changes, and impaired judgment. Whether the tumor is benign or malignant doesn't really alter the symptoms it causes. Its position within the skull is more predictive of symptoms produced and the outcome of potential surgical removal.

>> **Multiple sclerosis:** In this disease, the insulating outer coating of nerve cells, called myelin, is deficient in some parts of the nervous system, which means messages carried by the nerves aren't transmitted as well as they should be and may not get through at all. If the nerves affected are in the cortex of the brain, which is where most of the clever functions people perform are carried out, patients can develop cognitive symptoms including forgetfulness and difficulty with problem solving.

>> **Normal pressure hydrocephalus:** The brain and spinal cord are surrounded by cerebrospinal fluid, which supplies nutrients and acts as a shock absorber to protect the nervous system from damage during trauma. People with hydrocephalus have too much of this fluid, which accumulates and begins to damage brain cells because of the increased pressure. Normal pressure hydrocephalus usually begins to develop in people aged 55 to 60.

The damage that normal pressure hydrocephalus causes in the brain produces symptoms similar to those of dementia, accompanied by difficulties with walking and urinary incontinence. Treatment involves placing a shunt in the brain to allow the fluid to drain. If the treatment is carried out early in the disease process, the success rate for resolving symptoms is at least 80 percent.

» **Huntington's disease:** Huntington's disease is hereditary and is caused by a defect on chromosome 4. If one parent has the disease, a couple's children have a 50-50 chance of inheriting the condition because it's a dominant trait. Symptoms don't develop until middle age, but once they do, the disease progresses relentlessly until death. Alongside dementia, sufferers develop jerking movements of their limbs and changes in mood and personality.

Hormonal and nutritional causes

The following conditions are generally not as devastating as the neurological conditions described in the preceding section. Many of the symptoms caused by these conditions are reversible with the correct treatment. Hormonal and nutritional causes of dementia include the following:

» **Addison's and Cushing's diseases:** These conditions both affect the levels of a hormone called cortisol. In Addison's, not enough cortisol is produced; in Cushing's, too much. The effect of these altered cortisol levels is a corresponding upset in the levels of some of the minerals in the bloodstream, most notably sodium and potassium, which may lead to confusion. Thankfully, by treating the underlying cause, the confusion is reversible.

» **Diabetes:** One of the most common reasons for doctors seeing people who are acutely confused is that their blood sugar levels are either too low or too high. Neither situation is particularly good for people, but when their blood sugar is adjusted, their confusion quickly fades.

» **Thyroid disease:** Thyroxine is a hormone produced in the thyroid gland, which sits at the front of the neck. In simple terms, this hormone is involved in metabolism: too much and everything in the body is in a rush (the heart races, diarrhea develops, and people become agitated); too little and everything slows down (pulse is slow, people gain weight, skin becomes dry, hair falls out, and they can become constipated). Both an under and overactive thyroid can cause confusion. In both cases, doctors can reverse the confusion by treating the underlying cause and normalizing the level of thyroid hormone.

» **Hyperparathyroidism:** The parathyroid glands are pea sized and sit just behind the thyroid gland in the neck. The hormone they produce, parathyroid hormone, is involved in controlling levels of calcium, phosphate, and vitamin D.

If the gland becomes overactive, levels of calcium in the blood shoot up. Too much calcium can affect personality and consciousness, cause disorientation and, if not corrected quickly enough, coma. Treatment is curative.

>> **Vitamin B12 deficiency:** This vitamin, found in fish, poultry, eggs, and dairy products, is absorbed in the gut during digestion with the help of a protein called intrinsic factor. Some people either don't make enough of this protein or have a condition that destroys it. As a result, they don't absorb vitamin B12. One of the roles of this vitamin is ensuring healthy nerve function. A lack can cause numbness and tingling in the hands and feet and, if significant, mood changes and poor memory. Treatment by injection of vitamin B12 avoids the problem of lack of stomach absorption and can improve symptoms.

Alcohol-related causes

Indulging in more than the advised levels of society's favorite drug more often than recommended will reveal it to be the poisonous substance it truly is. The effects on the body are wide ranging, and it can damage several of our internal organs, but it's the problems it can cause in the liver and brain that mimic dementia.

>> **Cirrhosis:** Liver cells can be damaged by alcohol. A virus, such as hepatitis, and an autoimmune condition in which the immune system, rather than an infection attacks the body, can affect the liver. Such damage stops the liver from working as it should, which, among other things, leads to the build-up of toxic waste products in the blood. When these toxins build up they can damage brain cells, leading to encephalopathy, which encompasses a collection of symptoms like confusion, poor memory, personality change, and inappropriate behavior. Occasionally, treating the liver damage can reverse encephalopathy, but it can prove fatal.

>> **Korsakoff's syndrome:** Korsakoff's syndrome is most often seen in alcoholics in whom high alcohol intake stops the absorption of a B vitamin called thiamine. *Thiamine* is needed for normal nerve cell function, and insufficient levels commonly cause people to develop memory problems and changes in personality. This condition can be treated by quitting the booze and taking a thiamine supplement.

Infectious causes

Many infections can produce acute confusion, especially in the elderly. The direct effect of viruses or bacteria on the brain, the toxins they produce in the blood-stream, or the more general effects of infection on the body, from high temperature to dehydration, can all cause this confusion. The most common infections that can cause confusion or delirium are

>> Urinary tract infections such as cystitis (affecting the bladder) and pyelone-phritis (affecting the kidneys)

>> Chest infections, from bronchitis to pneumonia

>> Severe viral infections like influenza

>> Infections that directly affect the brain, such as meningitis (which affects the meninges covering the central nervous system) or encephalitis (which affects brain cells)

Prescription medication causes

Although doctors try to follow the age-old dictum "first do no harm," and medicines are designed to help people get better rather than make them worse, prescribing doesn't always work as planned. We're all different, and in an ideal world, all treatment would be individualized.

However, we don't live in an ideal world and so, despite doctors' best efforts, their prescriptions may make people, especially older people, feel worse than before they picked up their pills from the pharmacy. The following medicines can potentially make people acutely confused:

>> Benzodiazepines such as diazepam (Valium)

>> Narcotic painkillers such as tramadol (Ultram), codeine, morphine, oxycodone (Oxycontin), and hydrocodone (Vicodin, Norco, Lortab)

>> Steroids like prednisone (often used for chronic bronchitis and arthritis) as an anti-inflammatory

>> Anticonvulsants such as carbamazepine (Tegretol) and phenytoin (Dilantin)

>> Anticholinergics, including some hay fever and allergy tablets like diphenhydramine (Benadryl) and medicines used to treat an over-active bladder such as oxybutynin (Ditropan)

Other conditions that could be confused with dementia

You're probably asking yourself, what other conditions could possibly be confused with dementia? Well, believe it or not, we have a few more to discuss.

Because of the number of possible causes for dementia, your loved one's doctor will want to take a thorough medical history, including what drugs your loved one is taking and the start/stop dates for those drugs. Because so many different conditions can produce symptoms typically associated with dementia, the doctor must rule out all other potential causes and ensure that your loved one's symptoms fit the criteria for dementia (including Alzheimer's disease) before arriving at a diagnosis:

>> **Depression:** Severe clinical depression may be mistaken for dementia, which is why such cognitive problems in depressed patients are referred to as *pseudo-dementia*. People who are severely depressed can experience problems in thinking or memory, including difficulty concentrating, recalling information, and keeping track of dates or time, or they may complain that they can't stay focused on a task. They may report difficulty making decisions or starting or completing projects, and they may appear apathetic.

However, a person *can* have both depression and dementia at the same time. A good medical and neuropsychological evaluation is needed to determine if your loved one is experiencing one or possibly both of these conditions. If your loved one is suffering from depression and not dementia, you can expect his cognitive problems to respond to proper treatment for depression. If he is treated for depression and shows an improved mood but no improvement in thinking or memory, a diagnosis of dementia (possibly AD) may be appropriate. The bottom line is that your healthcare practitioner must assess whether your loved one is depressed before making a diagnosis of dementia.

>> **Delirium:** Another condition that can cause dementia-like symptoms is delirium. Delirium is suspected when someone shows a fluctuating change in alertness — particularly problems focusing, maintaining, or shifting attention — that usually starts within hours or days of another medical condition. This is unlike dementia that develops over months to years. In delirium, speech may be incoherent, and the individual may have problems staying awake or become agitated and restless in a fluctuating manner. Disorientation to person, place, or time; mood shifts; or hallucinations may also come and go.

Delirium is often caused by an illness (for example, an infection, such as a urinary tract infection or pneumonia, congestive heart failure, a metabolic disorder, such as dehydration, low sodium, or kidney problems; physical trauma like a head injury, or cardiac problems, such as a heart attack or congestive heart failure). Many drugs commonly used by older adults to treat pain, infection, inflammatory diseases, gastrointestinal problems, and more can also cause delirium. Delirium is a reversible condition if the underlying cause is properly diagnosed and treated.

Dementia or delirium can also result from alcohol or drug abuse, so you need to inform the healthcare practitioner if your loved one has a history of drug or alcohol problems, including abuse of over-the-counter medications or prescription drugs.

REMEMBER

As with depression, a person can have both delirium and dementia simultaneously. People who become delirious don't necessarily have dementia, but people with dementia are more susceptible to delirium than those without it.

2

Helping a Loved One Manage the Illness

Chapter 5

Receiving a Diagnosis

Very often, not knowing what's wrong with you, or someone you care for, is worse than actually knowing. That may sound a bit backwards because, you think not knowing you have a disease like cancer is surely a better state to be in than being told you have the disease. When you don't know, you're just a person with a few symptoms, but after you have a diagnosis, you're a cancer patient, with operations, chemotherapy, or radiotherapy ahead of you. Then you must pose the inevitable question: How long do I have?

But as many patients who have been given all manner of difficult diagnoses have testified, after your set of symptoms has a name, after you've been told that you have this or that disease, you and your family know what you're up against. In fact, people often say that the worry of not knowing what's wrong is far worse than the worry associated with knowing what's wrong.

With a label to your illness comes a treatment plan, the knowledge that physicians are going to do their best to care for you, and, if not make you better, then at least to help you manage your symptoms. Without a label, you often imagine even worse diagnoses than the one you're about to be given. Anxiety about the condition also makes the likely outlook seem worse, as you envision all sorts of catastrophic scenarios about symptoms and treatments.

And, of course, with many diseases, the sooner you get a diagnosis, the more likely it is that you can be cured. Sadly, with all types of dementia, there's no cure, no matter how soon the condition is picked up. But early diagnosis does mean that some medicines may help keep symptoms at bay for longer, and it certainly provides more time to plan for the long-term.

In this chapter we look at the initial steps that you need to take in order to find out whether you're dealing with dementia or whether something else is responsible for the symptoms you or a loved one are experiencing. (*Note:* We cover the specifics of diagnostic testing for Alzheimer's disease in Chapter 6.)

REMEMBER

Because this book is intended for readers throughout the United States, the steps for getting a diagnosis in different parts of the country may vary from those described here. However, as the government begins to place a higher priority on services for people with dementia, the hope is that these services will become more uniform across the United States, with better training for professionals dealing with the condition and greater access to both diagnostic tests and follow-up treatment and care. However, regardless of where you live in the United States, the first stop on your journey is an appointment at your primary care physician's office.

Finding Someone to Do an Evaluation

One of the most important decisions you'll make when you start looking for a conclusive diagnosis is whom to call for an evaluation. If you live in or near a large metropolitan area, you may be able to find an Alzheimer's disease or dementia program associated with a medical school, and that's a good place to start. These sections explain what's important for the evaluation.

WARNING

Before you seek a diagnosis of dementia or AD, get long-term care insurance in place for your loved one if you think it will be needed to pay for future care. You can always cancel the policy if it is not needed; however, if a diagnosis of AD or dementia on your loved one's medical records, he is no longer eligible to purchase long-term care insurance.

Enlisting help from your family doctor

The easiest place to start an evaluation is with the doctor who knows you and your loved one best: a primary care physician who is usually a family practitioner or general internist. Even though these doctors may not be specialists in memory disorders, they are most familiar with the health of their own patients. When a doctor has seen a patient regularly over many years, it's easier for her to pick up on subtle changes in behavior and personality that may signal a real problem. Someone who's never seen the patient before doesn't have this advantage because she doesn't have personal knowledge of this person over time.

Your loved one's primary care physician should have full copies of his medical records and can use this knowledge of his background medical history to make new diagnoses. Using the primary care physician to the best of your advantage is important, because seeing the wrong specialist, or the wrong combinations of doctors, can slow down the diagnostic process and lead to confusion for both patient and doctor.

Family practitioners generally have a network of specialists that they work with on a regular basis. They feel comfortable referring patients who need further assessment to these trusted colleagues. If the primary care physician suspects that your loved one may have dementia or AD, she may make the diagnosis herself or refer to a specialist for further evaluation. If you feel that your loved one's primary care physician isn't responsive to your concerns, don't hesitate to ask for a referral to a specialist.

WARNING

Unfortunately, research shows that, as a group, primary care physicians aren't always good at diagnosing dementia or AD, especially early on. One study showed an average of 30 months from time of onset of symptoms of AD until diagnosis by the primary care physician. Obviously, this is variable and dependent on the knowledge and experience of the doctor.

Picking a specialist

If you live in or near a large metropolitan area, you may be able to find an Alzheimer's disease or dementia program associated with a medical school, which is a good place to start. However, if you live in a smaller community, your area may not have such a program. Contact your local branch of the Alzheimer's Association. The office likely maintains a list of healthcare providers who treat people with memory disorders. See the section, "Tapping into other resources" later in this chapter for details on finding these programs.

Several types of healthcare providers specialize in the diagnosis and treatment of dementia and AD. In this chapter, we provide an overview to help you understand their different areas of focus. Armed with this info, you'll be able to ask savvy questions if your loved one is referred to a specialist for further testing. And remember that the title of geriatrician, neurologist, or psychiatrist doesn't automatically mean that the doctor is an expert in memory disorders. Go ahead and ask if you're not sure of a doctor's area of specialization or experience in working with AD and dementia patients.

>> **Geriatricians:** Geriatrics is the medical care of older people (usually those older than 65 years of age), and geriatricians are the physicians practicing this specialty. Geriatricians are either family physicians or internists who have taken additional training to specialize in the care of seniors. Because the incidence of AD increases so significantly with advancing age (from about 10 percent of adults at age 65 to almost 50 percent at age 80), geriatricians frequently diagnose and treat dementia and Alzheimer's patients. Although some geriatricians serve only as consultant specialists who will advise the primary care physician, others work as primary care physicians themselves and can assume full medical care in place of your loved one's family doctor or internist.

>> **Neurologists:** A neurologist is a physician specializing in the diagnosis and treatment of disorders of the nervous system, such as strokes, seizures, headaches, multiple sclerosis, other muscle and nerve diseases, nervous system tumors and infections, Parkinson's disease, and dementias.

TIP

If you're picking this specialist out of the phone book or an online listing, make sure you call a neurologist and not a neurosurgeon. A doctor specifically trained in the surgical treatment of brain and spinal cord disorders is called a neurosurgeon. If you end up in a neurosurgeon's office asking for a dementia evaluation, she'll refer you to a neurologist anyway, so save yourself some time and expense by starting out with the appropriate specialist.

>> **Psychiatrists:** Psychiatrists are medical doctors who specialize in the diagnosis and treatment of mental illness. Psychiatrists can determine whether a symptom such as agitation is indicative of mental illness or a manifestation of an underlying problem such as pain or infection, or is a sign of a neurodegenerative disorder such as dementia. Keep in mind that people with dementia may also suffer from psychiatric problems, such as depression or anxiety, that should be treated. Psychiatrists can diagnose dementia, but they limit their practice to mental health and don't provide full body medical care like your primary care physician.

>> **Psychologists:** Psychologists aren't medical doctors and, therefore, can't order diagnostic tests or prescribe medications. They specialize in the science of human behavior. Some psychologists specialize in counseling dementia patients and their families. Psychologists provide counseling to meet patient's emotional needs. They can also help family members/caregivers to learn how to deal with the challenges of caring for someone with dementia or AD.

>> **Neuropsychologists:** Neuropsychologists practice a specialty of psychology that assesses cognitive status, personality, and behavior. Neuropsychologists conduct a battery of diagnostic tests that can reveal patterns of cognitive changes that indicate various dementia disorders. The tests used are very specific and sensitive in determining the functional status of different parts of the brain. They then report their findings to physicians who will factor these findings into their diagnostic decision-making.

Try asking friends or colleagues who may have a family member with dementia or Alzheimer's for the names of their healthcare providers. Their advice can be particularly valuable because it's based on personal experience. Other patients and their family members have nothing to gain or lose by providing an honest assessment of a physician. Talking to people who've been down the road before you can save you time and money. Doing so may also help you to avoid wasting your time with a difficult or not very helpful doc.

Although a specialist such as a neurologist or psychiatrist may manage dementia, patients still need a generalist or primary care physician to manage their other health needs. As previously mentioned, some geriatricians can fulfill this primary doctor role. Realize that common problems such as upper respiratory infections may greatly increase confusion in patients with dementia or AD. A neurologist or psychiatrist won't feel comfortable treating this problem, which is why you still need a primary care physician. However, a specialist can work together with the family doctor in situations like this to provide optimum care for the patient.

Evaluating your choices

With so many choices, how do you know which doctor to select as the primary healthcare provider for your loved one? Although you must consider several factors, the most important one is to trust your own instincts. Still unsure? Ask yourself the following questions before making your choice. And remember, if you're not happy with the first doctor you choose, there's no law against switching to another doctor who may make you feel less rushed or do a better job of answering questions and calming your fears.

>> Do you like and trust the doctor?

>> Does she have experience in diagnosing and treating dementia and AD patients?

>> Does your loved one feel comfortable with her?

>> Does the doctor answer your questions and those of your loved one fully and treat you both with courtesy, compassion, and respect?

The answers to these questions are important because they can help you select a healthcare provider who keeps you informed and helps you both to feel comfortable and supported. Dementia and AD typically progress at a slow rate, so finding a doctor you can work with over a long period of time is essential.

Ensuring continuity

When you've decided on the doctor you want and are happy with her, stick with her. Continuity of care is crucial with a chronic condition such as dementia. This doctor has a working knowledge of the situation, a handle on the evaluations performed so far, and an individualized plan in her head about how to manage future concerns as they arise. A different doctor, without a thorough background knowledge of the situation, may manage problems differently, altering consistency of treatment. Seeing different physicians at different times may make managing your condition far more complicated and fragmented than it need be.

If you need to see a doctor for an unplanned appointment, try to wait for your own to be available rather than seeing a different doctor (unless it's an emergency, of course). This advice also applies to situations that occur outside of office hours, on the weekends, or on holidays if you have to call your doctor's answering service. Often there may be a doctor other than your family doctor on call who won't be familiar with your loved one's situation. Unless it's a medical emergency or something potentially life threatening, which requires an immediate trip to the emergency department of the hospital, try to wait to see your usual doctor.

But should this be necessary, remember an emergency doctor who usually doesn't have access to medical records is more likely to be overcautious about symptoms than someone who knows you (or your loved one). If you see a doctor who doesn't know you, you may be prescribed unnecessary medication, given tests you may not need or have already had, or, worse still, you may end up taking a precautionary trip to hospital to sit on a stretcher for the rest of the day or night.

Of course, if you're facing an emergency or aren't sure what to do, you must call for help. But always be mindful that, as is the case with cooks (too many cooks in the kitchen can spoil the soup), likewise too many doctors can mess things up and leave a bad taste in your mouth.

Tapping into other resources

If your family practitioner doesn't know a local specialist, try contacting the local branch of the Alzheimer's Association for a physician referral. Can't find the organization in your phone book? Go online to www.alz.org. Click on "In My Area" at the top left of the home page. Doing so will take you to a page entitled "In My Community." Enter your zip code in the space provided and click "search" to find the programs and services nearest to you. Volunteers with the local chapter of the Alzheimer's Association are happy to help you find an Alzheimer's specialist in your area.

Many Alzheimer's disease centers (ADCs), Alzheimer's disease research centers (ADRCs), and Alzheimer's disease clinical centers (ADCCs) don't require a physician referral for a patient to be seen. The National Institute on Aging funds these centers, which are located in major medical institutions and teaching centers across the country. Some maintain satellite facilities to serve rural and minority communities. Call your local Alzheimer's Association for information regarding the availability of such services in your area.

Wondering whether an ADRC or ADCC is located near you? Log on to www.nia. nih.gov/alzheimers/alzheimers-disease-research-centers and scroll down to the map on that page that shows the cities where these centers are located. Find the ADC nearest you and then call to see whether it offers any services close to your home.

The doctors and research scientists who staff ADC are devoted to better understanding the cause of dementia and AD and to finding effective new treatments. They're also searching for a cure and, better yet, a preventive measure like a vaccine that would spare future generations from the heartbreak of this devastating disease. Because the centers network together, researchers are able to collaborate on promising treatments; the resulting synergy is producing some exciting advances in the field of dementia treatments.

So what does all this mean for you and your loved one? If you're fortunate enough to live close to an ADC, you'll be able to take advantage of the latest diagnostic and disease management resources, as well as tap into a vast storehouse of knowledge and information about dementia and AD. In these centers, you may connect to support groups or even private counseling resources. In addition, your loved one may have the option to participate in a clinical research trial to evaluate new Alzheimer's drug therapies.

Before You Seek a Diagnosis: Collecting Medical History

If you've made up your mind to pursue a diagnosis for your loved one, you can do several things to help your doctor determine what's causing the symptoms. If you were a fly on the wall in any doctor's lounge, you'd discover that their number one complaint is that patients don't provide them with enough information to plan a targeted diagnostic assessment.

The first thing any doctor does when seeing a new patient is collect a medical history from that patient. You know those 28-page documents that your doctor's office forces you to fill out when you arrive with a sprained knee and are waiting to see an orthopedist for the first time? Those documents make you ask, "What does my history of gall bladder surgery have to do with my painful knee?"

Those are medical histories. These forms collect information on past illnesses and hospitalizations; previous surgeries, vaccines, medications, and supplements in use; and family history in addition to asking about current symptoms. It's most helpful to inform the doctor of any other health problems your loved one may be experiencing, particularly chronic problems such as diabetes or emphysema that require ongoing care and daily medications. It's also helpful for your doctor to know whether any other family members have ever suffered from any sort of dementia or brain disease, because there's a rare type of AD that is genetic and may be inherited.

Digging through your roots

When you compile your family medical history, you may have to search through old family scrapbooks or obituary clippings to find causes of death for older or deceased family members or even interview aunts or long-lost cousins you haven't seen in years. But this expedition through your family's medical history is important. Remember that dementia was referred to as "senility" in years past so if you learn about grandma being "senile," more than likely she had dementia. A little digging through your roots can produce some valuable clues to help your doctor narrow the scope of her diagnostic efforts by providing other possible causes or contributing factors for the symptoms your loved one is displaying.

A complete family medical history can suggest areas of interest to a doctor. For example, if your family has a tendency toward thyroid problems, perhaps low thyroid levels are causing your loved one's cognitive symptoms. If the doctor prescribes a thyroid supplement to reverse the low thyroid levels, that may help the cognitive symptoms to clear. Or your loved one could be suffering from sleep apnea, a sleep disorder that shuts off the airway, repeatedly depriving the brain of oxygen for periods as long as a minute throughout the night. This asphyxiation "in slow motion" can seriously affect memory and attention. Sleep apnea is also treatable.

TIP

Please don't hold any information back from your doctor because you think that it's too embarrassing to think about, much less write down. You know what we're talking about — things like psychiatric, gastrointestinal, urinary, or sexual problems. Details help to support or rule out a diagnosis of a particular disorder. For example, impotence in men is frequently caused by high blood pressure or diabetes leading to vascular disease, which may also have significant adverse effects on the brain. So tell your doctor everything you know about your loved one's medical history, even if you don't think it's relevant. You should also include any family's history chronic conditions like high blood pressure, diabetes, or heart disease that would require treatment if identified in your loved one.

On the other hand, if your loved one has no underlying health issues and other medical conditions have been ruled out with diagnostic testing (see Chapter 6 for more), the doctor may suspect dementia or Alzheimer's. But remember that the cognitive, functional, and behavioral problems you're reporting can only be diagnosed as dementia or AD after a complete workup. You don't want to jump to conclusions without evidence, and you certainly don't want the doctor to do so either.

After you've gathered as much family medical history as you can, construct an individual medical history for your loved one. Make it as complete as possible, which may mean collecting medical records from a number of doctors to build an accurate history. Although most doctors readily comply with requests for these records, occasionally, one will make it difficult and try to act like you can't have the information you're seeking. To be complete in your search for records, start by making a list all the doctors and hospitals that have provided inpatient or outpatient diagnostic tests or medical care for your loved one. You need to request records from each of these.

If a doctor's office gives you an attitude when you request medical records, remind the staff that while the records belong to the doctor, the information contained within those records belongs to the patient. As power of attorney (POA), you have a legal right to access them on behalf of the patient (more on this in Chapter 12).

The doctor's office or hospital may charge you a copying fee priced per page, which can really add up if there are a lot of records, but it can't refuse to provide you with copies of requested records. If you sign medical record releases at the doctor's office and ask the staff to gather medical records directly from the appropriate hospitals and other physician's offices, no fee is charged. Your doctor's staff will fax the releases to the appropriate sites and the pertinent records will be faxed or mailed back to your doctor, because such transfer of medical information directly between hospitals and physicians or between different physicians is considered continuity of care for the patient's benefit and as such should be without cost to the doctor assuming the care. If your loved one is still able to sign her name, then have her sign the releases. If not, then you as POA, or whoever is the POA, need to sign.

No matter how hard you search, some records may be impossible to find. For example, a doctor may have retired, passed away, moved to a different state, or even lost his records. If you can't find complete medical records for your loved one, try to fill in the blanks by talking to family members and close friends who may be familiar with prior medical history. Ask whether they can recall any details about your loved one's past that may help your current doctor make a good diagnosis.

Keeping a journal

When you first notice symptoms that make you suspect your loved one may be entering the early stages of dementia or AD, start keeping a journal. A journal can be something as simple as a 79-cent spiral notebook or a file on your computer (just remember to print it out before you visit the doctor). The most important thing is to record symptoms and events in the order they occur. Note specific instances of worrisome or uncharacteristic behavior, and accurately record the date, time of day, and any factors you believe may have triggered the incident and that may help the doctor in his evaluation. For example, record exactly what happened and what your loved one was doing just before and during the event and how long the event lasted or if it was recurrent or persistent.

This sort of information can be invaluable in helping a doctor determine a diagnosis. For example, if you record that your loved one is blacking out frequently, your doctor may begin looking at heart block, cerebral vascular disease, or seizures as the problem. A series of TIAs, or transient ischemic attacks, during which the blood supply to the brain is momentarily cut off, can produce neurological symptoms similar to those experienced by the AD patient. If your journal shows that your loved one's symptoms started soon after a new medication was added, the doctor may suspect that the medication may have side effects that could be triggering the altered behavior. This problem is very common in older people, especially if they're going to several doctors and taking many prescriptions, some of which may not be compatible. This problem also highlights the importance of all your doctors being in communication with each other to prevent situations where combinations of various drugs can cause cognitive problems or even actually be life threatening. Some drugs shouldn't be used simultaneously and their interactions can be very dangerous.

WARNING

If you don't record information in your journal as it happens, and you don't tell your doctor about significant events such as new behavioral changes or physical symptoms, you may put yourself and your family member through an expensive and unnecessary series of tests as the doctor strives to rule out possible causes for the symptoms.

Looking for other sources of information

While you're gathering records to compile your family member's medical history, don't forget dental history as well. Infections can spread from the teeth or gums to the heart valves. Such infection can then spread to the brain and may cause permanent damage that affects day-to-day functioning.

Other family members may be able to help if you can't get all the information you need to compile a complete medical history for your patient. If the patient is one of your parents, perhaps your aunts and uncles can tell you where to get additional information. Even an old family Bible that lists causes of death for deceased relatives can provide a valuable clue for your doctor in his search for answers.

Rounding up medication records

When you're compiling a medical history, don't forget to include a complete list of any prescription drugs, over-the-counter medications, vitamins, and herbal supplements that your loved one may be taking. This information is vitally important in order to identify potential medication side effects that could be contributing to the cognitive problems and to avoid a potential drug interaction when a medication is prescribed. Doctors must know all prescribed and over-the-counter medications. Certain pills may cause dementia-like symptoms as side effects that can clear if those pills are discontinued. This is especially true for psychotropic or mind-altering medications like narcotic painkillers, benzodiazepines (used for anxiety or as sleeping pills), certain antidepressants, and antipsychotic medications.

For example, if your loved one has blood clots in her leg or lungs, the doctor may put her on a blood thinner warfarin (Coumadin). But if you fail to inform your doctor that the patient is already taking aspirin or herbal supplements such as ginkgo biloba or vitamin E that can also thin the blood, mixing these pills could trigger bleeding problems that can be as serious as a bleeding ulcer or fatal stroke, or if the patient requires emergency surgery, a serious hemorrhage.

TIP

Most pharmacies today keep computerized records of their customers' medication histories. Ask the pharmacist to print out a copy for you to give to the doctor. Although some pharmacists may be willing to share this information with you especially if they know you're caring for your loved one, like other medical records, pharmacy records are personal health information. In a less familiar setting, you'll have authority to obtain these records only if you're the POA. But remember, these records supply only prescription drug information. You must supply accurate records regarding any self-prescribed over-the-counter medications like painkillers or sleeping aids, vitamins, minerals, nutritional supplements, or herbal regimens your loved one may be using.

Knowing What the Doctor Will Ask during the Appointment

Medical school professors teach that 90 percent of any diagnosis can be made from taking a good medical history alone. A thorough physical examination then almost clinches it, with blood tests and scans simply putting the icing on the diagnostic cake. So whereas doctors on TV may shout for X-rays the moment a patient walks through the hospital door, their real-life counterparts will want to ask a few questions first. The following sections outline what you and the physician will likely discuss.

Inquiring about the current situation

A bit like journalists getting the full scoop, doctors want to know the five Ws and an H that are crucial to a news story: who, what, where, why, when, and how? You can help your doctor with information gathering by writing things down and taking your notes to the appointment with you.

Specifically, the doctor wants to know the following:

>> **Why have you booked an appointment today?** What's changed or become worse and made you bring your loved one to see the doctor?

>> **What are the symptoms?** If your loved one is aware of the issues, this is his chance to have his say. However, most dementia evaluations are initiated by family members who have noted significant memory or thinking problems that are affecting daily function in their loved one. Don't worry about trying to use clever medical terms to describe what's happening; use your own words and don't sound like you've eaten a medical dictionary for breakfast. Tell her all your concerns, both cognitive and physical.

>> **When did the symptoms start?** The doctor wants an idea of how long your loved one has been struggling with these symptoms. Did they start suddenly or creep up gradually? Did they worsen steadily or change in a stepwise pattern? Tell the doctor what else was going on at the time symptoms started, such as a death of a close friend or family member or an accident involving a head injury. All this information is helpful in the diagnostic process.

>> **Who first noticed the symptoms?** With physical symptoms, usually the patient is the first to notice a problem like shortness of breath when climbing stairs, bowel changes, or a new lump. But where dementia is concerned, often a family member or friend notices changes like decreasing memory, frequently losing things, or getting confused during usual tasks.

>> **How are the symptoms affecting day-to-day life?** Dementia isn't just about memory; it can also lead to changes in ability to accomplish day-to-day tasks like bathing or paying bills. So tell the doctor if your loved one can no longer complete the cryptic crossword he previously whistled through without a hitch or how he can no longer properly dress himself.

The doctor then will follow up with more questions based on your answers to find out more about each issue. For example, if your loved one is having difficulty baking cakes, the doctor will want to know which parts of the process have become problematic. Is it remembering the recipe that she knew by heart, physically stirring the mixture, or setting an oven timer so the cake doesn't burn?

TIP

Because these things can be difficult to remember and express within the time constraints of a doctor visit, it's always a good idea to make a list of concerns and questions to take to the appointment. You may want to include another relative or friend who has a good understanding of the situation and can help you remember the doctor's answers and suggestions. Refer to the earlier section, "Keeping a journal" for more help. You can record all types of information in the journal about your loved one's condition.

Reviewing background history

Even with the medical history displayed on her computer screen, the doctor will ask background questions about the concerns at hand. Reviewing prior history is key because it enables the doctor to fill in gaps in the record.

The doctor will want to know about

>> **Family history of similar conditions:** These questions focus on how distantly related the affected people were and how often the problem has cropped up. The previous "Digging through your roots" section can provide more help.

>> **Social history:** These questions address smoking and alcohol use (both how much and how long), occupational history, hobbies, and living situation. For example, is your loved one a banker that can no longer write a check?

>> **Dietary history:** The doctor examines your loved one's diet. For example, does he drink two pots of coffee every day or eat only hamburgers while skipping all nutritious five-a-day fruits and vegetables?

Thinking about the Examinations and Tests the Doctor Performs

After the doctor has all the information she needs about symptoms and history, she'll move on to physical examination and tests. Memory problems and confusion have many causes and don't all herald dementia. Therefore, the doctor looks for specific physical findings and test results that can sort out these possibilities. The physical exam is an important head-to-toe check that can show signs of diseases that may affect memory. (You can find out more about the different parts of a physical exam and the different types of tests in Chapter 6).

Then your doctor will administer screening mental status tests (either the same day or at a future appointment). These tests are useful tools for the doctor to help identify and quantitate the extent of memory and other thinking problems. Then the evaluation moves on to diagnostic tests.

These sections examine the types of brain scans the doctor may order and what being referred to a specialist means.

Undergoing brain scans

Unlike a car, where you simply lift the hood and see what's going on with the engine, access to the brain is (thankfully) restricted by the hard outer casing of the skull. Fortunately, advances in imaging techniques now allow doctors to take a look at the brain's structures and some brain functions without having to physically lift the lid. And although these scans are only a piece of the diagnostic jigsaw and can give rogue results that are occasionally dismissed, they're a useful part of the investigation process.

Your doctor can choose one of five main types of scan. The choice is directed by what the doctor is looking for after she has analyzed your other results. Which tests are done also depend on insurance coverage. Because these scans are expensive, many insurance companies require prior authorization, meaning they want to be sure that appropriate medical criteria is in the doctor's record to justify payment. The staff of the doctor who ordered the test will complete this process. The choice of scans may also be defined by what technology is available in your locale. Whereas most communities now have access to CT scans, other scans may not be available.

CT scan

Computerized tomography (CT) scans are the most commonly available brain scan. You lie in a large, doughnut-shaped scanner and completely painless X-rays penetrate your body tissues. A computer records the resulting images in thin cross section slices from top to bottom. By and large, the CT scan is a simple and painless procedure that lasts up to half an hour, at most.

A radiologist (a doctor who specializes in interpreting X-ray tests) then analyzes these images for signs of disease. A scan of a normal brain has a classic appearance, so the radiologist checks the CT scan for changes from normal. Different types of dementia have different patterns on a CT scan. The radiologist looks for structural changes such as evidence of strokes, shrinkage of brain tissue, and brain tumors.

Sometimes, the radiology technician will inject intravenous dye into your bloodstream through a hand or arm vein to make some brain structures stand out more when scanned. This is important to do when a brain tumor is suspected because the dye will help it show up better on the CT scan.

MRI scan

Magnetic resonance imaging (MRI) scanners don't use X-ray radiation, like their CT scanner cousins, to capture images; instead, they use magnetic fields and radio waves to build a picture of your brain. An MRI scan shows blood flow in the brain better than a CT scan does, which can be useful if your doctor thinks you may have vascular dementia.

TIP

A patient is in the scan (a tunnel) for a long time, usually around 45 minutes. The experience is very noisy; the patient can wear headphones to try to drown out the mechanical din that these machines make. Sometimes, the technician plays soft music through the headphones to decrease the noise. Some people experience claustrophobia in the MRI scanner. If you think your loved one will be bothered, you can request the doctor ordering the test to also order a mild sedative ahead of time. You'll have to get this sedative prescription filled at the drug store before the MRI study. Administer the sedative pill at the prescribed time before the appointment so it'll be in effect during the MRI scan.

Another technique to lessen anxiety or claustrophobia during an MRI exam is to ask the technician to lay a pillow case over your loved one's eyes so he can't see the walls of the tunnel staring during the test. The radiology technician taking the images is in contact with your loved one at all times through the headphones and can quickly stop the test if problems arise.

Because MRI scans are made with huge magnets, they're not suitable for people with certain surgically implanted metalwork, such as pacemakers or metal clips. Other types of metal (that aren't attracted to magnets) are allowed in MRI machines. Tell the technician about any internal metal so she can determine whether it's safe to have an MRI scan.

SPECT scan

Single-photon emission computed tomography (SPECT) scans are able to look in detail at how blood flows into tissues. These tests are most likely to be arranged by specialists rather than primary care physicians. To get this sort of information, liquid containing a radiolabeled tracer is intravenously injected. This tracer is detected by the SPECT scan as it flows through the brain. The areas that light up more brightly on the scan images highlight the greatest brain activity, whereas those areas with less blood flow and therefore less brain activity show much lower levels of tracer.

The different patterns of low activity in various areas of the brain can then help doctors identify which type of dementia you have. So, for example, low blood flow is evident in the frontal lobes if you have frontotemporal dementia and in the middle of the temporal lobes, which are involved in memory, if you have AD.

DaTscan

DaTscan is another type of SPECT scan that involves having an injection of a radioactive liquid into a vein. This substance is used to show levels of a chemical transmitter in the brain called dopamine. Based on the concentration of dopamine on certain scan images, DaTscans may be used to differentiate between AD and the rarer Lewy body dementia. Due to this specific usage, only specialists and not primary care physicians are likely to request this scan.

PET scan

PET scans, or *positron emission tomography,* are another type of scan that evaluates brain function. This scan detects gamma rays that are emitted indirectly by a positron-emitting radionuclide tracer. One type of PET scan identifies areas of the brain with amyloid deposits. Scientists think that an increase in amyloid deposits is related to the development of AD. Although this finding isn't a guarantee of the diagnosis of the disease, it may provide your physician with important additional information. Another type of PET scan identifies decreased use of glucose (sugar) in brain areas important in memory, learning, and thinking in AD patients.

Being referred to a specialist

With the medical history and examination completed, blood taken, urine analyzed, brain scanned, and memory scores added up, doctors will now be pretty certain about whether your loved one has dementia.

If the diagnosis is straightforward Alzheimer's disease or vascular dementia, the primary care physician will manage it. If, however, the diagnosis still isn't clear-cut, and it appears that your loved one may have an atypical or less common type of dementia, the doctor may make a referral to a specialist such as a geriatrician or a neurologist (see the earlier section "Picking a specialist" in this chapter for details on these specialties). Often, your primary care physician's staff will arrange the specialist consultation appointment. After that consultation, the specialist will write a letter to the primary care doctor explaining any important findings and any further test results.

WARNING

You may have to wait several weeks (or months) for your loved one to see a specialist who treats memory loss. There are many more people with dementia than specialists who provide care for this condition. However, waiting to see a doctor who is well versed in dementia can be worth it.

The specialist will probably want to review details of your medical history for herself, so if anything has cropped up since the last visit to the primary care doctor or you realize you forgot to mention something, jot down the details so you can tell the specialist. If the specialist is a geriatrician or a neurologist, she will also do a physical examination. A psychiatrist doesn't conduct physical examinations but rather focuses on history, interview, and observation alone.

After this assessment, the doctor may order more specialized scans and even more detailed cognitive tests called *neuropsychological testing.* Make sure the specialist has the results of any tests done by the primary care doctor prior to referral, so she can make sure the battery of investigations is complete.

Sorting Out Follow-Up and an Ongoing Plan for Care

Now that dementia has been diagnosed, what happens next? First, you must decide whether to get a second opinion to confirm the diagnosis. Hopefully the primary care physician or specialist has spoken directly to your loved one to explain the diagnosis of a memory disorder. If not, then you must bring this up. The conversation may not be pleasant, but it needs to happen. Because dementia is a memory disorder, more than likely the person with dementia won't remember this discussion. Realize that you may have to remind your loved one of this diagnosis again if need be.

As far as care goes, unfortunately, no magic cure for dementia exists, whichever type your loved one has been diagnosed with. Fortunately, however, certain prescription medicines can help manage many of the more troublesome symptoms of dementia. Part IV discusses caregiver support as well as considering residential facilities when care needs become too much to handle at home. Read the following sections for more in-depth information.

Seeking a second opinion

A diagnosis of dementia or AD can be terribly upsetting for both the patient and his family, so wanting a second opinion is natural. Just be aware that you don't need your loved one to go through all the testing and evaluation again; you can simply bring the results of those tests to another doctor to review and confirm the findings of the first tests.

Both you and your loved one should feel comfortable with the diagnosis and with the healthcare provider who's given it to you. There's nothing wrong with looking around for a doctor who offers you the kind of comfort and support you need to survive the challenging road ahead. If you don't really like the doctor you started out with, by all means, switch to someone else.

TIP

Before you make your decision to either seek a second opinion or skip it, do a risk-versus-benefit analysis. What are the potential benefits if you do decide to get a second opinion and what are the potential risks? Identifying what you hope to gain from seeing another doctor may help you make the decision as to whether that step is truly necessary. If not, then skip the hassle and expense a second opinion will involve.

Letting the patient know

How you tell your loved one that she has dementia or AD depends on several factors, particularly his ability to understand the implications of the diagnosis. But remember, how and not if you should tell your loved one is the question. Most doctors believe patients have a right to know so they may participate in the decision-making process regarding their care (if they're able).

Although sharing the diagnosis with your loved one may be upsetting, it may also offer relief to the person with memory loss if he is able to understand the conversation. Because it gives him an explanation for the problems that he's been experiencing, knowing the diagnosis validates his experiences and dispels incorrect beliefs he may have, such as "I'm crazy." In addition, it gives him the opportunity to talk about the experience of having AD or dementia if he's still able to express himself.

Understanding what doctors can do

In addition to diagnosing dementia (or arranging appropriate referrals), your primary care physician will also provide support and care after the diagnosis. She knows what the specialists have concluded, because those doctors will send a letter detailing diagnosis and management suggestions as well as the most appropriate treatments to try and how to access other help that's available.

Seeing your primary care physician about two weeks after an appointment with the specialist is a good idea, because she'll be able to go through the details of the correspondence from the consultation, answer questions, and translate any medical terms used into plain English.

TIP

Don't be afraid to ask the doctor anything, however silly you may think it sounds. The physician is there to help and is extremely willing to do so. And if your doctor doesn't have the answer to your question, she'll know whom to contact to get the answer.

These sections focus on a few things your primary care physician and specialist can do based on your test results with your specialist.

Determining whether to prescribe medication

Sadly, there's no "pill for every ill," and that's particularly the case in relation to dementia. But pills are available that can help improve the symptoms and, in some sufferers, even slow the disease's symptomatic progression.

WARNING

Your specialist or primary care physician can advise about which medicines may help. Unfortunately, she won't just be able to hand you a prescription. Available medicines may not be suitable for your loved one, not because of their cost, (which can be an issue), but for clinical or safety reasons.

Reasons for not prescribing particular medicines include

>> **Unsuitability for your type of dementia:** No drugs are licensed for all types of dementia, and your doctor has to weigh the risk of side effects you may experience with the potential benefits the drug may provide. If the drug isn't for your type of dementia, the possibilities for harm obviously come out on top.

>> **Potential drug interactions with other medicines you're taking:** Drugs don't all get along with each other inside our bodies, and some interactions are potentially lethal. Thankfully, most aren't deadly, but they can still lead to some pretty serious physical side effects. Other interactions may mean that a pill you're already taking may not be effective when taken with the medicine. Conversely, the different medications taken together may heighten the effect of one or the other, making the interaction potentially toxic.

>> **Risk of making another medical condition you have much worse:** Very rarely do any pills act like magic bullets, targeting only the symptoms doctors want them to and not making mischief elsewhere in the body. That's because after you swallow a tablet or put on a patch, the drug is absorbed into your bloodstream and courses all around your body. Consequently, if any other body tissues are sensitive to the chemical in your medicine, they'll be affected too. Aspirin provides a good example. While preventing heart attacks and helping in vascular dementia, it can also cause stomach ulcers and potentially life-threatening hemorrhages in sensitive people. So you can see that aspirin isn't appropriate for everyone.

Don't believe everything you read or hear in the media. If your doctor won't prescribe a particular medicine for your dementia, it's not because you're too old and she can't be bothered with you or because it's too expensive and you're not worth it. Instead, your doctor recognizes that either that medicine won't help or, worse still, will give you other problems.

REMEMBER

All doctors practice according to the moral standard to "first do no harm," and that ethos guides all their decision-making.

Identifying suitable medication

Providing it's safe to do so and likely to help, your doctor may prescribe a number of groups of medicines to help with your dementia and its symptoms. Here is a quick run-through of the types of drugs available (Chapter 8 covers them in more detail):

>> **Drugs to treat dementia itself:** Four drugs are available at present (donepizil, rivastigmine, galantamine, and memantine), all of which have been designed specifically for use in people with AD. Unfortunately, they provide no benefit for patients with frontotemporal dementia or vascular dementia. These drugs are, however, sometimes used for people with a mixed diagnosis of Alzheimer's and vascular dementia, and can help a little in Lewy body disease. (Chapter 1 identifies the different forms of dementia.)

>> **Drugs to protect against further deterioration:** The Alzheimer's medicines previously listed may slow the progression of the disease for a while and are prescribed for this reason as well as to help with the symptoms of Alzheimer's. In vascular dementia, stopping further damage to blood vessels in the brain is very important. Doctors prescribe pills to make sure your blood pressure and cholesterol are well controlled to prevent further strokes. They may also give you aspirin or other blood thinners to prevent blood clots from forming in your circulation (which can also cause strokes).

>> **Drugs to help with troublesome symptoms:** Although not being designed to treat dementia specifically, several drugs nonetheless can help with the symptoms they can produce, which for some people can prove more disturbing than the condition itself. A common example of medicines in this category is antidepressants to help with anxiety and depression.

Providing monitoring and follow-up

Following diagnosis and the initiation of treatment, your doctors will want to keep an eye on you. They'll monitor the following:

>> Whether your treatment is helping

>> The development of any side effects from prescribed medications

>> The state of your symptoms, to assess whether you're improving or are at least stable, or to pick up any deterioration in your condition that may require a change of management plan

>> Your general physical health and the treatment of potential risk factors for your condition (blood pressure, cholesterol, diabetes, and such)

The timing of follow-up visits varies between primary and specialty care. Primary care physicians are likely to see your loved one more often than specialists, who lean toward periodic visits and send you back to your family doctor as soon as they're happy that your condition is stable. Most primary care physicians find monitoring patients every three months to be a particularly useful time interval.

Additional members of the healthcare team (nurse practitioners, physician assistants, home health nurses, or social workers) may see your loved one. They can consult the primary care doctor if any concerns that you or your loved one raises that are beyond their expertise.

Sorting out social supports

Medical treatment is unfortunately pretty impotent in relation to dementia; thus the mainstay of help comes from social support. Unfortunately, such support isn't typically covered under Medicare or other health insurance. However, remember that the Alzheimer's Association offers a wealth of resources and valuable support for patients and their caregivers.

Depending on your loved one's circumstances, a variety of social services may be available, although again this varies between in different areas of the country. Payment for these services is often out of pocket, although some insurances or government programs may pay all of some of these expenses based on financial need. These services can include

>> Home health aides, which can include assistance with shopping, cooking, cleaning, washing, and dressing

>> Meals on Wheels to deliver prepared meals to the home

>> Adaptations to the home such as handrails, walk-in showers, access ramps, and raised toilet seats to help patients live at home more safely despite increasing frailties

>> Help sitting up and/or remembering to take medication

>> Access to adult day care centers

>> Respite care (in adult day care, assisted living, or nursing homes depending on the level of care needed)

>> Support dealing with insurance and other money matters

Addressing practical issues

You also need to address some important practical issues for or with your loved one (depending on his stage of dementia and functional ability at the time of diagnosis), such as

>> Assessing driving ability and helping your loved one to hang up the keys when necessary.

>> Planning for future financial management for your loved one including bank accounts, savings, investments, and insurance policies (check out Chapter 13).

>> Establishing legal responsibility for ongoing care needs including when to invoke power of attorney (see Chapter 12).

>> Helping your loved one to make a will if he is still mentally able to do so if he doesn't already have one. Make sure you know where your loved one's will is located.

Chapter 6

Looking at the Tests Used to Diagnose Alzheimer's Disease

Perhaps you think there's a good chance your loved one is suffering from Alzheimer's disease (AD). Now you need to get a diagnosis so you and your loved one can start planning for the future.

This chapter provides an overview of standardized AD diagnostic criteria. In other words, we explain how a doctor diagnoses AD. In many ways, the diagnostic process is something like following a treasure map. The path may not be clear, but if doctors can follow the clues, they'll end up at the right destination.

We discuss the types of tests that may be performed to reach a diagnosis, including initial screening, a mental status evaluation, and neuropsychological tests that help to determine the patient's current level of cognitive and functional ability. We review the general physical exam, neurological evaluation, psychiatric examination, as well as various laboratory blood and urine tests, and brain imaging studies. (If you're looking for information about how to find a doctor who treats dementia and AD and what information to take with you to an appointment, flip back to Chapter 5.)

How Doctors Diagnose Alzheimer's Disease

There is no definitive, 100 percent sure way to diagnose AD other than by dissecting the patient's brain after death to look for the presence of characteristic neurofibrillary tangles and amyloid plaques in the brain. (Refer to the nearby sidebar for clear definitions of these terms.) However, by applying nationally recognized diagnostic criteria, doctors can and do make the diagnosis of AD with 90 percent or greater accuracy.

Diagnosis is a two-part process. First, doctors conduct a variety of tests to rule out what the patient doesn't have. For example, they need to determine that a patient hasn't had a stroke, doesn't have Parkinson's disease or multiple sclerosis, isn't suffering from low thyroid levels, and isn't clinically depressed.

Doctors use standardized diagnostic criteria that outline the behaviors, physical findings, and cognitive symptoms that are typical of AD sufferers to "rule in" a diagnosis of AD. If your loved one meets the criteria for AD established by the American Psychiatric Association DSM (Diagnostic and Statistical Manual) or the National Institute of Neurological and Communicative Diseases and Stroke/Alzheimer's Disease and Related Disorders Association and no other underlying cause for his symptoms is found during a physical examination, then your doctor should feel confident in making a diagnosis of AD.

GRASPING WHAT THE JARGON MEANS

Neurofibrillary tangles are abnormal deposits of a protein called *tau* along nerve pathways within the brain. The body normally uses tau to build and repair structures called *microtubules* that transport substances like nutrients and waste products into and out of brain cells. In AD, the microtubules collapse in tangles, which then prevents the brain cells from properly communicating with each other. As these neurofibrillary tangles accumulate, they prevent the brain from working the way it's supposed to. As a result, the Alzheimer's patient becomes less and less able to function normally.

Amyloid plaques are formed when a protein called *amyloid* divides incorrectly into beta-amyloid. *Beta-amyloid* is sticky and clumps together, gradually building up into amyloid plaques that group together and interfere with brain cell function. These plaques block the communication between brain cells and trigger inflammation. They ultimately accumulate and clog up the brain like the neurofibrillary tangles do. Both neurofibrillary tangles and amyloid plaques are seen in Alzheimer's patients' brains when examined under the microscope after death.

REMEMBER

Cognitive deficits have many causes. Something as readily identifiable as depression, a thyroid problem, dehydration, urinary infection, vitamin deficiency, or medication side effects can cause people to act in a cognitively impaired manner. It doesn't always have to be AD. Appropriate diagnostic tests can help your doctor determine the cause of your loved one's problem and the best course of treatment.

Understanding AD Diagnostic Tests

Not having a piece of paper with a definite diagnosis written on it can be unsettling. This is just one of the many frustrating things about AD: You can't be 100 percent sure that's what you're dealing with. But current diagnostic practices do offer a high degree of certainty. And researchers are working to develop new ways to quickly identify Alzheimer's patients through use of gene markers or other chemical flags.

BUT WHY IS A DIAGNOSIS IMPORTANT?

You're pretty sure that your loved one has Alzheimer's disease, so why waste time and money getting a diagnosis? What good is that going to do?

Getting an accurate diagnosis is essential because other medical conditions that are treatable and potentially reversible, such as depression, vitamin B12 deficiency, low thyroid levels, and certain medication side effects, can mimic the symptoms of Alzheimer's disease. If your loved one has such a look-alike but reversible condition and you just assume that it's Alzheimer's, the person won't get the treatment that could restore normal functioning. We discuss more about diseases that can be mistaken for Alzheimer's in Chapter 4.

Your doctor must perform a complete physical exam and comprehensive evaluation of your loved one's cognitive and functional abilities so he can give you the most accurate diagnosis and create a personalized treatment plan. Ultimately, finding out that your loved one actually has Alzheimer's relieves the stress of not knowing and allows you and your loved one to make reasonable plans for the future. If the diagnosis is early enough (in the mild stages of AD), it also gives the patient an opportunity to participate in decisions about her future care, which can go a long way toward relieving the anxiety and fear a person experiences when diagnosed with Alzheimer's. Finally, early diagnosis means early treatment, and early treatment gives your loved one the best chance of maintaining her cognitive abilities and usual functioning for a longer period of time.

In the following sections, we discuss the various diagnostic tools your healthcare provider may use to help diagnose your loved one. We tell you why that particular procedure may be used and what information it provides.

Screening for dementia and AD

To arrive at a diagnosis of dementia in general and specifically AD, doctors must evaluate multiple aspects of daily functioning through screening questions. In addition to an interview of the patient and family members/caregiver, mental status screening tests are conducted. Multiple different mental status examinations are available to screen for dementia/AD. Here are the most common:

>> **VAMC/SLUMS and MMSE:** Although somewhat different, these two screening tests — the Veteran's Affairs Medical Center-St. Louis University Mental Status test and the Mini-Mental Status Exam, also referred to as the *Folstein test,* are meant to look for cognitive impairment.

Both have a total possible score of 30 points. They evaluate orientation, memory, visuospatial skills, attention, calculation, and the ability to follow simple commands. Scoring is as follows:

- **Normal:** 27–30

- **Mild cognitive impairment:** 21–26

- **Moderate cognitive impairment:** 11–20

- **Severe cognitive impairment:** 0–10

>> **BIMS:** The Brief Interview of Mental Status (BIMS) is a quick screening test that focuses on repetition, time orientation, and recall.

>> **Mini-Cog:** The Mini-Cog is a simple two-part test that asks a person to complete two tasks:

- Remember three common everyday objects and recite them from memory after the second task.

- Draw a clock face and label it with all 12 numbers and put the hands on the clock showing a specified time. The ability to draw and label a clock face tests memory, visuospatial skills, drawing, and sequencing of numbers. These skills decline progressively in Alzheimer's patients, so drawing a clock is a helpful tool in diagnosing and staging AD.

These screening tests measure basic skills of short-term memory, orientation, concentration, language, and visuospatial skills. Doctors often repeat these tests at least annually to track cognitive changes. But remember these mental status tests are only screening tools and may not be able to detect early symptoms of memory or thinking problems, particularly in high-functioning people. As these skills decline with AD progression, your loved one's functional ability to manage daily life independently will simultaneously decline. Knowing this can help you to help your loved one as they become less able to care for themselves.

Furthermore, your loved one's doctor performs these screening tests to assess the following types of skills:

>> **Self-care skills:** These skills include the ability to get dressed, prepare and eat simple meals, move about safely without risk of falling, bathe, and perform other hygienic routines such as brushing teeth, driving, cleaning house, taking prescribed medications, and using household equipment and supplies appropriately.

>> **Communication skills:** These skills include a person's ability to make himself understood either verbally or in writing, and the ability to read and understand simple written instructions and comprehend and carry out oral instructions consistently.

>> **Simple math skills:** This category includes the ability to make proper change, write checks, pay bills, tell time, balance a checkbook, and manage personal finances.

These sections take a closer look at how your loved one's doctor tests for these skills and more.

Assessing your loved one's self-care skills

In order to assess your loved one's ability to care for herself, questions will be asked to determine whether she still is capable of functioning independently. Be sure to state whether you're already assisting your loved one with functional tasks (such as bathing, grooming, cooking, paying bills, and so on) so the doctor can determine how these tasks are being completed.

Possible questions include the following:

>> Does your loved one's appearance show attention to detail? Is she neatly groomed or disheveled? Is she dirty from lack of bathing? Is she wearing two different kinds of shoes? Is she dressed for winter in summer or vice versa?

>> Does she remember to eat regular meals or is she forgetting to eat and therefore losing weight?

>> Can she manage her personal hygiene or does she need help?

>> Is she paying her bills and income taxes on time?

>> Can she successfully and consistently perform necessary household functions, such as cooking and garbage removal?

>> Does she still know how to operate basic household equipment, such as telephones, wash machines, stoves, and faucets? Does food burn on the stove because she forgot to tend to the pan and turn off the burner?

Determining communication skills

Communication skills vary widely from one person with AD to the next. One person may retain the ability to engage in conversation for quite some time, whereas another may struggle to find words, express herself, or understand conversations earlier in the disease. As AD advances, the ability to communicate declines. This loss is most often gradual and like all other symptoms, it varies from patient to patient.

No one can predict how any given patient will be affected as the disease progresses, but speech and communication skills offer a measure to assess a patient's current level of cognition. Although the doctor will observe your loved one's communication skills in conversation, be sure to tell whatever you know about the following:

>> Is her speech normal in tone and pacing?

>> Does she speak in a louder than normal tone of voice?

>> Does she have problems reading? Does she read the same news article over and over?

>> Does she repeat the same statements, questions, or stories over and over?

>> Can she listen to and follow instructions?

>> Does she have difficulty expressing herself or finding the right word?

>> Can she follow and participate in a normal conversation, or does she quickly lose interest?

>> Are her facial expressions relaxed and friendly or guarded and worried?

>> Does she look you straight in the eye or avoid eye contact?

>> How is her mood? Is she depressed? Anxious? Angry? Irritable? Uninhibited? Inappropriately giddy?

Assessing simple math skills

You may be wondering why math skills are important in assessing the ability to live independently. But think about how many times in the course of your day you use math. Every time you get change from a $20 bill for lunch, calculate a tip, or figure out how much time you have before a meeting, you're using basic math skills.

In the early stages of AD, difficulty with math skills is one of the first signs that your loved one is having problems. Determining your loved one's ability to perform simple practical math problems can give your healthcare provider a surprisingly accurate measurement of the degree of impairment.

Here are some things to watch for that you'll want to report to the doctor:

>> Does your loved one have difficulty tracking time?

>> Can she write a check, balance a checkbook, make change, or calculate a tip?

>> Can she follow a complex train of thought or perform activities that have many sequential steps, such as cooking?

>> Does she pay her bills on time?

REMEMBER

The observations that you share with the doctor will help construct a profile of the patient's current level of cognitive functioning. Regular assessments of these skills can help you and the doctor to decide when your loved one requires additional care or monitoring. Ongoing reevaluation of cognitive functioning is critical to provide the best possible care for your loved one, so regular follow-up with the doctor is essential.

Evaluating memory

The doctor will want to know whether your loved one is suffering from memory problems, the extent of those problems, and whether they affect immediate memories, recent memories, remote memories, or all three. Does your loved one have trouble remembering recent events and conversations and a tendency to misplace objects? Frequently, Alzheimer's patients become quite agitated if they can't immediately put their hands on something, such as their purse or wallet. Even if it's in plain sight, they may not recognize it for what it is.

WARNING

Don't be surprised or get upset if your loved one accuses you of stealing from him. Although it's distressing, this behavior is common for Alzheimer's sufferers. Think how frustrated you would feel if you could never find your wallet. You might start to assume some sort of conspiracy was afoot, too. A little humor can help to defuse these situations, but they can be tiring especially if they happen frequently. For tips on how to take a mental health break from caregiving, see Chapter 16.

Gauging judgment and reasoning skills

The doctor may present your loved one with a series of everyday problem situations and ask what she would do if that situation occurred. Here are some examples:

>> If your bathroom flooded, what would you do? A person with normal cognitive functioning would lay down towels to clean up the water, and then call a plumber. A cognitively impaired person may offer a solution but not the best one; for example, she may say she'd call her doctor. Or she may offer no response at all, look away, and appear to be disinterested, or she may exhibit an inappropriate response, such as loud giggling or anger.

>> If a man rang your doorbell and told you that your roof was damaged but he could repair it if you lent him your debit card to buy materials, what would you do? A cognizant person would recognize an obvious scam and either chase the man off or call the police. A person with impaired cognitive functioning might freely hand over her debit card, if she could remember where it was. If she couldn't remember its location, she may even go so far as to invite the person in to help her look!

As reasoning and judgment skills deteriorate, you can see how an Alzheimer's patient can become an easy target for rip-off artists. See Chapter 13 for ways to protect your loved one from fraud.

Assessing orientation

People in the early stage of AD have trouble managing time and keeping their appointments. People in the advanced stage often show classic signs of disorientation. They may not know where they are or why they're there, and they may not have any idea of the time of day, or day of the week, month, or year. In advanced AD, some patients actually get lost in their own homes, unable to find their way from the bedroom to the kitchen or to the bathroom. If they leave their homes, they may quickly become disoriented and get lost.

This disorientation may make AD patients fearful, inattentive and easily distracted, or confused. They may show overt signs of confusion by repeatedly asking where they are or what time it is.

WARNING

This loss of ability to remain oriented puts your loved in danger of getting lost. Alzheimer's patients are at greater risk for wandering. If this becomes a problem, you must adjust your care arrangements by increasing supervision to keep your loved one safe. Often family caregivers become overwhelmed with wandering AD patients. If this happens, then admission to a locked unit of an assisted living facility or nursing home (depending on the AD patient's overall behavior and other health considerations) may be needed to keep the person from wandering and getting lost in unsafe settings like busy highways or isolated forests.

Evaluating eye-hand coordination skills

Eye-hand coordination is another basic skill that everyone takes for granted. You may be asking yourself, but what that does that have to do with anything? Well, think about trying to feed yourself if you couldn't make your hand pick up and correctly hold your fork whenever you wanted. Or, if you did manage to pick up the fork but couldn't figure out how to use it to get food from your plate to your mouth. Or maybe you forget how to comb your hair or brush your teeth. That's the state your loved one may find herself in as AD slowly advances and robs her of eye-hand coordination.

Share with the doctor your observations, such as the following:

>> Can your loved put on her clothes properly? Comb her hair?

>> Can she tie her shoes and consistently put the left shoe on the left foot?

>> Can she button her shirt or use a zipper?

>> Can she handle utensils with enough skill to feed herself?

The doctor may ask your loved one to demonstrate some of these eye-hand coordination skills during the evaluation.

Evaluating motor skills

The doctor may also want to know about motor skills such as the following:

>> Can your loved one walk steadily on her own, or is she shaky and disoriented?

>> Can she sit down and get up again without assistance?

>> Is she steady on her feet?

>> Can she get in and out of the shower or tub safely?

>> Can she use her cane or walker properly to maintain balance?

As motor skills start to fail, Alzheimer's patients tend to become more and more sedentary. Family members should try to keep their loved ones up and moving for as long as possible because even moderate activity helps to decrease the incidence of other health problems, such as diabetes, heart disease, and blood clots. In addition, after an Alzheimer's patient loses the ability to walk, cognitive losses seem to accelerate.

Neurological assessment

Some people mistakenly think that a neurological assessment looks only at what's going on inside an Alzheimer's patient's brain. People hear the word *neurology* and tend to think "head." Even though the damage caused by Alzheimer's takes place in the brain, it eventually affects the entire body because the brain controls the body. A neurological assessment helps the doctor determine how Alzheimer's affects other bodily functions such as muscle strength, reflexes, coordination, speech, and sensation.

Checking muscle tone and strength and reflexes

If Alzheimer's sufferers become sedentary, they lose a significant amount of their muscle tone and bodily strength. A loss of muscle tone can then lead to incontinence, breathing trouble, or cardiovascular difficulties. Decreased strength affects the person's ability to get around safely and may lead to falls.

Doctors check strength with a simple grip test and muscle tone using a hands-on pull back in the office. For example, the doctor may lightly hold a patient's wrist and ask the patient to pull against his grip as hard as he can and then push against his hand to evaluate another set of muscles.

In advanced stages, AD patients develop *primitive reflexes* that are like those seen in babies, which include the *suck reflex* (mouth makes a sucking movement when the closed lips are touched) and the *glabellar reflex* (repeatedly tapping the forehead causes the AD patient to repeatedly blink as each tap is perceived as a new stimulus) With this reflex, the patient has forgotten the prior tap, whereas a healthy person remembers and perceives the next tap as repeated and keeps his eyes open with repeated tapping.

Evaluating coordination and eye movements

One of the most baffling things about Alzheimer's disease is that even though motor function remains intact, the damaged brain can't organize the series of commands required to execute a complex activity like walking. Ultimately, the brain can no longer tell the leg muscles how to function. Consequently, as AD patients decline, they lose their ability to walk.

This loss of coordination between the brain and the body is so profound that it even affects eyesight. As Alzheimer's disease progresses, it becomes increasingly difficult for sufferers to track moving objects with their eyes.

Doctors test eye coordination by holding up a finger and asking their patient to track the finger with her eyes as it moves. They check physical coordination by having the patient walk so they can observe any abnormalities in the patient's gait or balance. They may also ask the patient to pretend to perform a routine task, asking, "Show me how you would throw a ball, brush your teeth, comb your hair," and so on because difficulty in imitating these everyday activities may indicate a breakdown in executive functions.

Checking speech

Speech is a complicated activity that requires the brain to coordinate the movement of lips, tongues, teeth, and vocal cords to produce intelligible sounds. Alzheimer's sufferers often exhibit symptoms of *aphasia*, or the inability to use or comprehend words correctly. After other potential physical causes, such as a stroke, are ruled out, language disturbances are a good indication that someone may be suffering from AD.

In addition to neurological testing, which looks at several areas of language, doctors evaluate patients' ability to understand language and express themselves by asking them questions and observing their responses. They're looking for problems in understanding commands (for example, "Take this piece of paper, fold it, and place it on the table"), following directions, and finding the correct word when speaking. In other words, is the patient's speech fluid and cohesive, or does she use words incorrectly or have problems finding the right words?

Checking sensory abilities

Sensory abilities help people make sense of the physical world around them. Alzheimer's patients suffer a disruption of their sensory abilities that's similar to the language disruption that we describe earlier. They may see a common item and yet be unable to tell what it is. Tests that reveal an inability to recognize familiar items despite the fact that the five senses are still working perfectly may also point to a diagnosis of AD.

Doctors must first confirm that the patient's difficulties in identifying common objects aren't caused by an actual physical impairment, such as failing eyesight or hearing. Standard visual and hearing checks will rule out this possibility. Be sure to tell the doctor if you're aware of any problems with vision or hearing in your loved one. In addition, be sure your loved one is wearing both his eyeglasses and hearing aids at the appointment if required. Otherwise responses to questions may be inappropriate due to vision or hearing deficits. By having glasses on and hearing aids in, the doctor can more accurately assess your loved one's vision and hearing.

Physical exams and diagnostic testing

A physical exam is one of the most important parts of evaluating a person for a possible diagnosis of AD because it can rule out other diseases and conditions that may be causing the suspicious symptoms. Here are some areas that your loved one's doctor more than likely will pursue.

Ruling out other physical causes

The primary purpose of the physical exam is to rule out other possible causes for the symptoms your loved one is displaying and to check for any other underlying illness that may require treatment. The exam should include the following:

>> A blood pressure and pulse reading

>> Eye exam (looking for cataracts and other eye abnormalities)

>> Ear exam (checking for wax blockage and hearing impairment)

>> Mouth exam (checking teeth and throat)

>> Neck and thyroid gland exam (looking for lumps and inspecting carotid arteries for narrowing that can increase risk for stroke)

>> Heart exam (listening to heart sounds with stethoscope to check for rate, rhythm, and murmurs)

>> Lung exam (listening to breath sounds with stethoscope to assess lung function)

>> Abdominal and rectal exam (checking for bowel sounds and feeling for masses)

>> Neurological exam (checking for sensation, muscle function, and coordination)

>> Skin exam (inspecting for skin cancers, lumps, rashes, and bedsores)

>> Foot exam (checking for pulses in feet and seeing whether toenails are being cared for properly)

REMEMBER

Many times dementia patients neglect foot hygiene and toenail care due to forgetting or an inability to manage to accomplish these personal tasks.

WARNING

High blood pressure is a leading risk factor for stroke. If your loved one has significant high blood pressure, she may have suffered a stroke that could explain her symptoms. Thyroid disease (high or low thyroid function) can cause confusion. Lung disease can cause thinking problems if the lungs are unable to take in enough oxygen. A person with an irregular pulse may have heart block that can cause dizziness or atrial fibrillation, which can cause strokes. Cancers of many organs can metastasize to the brain and cause altered cognition. The neurological exam may show evidence of prior strokes, Parkinson's disease, or other nerve damage. The skin and foot exam may show evidence of poor hygiene and self-neglect, both common issues in dementia and AD.

Undergoing diagnostic tests

After performing a physical examination, the doctor will decide on what diagnostic tests to order to check for other underlying conditions that may be present that could mimic AD symptoms or be affecting your loved one in addition to AD. These may include blood and urine laboratory tests and radiology studies including the following:

>> A complete blood count

>> Blood chemistry tests to determine calcium, glucose, and electrolyte levels, and to assess kidney and liver function

>> Vitamin B12 level

>> Thyroid function blood tests

>> Syphilis blood test

>> Urinalysis (and urine culture if indicated)

>> Drug levels of certain medications including digoxin and seizure medicines if in use (blood test)

>> Heavy metal and toxicology screening blood test (if indicated by history of occupational or other exposure previously)

>> Electrocardiogram (EKG) to check electrical function of the heart

>> Magnetic Resonance imagine (MRI) or Computerized Tomography (CT) scans of the brain (brain imaging)

>> Positron Emission Tomography (PET) scan of the brain

Both kidney and liver disease can alter body chemistry and produce symptoms of dementia, as can variations in blood sugar (glucose), calcium, and vitamin B12. Even an electrolyte imbalance can mimic AD, such as high or low sodium levels. Certain thyroid conditions and even syphilis can produce similar symptoms. EKGs can find heart abnormalities like heart block or atrial fibrillation that alter brain function. The good news is that most of these conditions can be treated successfully with reversal of their symptoms.

MRI or CT scan brain structural imaging can reveal areas of brain atrophy, stroke, tumors, or swelling. PET scans provide functional imaging, meaning that these scans can identify decreased use of glucose (sugar) in brain areas important for memory, learning, and problem solving in AD patients. However, at present, none of these scans can detect the microscopic amyloid plaque deposits or neurofibrillary tangles that are the hallmark indicators of AD. Those markers can only been seen when brain tissue of AD patients is examined under the microscope after death.

Ruling out psychiatric causes

Don't get offended when the doctor asks questions about your family member's mental health; no one is suggesting that the person is crazy. But many psychiatric conditions can mimic or contribute to symptoms of dementia and can be treated successfully.

Early-stage Alzheimer's is frequently accompanied by clinical depression. In these cases, patients can benefit greatly from appropriate antidepressant medication. AD patients with more advanced disease may present with psychosis. You want to make sure that these problems are identified if present in your loved one. Doing so can enable the doctor to prescribe appropriate treatment for these treatable psychiatric conditions, which can greatly improve the person's quality of life. Depending on the complexity of psychiatric issues, the primary care physician may refer your loved one to a psychiatrist for a more detailed exam to rule out other potential causes for his symptoms

Your loved one may also show signs of *apathy*, a lack of interest, enthusiasm, or concern, which may be mistaken for depression. Apathy is common in Alzheimer's patients and interferes with his ability to organize, plan, and carry out normal activities. Doctors hear caregivers say, "He just doesn't do anything anymore. He won't do his hobbies. I keep telling him to get a new hobby, but he won't." Apathetic patients often withdraw socially.

REMEMBER

Psychosis is a profound disruption in an individual's ability to perceive and interpret events. People with psychosis may have *hallucinations* (they see or hear things that aren't real) or *delusions* (they have false beliefs). Common delusions in AD patients include a strong belief that they're being robbed of belongings despite the fact that they have misplaced these items and can't find them. Another common delusion occurs when AD patients no longer recognize family members and think that a stranger is present in their bed instead of their spouse. Psychosis in AD patients can lead to behavioral problems and agitation, which can make caregiving more difficult.

Mental capacity and competency

We must make it clear that mental capacity and competency are legal terms and not medical terms. The doctor's primary concern is the wellbeing of patients, not their legal status. But healthcare providers are the ones who perform the evaluations that lawyers and courts use to make judgments about mental capacity and competence, which can define the need for a legal guardian. Therefore, your loved one needs a doctor who's skilled and experienced to assess her mental capacity to provide food, clothing, or shelter for herself; to care for her physical health; and to manage her financial affairs. Having *mental capacity* means your loved one can handle the daily activities necessary to care for herself and stay safe. People suffering from AD lose their mental capacity and therefore their competency as their dementia progresses.

Competency is a legal term referring to the degree of mental soundness necessary to make decisions about a specific issue (such as whether to consent to surgery to amputate a gangrene-infected leg) or to carry out a specific task (such as signing a will). A person may be competent to say who she wants to manage her finances, but not be sufficiently competent to properly file her own income taxes. A competent person uses good judgment and exercises her ability to reason in order to make appropriate decisions for the situation at hand.

AD impairs memory, judgment, and reason, which, in the eyes of the law, are necessary for a person to be considered competent. These progressive impairments in AD patients mean that they can't remember why they're not supposed to do something so they'll do it over and over again and continue to be surprised at the repeated negative outcome.

WARNING

When AD patients can no longer remember basic concepts such as "I should not put my hand on the stove because it's hot," their safety is at risk. In that situation, you must promptly make appropriate arrangements for increased care and monitoring of your loved one.

Chapter 7

Understanding the Stages of Dementia and Alzheimer's Disease

Over the years, doctors and researchers have come up with a variety of ways to classify degenerative dementias including Alzheimer's disease (AD) as they progress. Healthcare professionals have found that using stages is a helpful way to describe the expected course a particular illness may take and the array of symptoms that can appear along the way.

People know that dementia, in all its manifestations, is a progressive disease. Although this decline is most often seen as a continuous process, dividing up its course into stages to get a better idea of how symptoms change over the course of the disease is useful.

Staging a disease not only provides a shorthand that everyone in the medical profession instantly understands, but it also helps to explain the progression of various conditions to patients and their families. It's a way to let them know what they can expect in the way of symptoms at various points during the course of an illness.

This chapter provides an overview of the staging classifications of dementia and AD for informational purposes. You can use the information in this chapter to help you better understand the symptoms that your loved one may be displaying and get a better idea of what stage you are dealing with as his dementia progresses. However, recognize that these classification systems aren't set in stone. They're meant only as a general guideline to determine the severity of dementia.

REMEMBER

Even though Dr. Alois Alzheimer in Germany first discovered AD in 1906, it wasn't widely recognized or diagnosed in clinical practice until the late 1970s and early 1980s.

Picturing Retrogenesis: The Opposite of Normal Human Development

Dr. Barry Reisberg, a geriatric psychiatrist and leading expert in AD at New York University School of Medicine, identified a basic biologic process that he termed retrogenesis. He defined *retrogenesis* as the reversal of normal human development illustrated by the progressive cognitive and functional losses seen in AD and other dementing disorders.

Think about retrogenesis as the opposite of normal childhood development. A baby develops both cognitively and functionally in a pattern with simple actions progressing to more complex actions. A baby first utters one word, and then over time, learns to speak in sentences. Likewise he sequentially learns to roll over, raise his head, crawl, stand, and ultimately walk. And of course, you celebrate a child's graduation from diapers to using the toilet.

However, the opposite occurs in advancing dementia: A person loses function and experiences reversal of childhood development. As dementia progresses, speaking becomes more difficult. First, finding the right word becomes difficult. Then sentences become more jumbled and disconnected as the person with dementia takes longer to express a thought. Speech then lessens to one or two words at a time, and finally in very advanced dementia, the patient loses speech all together. Likewise, as time passes, a person with dementia loses the ability to walk, maintain urine and bowel continence, and bathe and dress independently in a pattern of declining function.

Knowing How to Use the Classifications

Staging systems provide guidelines that can help patients and caregivers make critical decisions regarding independence, financial and legal issues, and the type of care and supervision that may be required at any given point. However, the edges of the stages, regardless of the classification used, are blurred.

Although created specifically to stage AD, the most common staging systems are also utilized to stage other forms of progressive dementia, as the patterns of cognitive and functional loss are similar with all dementia progression.

All dementias including AD develop in an unpredictable fashion that can vary from patient to patient, but a basic progression is usually seen. Your loved one may never exhibit certain symptoms or cycle through all the expected stages; on the other hand, she may experience a textbook progression of symptoms. People develop dementia as individuals. Realize that not everyone will experience the same symptoms or progress at the same rate.

Each individual will experience dementia differently depending on pre-illness personality, other medical conditions, and level of support. No one can say for sure how the disease will affect specific individuals. For example, if your mother is 93 years old when she's diagnosed, she'll probably pass away before she reaches the final stages. Or if your husband has had severe heart disease well before his AD diagnosis, that condition may take his life while he's still in the earlier stages of cognitive and functional impairment.

WARNING

Dementia symptoms don't appear in clockwork order. You may find your loved one displays some Stage 4 symptoms when, according to his level of functioning, he's actually still in Stage 3. Every person's dementia is different, so don't get hung up on staging or read too much into it. Dementia including AD is far too complex a topic. *Note:* There is still so much about these conditions that researchers don't understand to be able to make any blanket statements about the exact progression in any given patient.

Many types of dementia staging systems are in use in the medical world, but to keep away from overwhelming you with technical details, in this chapter we focus on the three most commonly used scales:

>> The Global Deterioration Scale for the Assessment of Primary Degenerative Dementia (GDS) divides the disease process into seven stages based on the amount of cognitive decline.

>> The Functional Assessment Staging Tool (FAST) is a seven-stage system based on level of functioning in daily activities.

>> The Clinical Dementia Rating (CDR) scale is a five-stage system based on both cognitive (thinking) and functional abilities. The CDR is commonly used to define stages in dementia research.

Focusing on GDS

The idea of classifying dementia including AD into stages evolved over time, but the various classifications are simply different interpretations of the same information. For example, a group of psychiatrists led by Dr. Reisberg developed the *Global Deterioration Scale for Assessment of Primary Degenerative Dementia (GDS)* and first published it in *The American Journal of Psychiatry* in 1982. It lists the following seven different stages, but Stage 1 is "Normal with no cognitive deficits." People who omit Stage 1 end up with a six-stage model.

>> **Stage 1:** No cognitive decline; normal functioning. No deficits at all.

>> **Stage 2 or Forgetfulness Stage — Possible Mild Cognitive Impairment:** Very mild cognitive decline. Patients begin to forget names of family members, friends, and common objects. They still function well in social and work situations. They may express worry about symptoms. Subjective functional deficit.

>> **Stage 3 or Early Confusional Stage — Mild Cognitive Impairment (MCI):** Earliest clear-cut deficits. Memory problems become noticeable with difficulty handling complex problems. People may get lost traveling to unfamiliar locations and try to hide or deny their deficits. They may act defensively and minimize their difficulties. Problems with finding the right word may arise. They misplace items, can't concentrate, and have some difficulty retaining new information. Mild anxiety symptoms may develop with lower tolerance for frustration. (See Chapter 1 for more details on MCI.)

>> **Stage 4 or Early Stage or Mild Dementia:** Cognitive decline continues with decreased recall of recent events; patients may lose memories of some of their own personal histories. They have trouble handling their own affairs, especially finances, and can no longer manage complex tasks. They're still oriented to time and place, and recognize themselves and familiar people and places. They may become very defensive about increasing cognitive deficits and deny vehemently that anything's wrong. They may withdraw from challenging situations rather than try to cope.

>> **Stage 5 or Early Middle Stage or Moderate Dementia:** Cognitive decline becomes more severe. Patients require assistance to function and can't recall

or may make up basic facts about their own lives, such as where they live and work, or the names of friends and more distant family members. They still know their own name and names of close family members such as their spouse and children. Math abilities decline sharply. Patients may still feed and dress themselves and use the bathroom without assistance, but due to impaired judgment, they may require close supervision such as in selecting appropriate attire.

>> **Stage 6 or Middle Stage or Moderately Severe Dementia:** Patients exhibit severe cognitive decline. They no longer remember names of close family members, but can still distinguish familiar people from strangers. They need help with all activities of daily living. They have a total lack of awareness of current events but may still exhibit some memory of their distant past. Patients may become incontinent; both bowels and bladder may be affected. They show severely impaired judgment and may exhibit dramatic personality changes with episodes of delusion, anxiety, obsessiveness, aggression, and even violent outbursts that are completely contrary to their original personalities. They may have *sundowning* (when symptoms worsen later in the afternoon when the sun sets) and *day-night reversal* (where they tend to sleep during the day and stay awake at night) due to disturbance of normal sleep-wake cycle.

>> **Stage 7 or Late Stage or Severe Dementia — Failure to Thrive:** Patients show very severe cognitive decline. They can't speak or understand speech and can no longer follow basic instructions. They're incontinent and require round-the-clock total care and supervision. They lose basic motor skills, including walking and the ability to sit up.

Staging with FAST

The GDS has considerable overlap with the Functional Assessment Staging Tool (FAST). Reisberg also developed FAST, although it was intended to more specifically describe the progressive stages of AD. FAST also divides the disease progression into seven stages but then further divides Stage 6 and 7 into more detailed substages to demonstrate specific losses as follows. We list the developmental age at which a child gains the listed skill that is being lost at each AD substage, another illustration of retrogenesis (refer to the earlier section, "Picturing Retrogenesis: The Opposite of Normal Human Development" for more specifics about retrogenesis).

Here are the substages of Stages 6 and 7 in FAST:

>> **Stage 6:** Moderately Severe Dementia

- **6a:** Needs help putting on clothes (developmental age 5 years old)

- **6b:** Needs help bathing (developmental age 4 years)

- **6c:** Needs help using the toilet (developmental age 3–4 years) (removing clothing, wiping, disposing of tissue, flushing, redressing)

- **6d:** Urinary incontinence (developmental age 2–3 years)

- **6e:** Bowel incontinence (developmental age 2–3 years)

>> **Stage 7:** Severe Dementia

- **7a:** Speaks 5–6 words in a day (developmental age 15 months)

- **7b:** Speaks only one word clearly (developmental age 1 year)

- **7c:** Can no longer walk (developmental age 1 year)

- **7d:** Can no longer sit up without assistance (developmental age 6–10 months)

- **7e:** Can no longer smile (developmental age 2–4 months)

- **7f:** Can no longer hold head up by self (developmental age 1–3 months)

In order to qualify for hospice services, an Alzheimer's patient has to be at FAST stage 7c or beyond to be considered to have less than a six-month life expectancy.

Current Thinking: Assessing Stages via Cognitive and Functional Impairment

Researchers, doctors, and clinicians often classify AD according to the level of cognitive and functional impairment that the patient displays using the Clinical Dementia Rating (CDR) scale. Originally published in the *British Journal of Psychiatry* in 1982, this scale measures performance in six areas: memory, orientation, judgment and problem solving, community affairs, home and hobbies, and personal care.

Cognitive skills relate to a person's ability to think, make, and carry out reasonable plans; make judgments; be aware; and learn and retain new information.

Functional skills relate to a person's ability to take care of oneself and carry out the activities of everyday life. Doctors and researchers use cognitive and functional skills as a way to classify dementia and AD patients to provide a more reliable indication of where a patient is in the course of the illness and make assessments of a person's current needs. Patients may show a notable decline in cognitive skills but still display a relatively normal range of functional skills or vice versa. No one can say for sure how your loved one's illness will progress. No one can accurately predict the rate of decline because experts still don't know what causes progressive dementias including AD. Doctors also don't know what factors contribute to either an accelerated or relatively slow rate of decline.

Here is an overview of the CDR stages that commonly are used to classify dementia including AD, by the degree of cognitive and functional impairment that the patient exhibits. After this overview, you can find sections that provide more detail of mild, moderate, and severe impairment stages:

>> **Stage 0 — No impairment:** No memory problems; fully oriented to time and place, normal judgment and problem-solving ability, full function socially in the community and at home, and total ability to manage personal care.

>> **Stage 0.5 — Very Mild Impairment:** Slight memory problems, may have difficulty with complex problem solving, may show some impairment when engaging in social activities or with home tasks but have full ability to manage personal care without assistance. This stage is now termed Mild Cognitive Impairment (MCI) and may or may not progress to more advanced stages.

These sections examine Stages 1, 2, and 3 in greater depth.

Stage 1: Mild Impairment

During Stage 1, early dementia has two main effects on someone: change and loss. Identifiable changes in memory, mood, personality, and ability to manage day-to-day living will be evident. Not only does a person with early-stage dementia physically lose objects and bits of his memory, but you also notice that you're losing something of your relationship with him, as well as him losing aspects of what made him the person he is.

Expecting the unexpected is wise, because you can never be 100 percent sure how dementia will announce itself. Symptoms are likely to develop in a different order and at different speeds in different people.

Early symptoms of dementia may go unnoticed because patients can be quite adept at covering up any problems they're experiencing. Patients may exhibit the following symptoms:

>> **Memory loss:** This is the reason why most people are taken to see their doctor. Forgetting names, faces, dates, appointments, directions to familiar places, and details of recent events is generally the problem.

>> **Problems in conversation:** People regularly notice that their relative, friend, or spouse has begun to have trouble following the thread of conversations when talking to him and/or that he keeps saying the same things over and over again, as if for the first time, or repeating the same questions.

>> **Difficulty managing change:** Any deviation from normal routine can become a struggle to deal with, as can adopting new ideas. This change is most noticeable in people who've always been up for a challenge or adaptable in relation to trying new ways of doing things. Likewise, stick-in-the-muds can become even more stuck and set in their ways. Another early sign may be taking longer to make decisions such as choosing between two items to buy when shopping, what to have from the menu in a restaurant, and which clothes to wear.

>> **Losing things:** This behavior can become the rule rather than the exception in early dementia and can include regularly misplacing items like keys, reading glasses, cell phones, and television remote controls.

>> **Poor judgment:** Simple monetary transactions can become confusing, and people with early dementia are also more likely to fall for a scam or sign up for an insurance policy or mobile phone contract they don't need.

>> **Alteration of mood:** Low mood, anxiety, uncertainty, mood swings, irritability, and a withdrawal from usual social activities can all be early symptoms of dementia. It includes loss of interest in normal daily activities and hobbies. The patient may exhibit uncharacteristic rudeness or lack of social graces.

REMEMBER

People can exhibit dramatically different early symptoms. Some people show symptoms that initially baffle their doctors and are medical mysteries for some time before the diagnostic shoe drops (often because their symptoms could easily be due to a host of other conditions). Likewise, others show symptoms during a simple visit to their doctor's office and may as well have the diagnosis tattooed on their foreheads it's so obvious.

Stage 2: Moderate Impairment

In Stage 2, the symptoms that have sporadically appeared and perhaps fluctuated in the first stage become more permanent and their arrival also gathers speed.

As a result, people in this stage regularly have memory problems, develop difficulties with day-to-day functions like cooking, shopping, and dressing, and demonstrate much more obvious changes in their mood and behavior.

It becomes increasingly obvious that these changes can't simply be put down to senior moments or the perceived inevitability of a progression toward eccentricity and increased grumpiness with advancing age. At this stage, it's clear that something's wrong, and medical advice about what's going on and what can be done to help is now essential.

The majority of dementia diagnoses are made when a patient has reached this stage. The symptoms demonstrated in the first stage now become more extreme, and the following may be more likely:

>> **Memory loss:** This symptom becomes more severe, and sufferers regularly forget names of family members and friends, miss appointments, and often put themselves and others at risk by, for example, leaving pans cooking on the stove, eating food that's well out of date, going out and leaving the front door open, forgetting to take medication, and leaving wet clothes to mildew in the washing machine.

>> **Problems in conversation:** Repetition and rambling speech can become the norm in conversation, or people in this stage of dementia may not bother to join in, because they simply can't follow what's been said. They may have increasing confusion about recent events. They may also have trouble finding the right words for things, so describe them instead; thus a watch, for example, becomes "the time-telling thing on my arm." People at this stage are also prone to *confabulation* — filling in memory gaps with false details that they believe to be true. If asked what they did over the weekend, for example, they provide a description of events that bears no resemblance to the truth, but is nonetheless a plausible reply.

>> **Losing things:** In this stage of dementia, the most common things to become lost may well be the dementia sufferers themselves. Wandering is common and leads to people being unable to find their way to their proposed destination or their way home. Getting lost even in familiar settings (including their own home) becomes more common. Losing track of whether it's day or night isn't unusual, and heading outside in pajamas at night may be a regular occurrence.

>> **Alteration of mood:** Depression, anger, and irritability can be more prominent, as can elated and disinhibited behavior. Poor impulse control can lead to the person making inappropriate and even sexual suggestions to strangers. Verbal or physical aggression can develop. Anxiety is also seen in this stage,

most often manifested in following loved ones around and constantly seeking reassurance from them. Some people may experience confusion that becomes worse in the evening.

REMEMBER

For unknown reasons, many AD patients in the moderate stage of cognitive and functional impairment become increasingly confused as evening approaches. This phenomenon is known as sundowning.

>> **Suspicious minds:** Paranoia and suspicion are frequent features of this stage of dementia, often leading to aggression toward others who are believed to have stolen things from the sufferer or to be out to get him.

>> **Self-care:** Personal hygiene often suffers in this stage of dementia, and people need to be prompted to change dirty clothes, wash and shower, and brush their teeth. They may also begin to develop incontinence, which compounds the problem of staying clean and tidy.

Stage 3: Severe Impairment

By the time a patient enters the severe stage of AD, her care needs may become so overwhelming that her family may need to put her in a nursing home or other long-term care facility due to increasing difficulty caring for her at home.

At this point, the person with dementia succumbs to the full force of the effects of the disease, completely dispelling the myth that dementia is simply a memory problem. In this final stage, a severe loss of memory is definitely evident and all the other thinking and physical functions, including speech, orientation, judgment, problem solving, mobility, and display of emotions are eroded. At this stage, much of the capacity to meaningfully exist as an independent human being occurs. Ultimately, the result is an existential loss of self.

REMEMBER

Unfortunately, intellectual effects aren't the only signs of this stage of dementia: It also plays havoc with the sufferer's physical capabilities too. Not only are sufferers often incapable of carrying out the most basic activities of daily life, but they also become physically frail and are at high risk of falls and increasingly susceptible to serious infections.

Again, exceptions to this pattern of deterioration always exist, but for most people in the late or severe stage of dementia there is a precipitous loss of any faculties that haven't already shut down. This change manifests itself in a number of ways:

>> Physical frailty may lead to difficulty getting into or out of a chair, problems walking, and ultimately confinement to, initially, a wheelchair and, ultimately, to bed.

>> Feeding can be a problem, compounded by swallowing difficulties, and severe weight loss may result as well. Pneumonia becomes a risk due to aspiration of bacteria into the lungs resulting from trouble swallowing effectively.

>> Memory is significantly limited, and although occasional moments of clear reminiscence may occur, it's more common for people in this stage to have little recollection of day-to-day events, names of objects, and, most upsetting for families, names of their nearest and dearest. The patient may even forget her own name.

>> Speech can be lost, so that people with severe dementia may only utter individual words and sounds, often repetitively. They also lose the ability to understand the words of others, and meaningful conversation thus becomes impossible.

>> Agitation and irritability can be common, with refusal to cooperate with caregivers being a frequent issue. Shouting, lashing out with hands and fists, pulling hair, and biting are possible responses to well-intentioned offers of help. It's not unusual for family members and spouses to find this extreme rejection of their best efforts to reach out to their loved one very upsetting and particularly difficult to deal with emotionally.

>> Hallucinations, delusions, and paranoia become more common as patients lose touch with reality and have difficulty interpreting what they see, hear, or feel.

Profound, terminal, advanced, or end-stage dementia

Although not a formal stage in the CDR scale, as the severe impairment progresses further, the sufferer enters the profound or terminal stage of dementia. This is the last or end-stage stage in which patients lose the ability to communicate, walk, swallow, and maintain continence of bladder and bowel. At this stage, patients suffer from an increasing variety of physical problems. They're more susceptible to certain health issues than are people of the same age who don't have dementia. One study of end-stage dementia patients showed a death rate in the six months following hospitalization for pneumonia at 53 percent compared to 13 percent for cognitively normal patients. Likewise, in the case of hip fracture, 55 percent of end-stage dementia patients died within six months of the fracture compared to 12 percent of cognitively normal patients.

Not all patients reach this stage, particularly those who have other significant underlying disease processes or who were diagnosed at a much older age. Patients with end-stage dementia including AD will likely exhibit the following:

>> Complete lack of awareness of surroundings

>> Total dependence on caregivers for feeding, hygiene, and everything else

>> Complete bladder and bowel incontinence

If the patient is otherwise healthy, death may result from a number of causes, such as

>> Falls leading to fractures, plus poor healing and/or complications following surgery to repair such fractures. Stress experienced as a result of the trauma and being in the hospital may also prove fatal.

>> Infections such as pneumonia, urinary-tract infections, or skin infections can occur. If untended, bedsores can develop and progress to serious infection.

>> Progressive deterioration in general health with increasing weakness and debility.

Although death is likely to be hastened by any of the causes listed, it's also extremely common for people with dementia including AD to simply pass away peacefully as a result of increasing frailty.

LIFE EXPECTANCY AFTER A DIAGNOSIS OF DEMENTIA

The big question on everyone's lips when they're diagnosed with a life-limiting illness is, of course, "How long have I got, Doc?" And it's a question physicians hate having to answer, not only because their estimates may be a lot shorter than the timescale patients are hoping for, but also because doctors' estimates are invariably wrong. Although doctors recognize when a person is nearing death, specific predictions are unreasonable. Humans rarely play by textbook rules because so many factors can play a part in determining each individual's outcome.

Human have evolved mechanisms to ensure survival. So it's never as simple as saying, "If you have diagnosis A, you'll therefore live X number of months or years," because so many other factors come into play, including

- The stage the condition has reached before it's picked up.

- Age at diagnosis (In the case of dementia, older age usually means shorter survival.)

- Other health conditions occurring simultaneously (In the case of dementia, diabetes, congestive heart failure, emphysema, cancer, and heart rhythm irregularities are associated with shorter survival rates.)

- Tolerance of treatment provided for the condition.

- Psychological impact and the patient's general state of mind.

- The strength of the patient's immune system.

- Social circumstances and levels of deprivation.

A cancer patient may be told her condition is so severe that she has just a few weeks left to live. Then after one last throw of the dice in the form of a final dose of chemotherapy, she is miraculously cured. In contrast, another patient given a much less severe diagnosis, may take to his bed, shutting himself off from friends and family, and die in his sleep not long after.

Dementia is no different because people's responses to it vary. But having a rough idea of what to expect can be helpful in planning for the future. That is why the "How long does she have?" question is so commonly asked by families as they see dementia progress. Generally, the outlook isn't good. Looking at all, the average life expectancy from the time of diagnosis is about 8 years. However, the range can be as little as 2 years from diagnosis at its shortest to 20 years at its longest, with people who are older when diagnosed being at the lower end of the scale.

Bearing in mind that the period from development to diagnosis spans an average 2.8 years, an actual figure is, unfortunately, always hard to predict. However, research has shown that being male, having difficulty swallowing, weight loss, seizure development, and bedsore development are all factors associated with shorter survival in patients with dementia.

Chapter 8

Eyeing Medical Treatments

Medical science has made enormous advances over the past century, and people now benefit from treatments for diseases affecting every system in the body, from infections to insomnia and headaches to heart disease. But still no pill exists for every illness, and for some conditions, a cure seems to be a ways off.

Unfortunately, dementia and Alzheimer's disease (AD) are in that category. No medicines on the market can treat their cause or cure them. However, a handful of drugs appear to slow down the progress of AD and improve symptoms, if only temporarily. In addition, other drugs can help manage some of the more difficult symptoms that memory disorders can cause, such as sleeping difficulties, hallucinations, and depression.

But because each person is unique, not all these medicines help all people. In some cases, although doctors prescribe medicines with the best of intentions, these drugs can actually be harmful. This may be because they cause documented or unique side effects, or because they interact with medication the person is already taking.

So with these warnings in mind, this chapter takes a look at the drugs that are available to help with AD and their troublesome symptoms and discusses some of the unfortunate limitations they can have.

Identifying the Medicines

When you scan the pharmacy shelves or browse in the supermarket's medicines section, you see box after box of different pills designed to relieve all sorts of human ailments. Usually, you see a dozen or so treatments for indigestion alone, a bunch of headache remedies, multiple different drugs to stop diarrhea, and even more laxatives to treat bowels that need unblocking from constipation. Sadly, when it comes to Alzheimer's disease drugs, the choice is nowhere near as extensive. These drugs are approved by the U.S. Food and Drug Administration (FDA) to treat AD specifically, and some are also approved to treat other dementias. In fact, just four medicines are available.

Dementia is finally at the forefront of government health policy, and it often makes headlines in the media. So we hope that investment into research by scientists and drug companies will continue, and the research will begin to bear fruit. But for now, here's a guide to what your doctors may have up their sleeves.

REMEMBER

These medicines can help the symptoms of AD, but they're not a cure for it. All patients with AD will worsen over time, even with the use of these medications. These drugs may slow AD progression for a limited period of time, but they don't return a person with AD back to normal nor do they prevent the disease from ultimately taking its toll.

The medicines that doctors prescribe for AD have been designed to lessen the rate of progression of cognitive loss over time. Patients taking these drugs may experience some cognitive improvement, but they don't return to their former baseline brain function. Sometimes these medications can benefit mood and behavior issues in AD patients as well. They're available in a variety of formulations to help make them easy to take including pills, patches, liquids, and soluble tablets.

As with all drugs, AD medicines have a so-called *generic name,* which all manufacturers must use, and a *brand name,* which is the specific name a particular drug company gives to them. Here's an example with a well-known drug: Ibuprofen is the generic name, and Motrin is the brand name for the drug manufactured by one pharmaceutical company, and Advil is the name for the same drug by another pharmaceutical company. The more companies that make the drugs, the more brand names you find on the market for that medication.

Here are the four AD drugs, with their generic names first, followed by their brand names in brackets:

>> Donepezil (Aricept)

>> Rivastigmine (Exelon)

» Galantamine (Razadyne)

» Memantine (Namenda)

Understanding How Alzheimer's Disease Drugs Work

The four medicines divide into two groups according to the different ways in which they work:

» **Acetylcholinesterase inhibitors:** Donepezil, rivastigmine, galantamine

» **NMDA receptor antagonist:** Memantine (a very small and lonely group of one!)

Here's a quick guide to their different mechanisms of action.

Acetylcholinesterase inhibitors

Scientists have found that in AD, the most common form of dementia, patients lose nerve cells in the brain that communicate with each other using a chemical neurotransmitter called *acetylcholine* (you can find more detail about the way these transmitters work in Chapter 3). As a result, communication is blocked, and messages can't easily flow from one part of the brain to another. That means the person can't form new memories or recall them, and will develop other cognitive, behavioral, and functional changes that are characteristic of AD.

The drugs in this group work by blocking the effect of an enzyme (enzymes are proteins in the body that promote chemical reactions) called *acetylcholinesterase* that breaks down acetylcholine. Acetylcholinesterase inhibitors therefore boost the level of acetylcholine, allowing the brain cells to communicate better.

Memantine

Glutamate is one of the brain's main activating chemical neurotransmitters involved in the processes underlying learning and memory. Researchers believe that the overexcitation of the NMDA (short for N methyl D aspartate) receptors by too much glutamate causes too much stimulation in brain cells, which causes their dysfunction and eventual cell death that occurs in the brain of AD patients.

Memantine is an *NMDA receptor antagonist,* meaning that it binds to the NMDA receptors on brain cells thereby stopping too much glutamate from attaching to these receptors and triggering this damaging chain of events. The important thing is that memantine still lets the proper amount of glutamate attach to the NMDA receptors on the brain cells, allowing more normal brain cell function. This, in turn, helps protect the brain cells from excess stimulation and thereby slows the progression of the damage seen in AD.

Knowing When to Start Taking the Drugs

The decision about when to start taking any medicine for AD is dependent on the stage of AD your loved one is experiencing at the time of diagnosis. None of these drugs is appropriate to use before a formal diagnosis of AD is made. Furthermore, none of these medications is meant for the prevention of AD and shouldn't be used by those individuals who experience a little forgetfulness with the hope of warding off dementia.

REMEMBER

Timing of when to start treatment determines the type of drug(s) that a doctor will recommend:

>> **Acetylcholinesterase inhibitors:** National guidelines recommend that doctors give these medicines to people who have a diagnosis of mild to moderate AD. Donepezil is the only one of these drugs FDA-approved for use in all stages of AD (mild, moderate, and severe). Rivastigmine can also be used to treat symptoms in people who have Lewy body disease or Parkinson's disease dementia. Those who have mixed vascular dementia and AD may also benefit. Although these drugs aren't formally approved to treat vascular dementia, they may be helpful in this setting as well because there is often an overlay of AD with vascular dementia.

Given the financial constraints that patients may have, doctors may try the cheapest drug first (or the one best covered by the patient's drug plan), providing they think it's safe and will be effective. Another consideration is how often the drug has to be taken because some are taken once daily and others are twice daily. Doctors start at a low dose and then increase it if the patient tolerates the med to the full dose. Then the dose is altered if needed, depending on response to treatment and any side effects that may develop.

>> **Memantine:** Doctors don't normally give memantine as a first-line treatment, but reserve it for use in people who either don't do well with acetylcholinesterase inhibitors because of side effects or reactions, or who don't seem to

respond to them. It's approved for use in moderate to severe AD, so it's a logical next step if symptoms are more severe. If a person is first diagnosed at a more advanced stage of AD, it may be started at the time of diagnosis. And some research evidence suggests that continuing a previously prescribed acetylcholinesterase inhibitor and adding memantine can be beneficial.

Seeing How to Take the Medicines

Drugs to treat AD come in a variety of formats. They're started at the lowest dose first, and then the doctor can increase the dose if the drug is tolerated without side effects to the maximal dose advised if needed as time goes on. Table 8-1 lists the formats, doses, and administration of each of the four drugs.

TABLE 8-1   **Taking Dementia Medicines**

	Formats	Dose	Administration
Donepezil	Ordinary and melt-in-the-mouth tablets	Once per day: 5 mg initially; increased after 4–6 weeks to 10 mg if tolerated. Can be increased to the 23 mg dose after the 10 mg dose has been used for three months (but there may be no clinical benefit of increasing beyond 10 mg per day, and the 23 mg dose is much more expensive and has a significant increased likelihood of side effects).	Once daily, the same each day; ideally in the morning with or without food. Avoid giving at bedtime, as it can increase the incidence of nightmares.
Rivastigmine	Tablets and patches	**Tablets:** 1.5 mg twice daily; can increase every two weeks in increments of 1.5 mg twice daily up to a maximum of 6 mg twice daily. **Patches:** Start at 4.6 mg every 24 hours; can be increased after four weeks to 9.5 mg every 24 hours. After an additional four weeks can be increased to maximal dosage of 13.3 mg patch daily.	**Tablets:** Twice per day — morning and evening taken with food or milk. **Patches:** Once daily: applied to nonhairy skin on the upper arms, chest, or back; must be changed to a different position (rotate sites of patch application) at the same time every 24 hours. Make sure to remove the old patch when applying the new patch.

(continued)

TABLE 8-1 *(continued)*

	Formats	Dose	Administration
Galantamine	Immediate-release tablets and liquid Extended-release capsules	**Immediate-release tablets and liquid:** 4 mg once daily for at least seven days; then 4 mg twice daily for at least four weeks; then can be increased to a maximum of 8 mg twice daily. **Extended-release capsule:** Start at 8 mg on alternate days for seven days; then 8 mg once daily for four weeks; then can be increased to 16 mg daily; then after four more weeks can increase to maximum of 24 mg per day.	**Immediate-release tablets and liquid:** Should be given at the same time each day — ideally morning and evening. **Extended-release capsules:** Should be given once daily with the morning meal.
Memantine	Extended-release tablets (Immediate-release tablets and liquids were discontinued in 2014 in United States.)	Extended-release tablets are started at 7 mg once daily and increased by 7 mg increments every week up to a maximum of 28 mg daily as tolerated.	Extended-release tablets should be given once per day at the same time each day with or without food.

TIP

If you miss a dose, don't take two the next day to make up for it; simply take the next day's dose as normal. Remember not to cut or chew any extended release medications because doing so can cause too much drug to be released into the body at once. Extended-release drugs have a special formulation to let them release medication slowly over a whole day to avoid the twice daily dosing needed for immediate-release drugs.

These medications can be taken for as long as they're providing benefit. The Alzheimer's Association believes about 40 to 70 percent of the people who take acetylcholinesterase inhibitor medications get some benefit from them. The drugs may delay worsening of symptoms temporarily for between 6 and 12 months, but then over time their effect wears off. The benefit may last longer in some people. Practical benefits of these drugs may include decreased anxiety, increased motivation, improved memory and concentration, and better functional ability to do daily activities like personal care and dressing. In some patients, these drugs may lessen agitation or aggression.

Considering the Side Effects and Risks

No medicine comes without its possible side effects, and unfortunately, not all drugs are suitable for everyone who may benefit from them. Take into account the following points about AD drug side effects.

Every box of pills obtained from the pharmacy comes with a package insert detailing all the possible side effects to look out for when taking the medication. Some lists are longer than others, and if you studied them in microscopic detail, you'd never swallow anything your doctor ever prescribed, for fear that the cure was worse for you than the illness itself. These package inserts must list *all* side effects experienced by subjects during the drug research studies. So, you can see that a list can be quite long although many of the side effects listed may occur infrequently. The most common side effects of a medication are listed first.

So although reading the leaflet is always a good idea, remember that the side effects listed are only possible and not definite, and the ones lower down the list are rare. Side effects are also less likely when beginning treatment at the lowest possible dose and adjust the dose up slowly as tolerated. That is why doctors are taught to "start low and go slow" when prescribing medication.

TIP

Side effects often wear off after a few days when you get used to taking the medication. So unless they're severe, persevere for a week or so to see whether the side effects resolve.

Most people take these drugs with very little trouble at all. The side effects of memantine are less likely to occur and generally less severe than for the acetylcholinesterase inhibitors. Here are some side effects to be aware of for both groups of drug:

>> **Acetylcholinesterase inhibitors:** Loss of appetite, weight loss, nausea, indigestion, abdominal pain, vomiting and diarrhea, muscle cramps, headaches, dizziness, tiredness, insomnia, slow heart rate, fainting, frequent urination or urinary incontinence, abnormal dreams (less when taking dose in morning), tremor, increased salivation (spit production), skin reactions from patches

>> **Memantine:** Headache, dizziness, and tiredness; abdominal pain, diarrhea, or constipation; shortness of breath; back pain; anxiety; weight gain; raised blood pressure

WHY DO DRUGS HAVE SIDE EFFECTS?

All drugs can have potential side effects because in essence when you take a medicine you're putting a dose of an unfamiliar chemical into your body that has the potential to disagree with you. Thankfully, given the number of prescriptions issued by doctors each year, very few side effects turn out to be serious. But even the mildest and most temporary (as most of them are) can be quite a nuisance.

People experience side effects for a variety of reasons. Some have to do with individual constitutions and some with the chemical make-up of the drugs themselves.

Here are some constitutional reasons:

- **Allergy:** These can cause the most severe side effects and can potentially be life threatening.

- **Intolerance:** This is milder than an allergy but can still cause the body to react against the medication. Intolerance usually leads to stomach upset, bowel trouble, or headaches.

- **Different rates of drug metabolism:** Some enzymes in the body are protein molecules that help break down and dispose of anything you take into your body, from pills to puddings. Some people have less effective systems than others, which means that doses of medicines may end up being higher than they need to be, which causes side effects.

- **Other medical conditions:** Breakdown in the liver and excretion by the kidneys removes drugs from the body. If these organs are working below par, drug levels in the bodies are higher than needed.

- **Age:** As you get older, the body's methods of breaking down and removing drugs become less efficient.

Sometimes side effects are caused by the drug's interactions in the body:

- **Collateral damage:** The drugs in this chapter work on receptors for chemical transmitters on cells especially brain cells where they can be beneficial. Unfortunately, these receptors aren't just on the brain cells that you want to affect; they're on cells all over the body. And as drugs travel throughout the bloodstream, they affect these receptors wherever they find them. This causes unwanted effects.

- **Interactions:** Drugs don't all get along with each other, and when you take more than one medicine, they may interact with each other, causing side effects.

Who shouldn't take these drugs? Here's the lowdown:

>> **Acetylcholinesterase inhibitors:** Other than breast-feeding mothers (who very rarely develop dementia), no groups of people exist who absolutely shouldn't take these drugs. Doctors do, however, prescribe them with caution to people with established heart, liver, lung, or kidney disease or active peptic ulcer disease, anyone who has a medical history of having seizures, and pregnant women.

>> **Memantine:** Not ideal for pregnant women or those individuals with epilepsy or other seizure disorder. Also avoid use if you have elevated blood pressure; heart, kidney, or liver problems; or had a recent heart attack.

Recognizing Drugs That Interact with the AD Medicines

Some other medications have interactions with these AD drugs. If your loved one is taking one of the four medications for AD that we discuss in this chapter, be aware of drug interactions. If your loved one is taking one of these medications, check with the doctor. Taken with an AD drug, the following meds can cancel out each other, eliminating any benefit from either medication (you don't want to pay for two expensive medications if neither one will work):

>> Certain anesthetics

>> Antihistamines (allergy pills)

>> H2 blockers (ranitidine used for indigestion/reflux)

   If used with beta-blocker heart medicines (like metoprolol or atenolol) or digoxin, these drugs can cause significant slowing of the heart rate.

WARNING

>> Muscle relaxants

>> Tricyclic antidepressants

>> Drugs used to treat urinary incontinence

Furthermore, certain medications can have other effects. When used simultaneously with the following Alzheimer's drugs, you can expect interactions:

>> **Donepezil:** Ketoconazole (an antifungal) and quinidine (a heart medicine) can increase donepezil levels and thereby side effects. Whereas, antiseizure drugs carbamazepine, phenobarbital, and phenytoin, rifampine (an antibiotic), and

dexamethasone (a steroid) can decrease levels of donepezil and thereby lessen their effect.

>> **Galantamine:** Levels are increased and may become toxic unless dosed down when used with paroxetine (an antidepressant), ketoconazole, and erythromycin (an antibiotic).

>> **Memantine:** Don't use it with other NMDA receptor antagonists, such as amantadine for Parkinson's disease or dextromethorphan (a common cough syrup) to avoid toxicity.

Looking at Other Drugs That Help Alleviate Symptoms

Doctors often prescribe medicines designed for other conditions to help deal with some of the troublesome symptoms that dementia and AD can cause. These other drugs have their downsides, and not all are suitable for all four main types of dementia. The following sections tell you what you need to know.

Antidepressant drugs

Depression is extremely common in society as a whole, and people with dementia frequently suffer from it. Its symptoms include

>> Irritability

>> Loss of interest in doing things

>> Low mood

>> Poor concentration and memory

>> Poor sleep and appetite

>> Tearfulness

>> Thoughts of death and perhaps even suicide

Depression can also provoke feelings of anxiety and worry.

REMEMBER

Dementia plus depression is an unfortunate double whammy that can make the symptoms of the dementia worsen more quickly than in normal disease progression. Treating the depression can therefore make a big difference to the person's wellbeing.

Understanding how antidepressants work

Antidepressant medications increase the levels of neurotransmitters in the brain that are thought to dip when you have depression. The main transmitters affected are serotonin and norepinephrine. These pills don't provide a fake dose of these neurotransmitters but increase depleted levels by preventing their breakdown.

Most people find that antidepressants begin to help after a couple of weeks, during which time early side effects may resolve. However, they may take four to six weeks to have maximal effect. Initially they're continued for 6 to 12 months and then weaned off as a trial. If depressive symptoms return off the antidepressant, then they can be restarted and taken for a longer time. They're not addictive.

Knowing when doctors prescribe antidepressants

Doctors suggest starting these medicines if significant symptoms of depression have persisted for a period of weeks. These prescription antidepressants aren't appropriate to use in someone who has just been down in the dumps for a few days.

Alongside their usefulness in treating depression, antidepressants also can help with symptoms of severe anxiety and worry. And evidence suggests that in dementia particularly, they can help reduce agitation and also improve motivation if your loved one has lost interest in life.

Being aware of the side effects and risks of antidepressants

Side effects depend on the type of medication used. Nowadays, doctors most commonly prescribe the SSRIs (selective serotonin reuptake inhibitors) for dementia patients. The main possible side effects of SSRI drugs include the following:

>> Nausea, indigestion, stomach ache, diarrhea or constipation, loss of appetite, weight loss or gain, dry mouth, rash

>> Headaches, tiredness, insomnia, loss of sexual desire, erectile dysfunction in men, and inability to have orgasm in women

>> Less commonly but potentially serious include easy bruising, stomach bleeding, blood in the stools, confusion, tremor, hallucinations, urinary retention

WARNING

Doctors use them cautiously in people with epilepsy, heart disease, diabetes, and any history of bleeding into the bowel. SSRI drugs can have serious interactions (which can be fatal) with some strong painkillers such as tramadol, so these drugs should never be used at the same time.

Sleep aids and sleeping pills

Unfortunately, disturbed sleep patterns are a common and serious symptom of dementia. The person with dementia is at risk of falls at night when lighting is less, not to mention daytime exhaustion, and caregivers are at risk of never getting any sleep themselves. The difficulty can be either with nodding off in the first place or waking frequently through the night. And some unlucky people struggle with a bit of both.

Often people with dementia and AD experience *day-night reversal*, meaning that they tend to be awake at night and sleep during the day. Clearly this poses many risks and challenges for both the patient and the caregiver. Such alteration in sleep patterns can cause exhaustion in both.

Understanding how sleep works

Three main groups of prescription sleeping pills exist, and each has a slightly different chemical make-up:

>> **Benzodiazepines:** Hypnotics, such as clonazepam (Klonopin), diazepam (Valium), temazepam (Restoril), estazolam (Prosom), alprazolam (Xanax), and lorazepam (Ativan)

>> **Nonbenzodiazepines:** Hypnotics, such as zolpidem (Ambien), zaleplon (Sonata), and eszopiclone (Lunesta)

>> **Sleep-wake cycle modifiers:** Ramelteon (Rozerem)

The first two work by increasing the level of the neurotransmitter gamma-aminobutyric acid (GABA) in the brain. This in turn increases drowsiness and triggers sleep. Remalteon stimulates melatonin receptors in the brain that control the sleep-wake cycle.

Doctors sometimes prescribe other medicines that aren't officially sleep aids but cause sleepiness as a side effect. Some of them are antidepressants, such as trazodone. Others are over-the-counter antihistamines, such as diphenylhydramine, which is the PM component in all the over-the-counter medications that are marketed to help sleep, such as Tylenol PM. All these drugs can have significant side effects (called *anticholinergic side effects*) of increased hangover drowsiness the next day, confusion, dry mouth, constipation, and urinary retention, however, so they shouldn't be used in older people, especially those with dementia.

Finally, melatonin is a naturally occurring hormone made by the pineal gland in the brain. It's involved in sleep-wake cycles and the regulation of the body clock. A dose of melatonin taken an hour before bedtime can help trigger sleep. It's available over the counter as a supplement. Melatonin can sometimes cause grogginess in the morning as well as vivid dreams, but many people find it to be a useful and non-addicting sleeping aid.

Knowing when doctors prescribe sleeping pills

Sleeping pills are a last resort for treating sleep disturbances and are meant only for short-term use. So doctors only consider prescribing them when patients have tried and failed to improve sleep with simple measures like increasing daytime activity, cutting down on napping, reducing daily caffeine intake, and taking *bright-light therapy* (which involves using light boxes to reinforce a person's sense of day with light thereby helping them to sleep at night).

Being aware of the side effects and risks

Sleeping pills are notoriously addictive, and as a result, no one should take them for more than two weeks at a time. So they're not a long-term solution to night-time problems.

WARNING

The drowsiness effect of all sleep aids and sleeping pills can make incontinence and toileting mishaps more likely (especially in those with dementia who may already have incontinence difficulties). They can put people in danger of having falls because of unsteadiness. They can also suppress breathing, so people with lung diseases or sleep apnea shouldn't take them.

Antipsychotic drugs

These medicines were initially developed to treat people who suffer with severe mental health conditions like schizophrenia. They were the first pills to help rid patients of disturbing symptoms like delusional ideas, paranoia, and hallucinations. These pills enabled sufferers to live more normal lives in the community rather than be admitted into asylums to be forgotten about.

WARNING

As a result of a patient's actions, antipsychotics may be prescribed to treat hallucinations and delusions that may develop in more advanced dementia as well as to settle aggression and agitation. However, in 2008, the FDA issued a *black box warning* (that is, a serious warning to all healthcare professionals), stating that all antipsychotic medications are associated with an increased risk of death in dementia patients being treated for agitation or psychotic symptoms including delusions, paranoia, and hallucinations. The risk of death in dementia patients taking these drugs was 1.6 to 1.7 times that of dementia patients taking a placebo. Most deaths were due to heart failure, sudden death, or infection such as pneumonia. The FDA instructs physicians who prescribe antipsychotic medication to dementia patients to discuss this risk of increased mortality with the patients' families and caregivers.

Understanding how antipsychotic drugs work

Two main groups of antipsychotic medications exist, separated chronologically into older or conventional antipsychotics (such as chlorpromazine and haloperidol) and newer or atypical antipsychotics (like risperidone and olanzapine). The newer drugs, developed since the 1970s, have fewer side effects than those made earlier.

Antipsychotics work on neurotransmitters. They affect serotonin, noradrenaline, and acetylcholine, but the majority of their action comes from their particular role in blocking dopamine.

Knowing when doctors prescribe antipsychotics

Every effort should be made to first address other potential causes of a patient's behavioral issues. Antipsychotic medications should only be used to treat specific disturbances that don't respond to environmental modifications or reductions in other medications. They shouldn't be used as a de facto chemical restraint.

Doctors keep these drugs in reserve and use them only when people have really serious and distressing behavioral or psychological symptoms. However, as per the FDA warning, these drugs should only be used after the physician has reviewed risks and benefits with the patient's family and caregivers and only if they agree to that use. Patients on these drugs must be monitored closely for severe side effects.

Being aware of the side effects and risks

The side effects of antipsychotics are quite wide ranging because the drugs affect so many different neurotransmitters in the brain. Dopamine is involved in movement (people with Parkinson's disease have low levels in their brains), so shakiness (tremor), muscle stiffness, and unsteadiness are common side effects especially with the older conventional antipsychotics. These drugs can cause abnormal uncontrollable movements of the mouth and tongue called *tardive dyskinesia.* They can cause drowsiness and a greater risk of falling. Antipsychotics can also cause headaches, weight gain, diabetes, and stomach upset.

WARNING

Antipsychotics should never be given to people with Lewy body disease. Half of people with this condition have a severe sensitivity to antipsychotics that can worsen symptoms and even, in some cases, be fatal.

Chapter 9

Considering Nonmedical Treatments

Many treatments are touted for dementia that aren't dashed off on a prescription pad by the doctor. Known variously as *complementary* or *alternative therapies*, some are more valid and useful than others. Unfortunately, a lot of nonsense is out there as well. Type "alternative medicine and dementia" into a search engine, and you'll be introduced to potential treatment cocktails that seem more like something dreamed up by JK Rowling for a potions class than medicines to treat a neurodegenerative brain disorder.

You probably know people who swear that this or that herb or dietary supplement has had a genuinely positive effect on the cognitive functions of someone they know. And most people are open-minded enough not to dissuade anyone from trying a treatment that may work for their loved ones, even if the evidence for its efficacy is flimsy (unless the treatment is known to be downright dangerous).

In this chapter we provide an open-minded but honest appraisal of the most commonly cited complementary therapies advertised as treatments for the symptoms of dementia. Some of these use herbs or vitamins, or cocktails of the two, whereas others are more physical, interactive therapies. We also introduce you to some of the most widespread scams related to Alzheimer's disease (AD). And because snake oil salesmen are slippery, we also clue you in on some savvy tricks to figure out if a new treatment holds real promise or is yet another scam.

The scientific evidence for the effectiveness of many complementary treatments is either nonexistent or at least not as robust as that for prescription medicines. And although we would never deter anyone from trying something as long as it isn't known to be dangerous, we don't believe it's a good idea to stick exclusively to alternative herbal or homeopathic remedies in place of mainstream medical treatment.

Eyeing the Different Vitamins and Herbal Remedies

Plants, herbs, and the vitamins they contain have been used as remedies for human ailments for millennia. And even in the 21st century, there's still a large market for these more natural pharmaceuticals. A few of these are touted as treatments for the symptoms of dementia, and the following sections cover some of the most frequently mentioned herbal remedies with details of where they come from and what they are supposed to do and a review of their effectiveness.

Recognize the following concerns about herbal remedies or dietary supplements:

>> FDA approval isn't required for herbal or dietary supplements in the United States.

>> Purity is unknown and not regulated. Herbal remedies and dietary supplements may contain variable amounts of active substances.

>> Herbal remedies and dietary supplements can have side effects and serious interactions with prescription medications.

REMEMBER

Just because a treatment is labeled as *natural* doesn't mean that it's safe or that it doesn't have potential side effects and won't interact with other medicines you're on.

UNDERSTANDING SOME IMPORTANT POINTS ABOUT ALTERNATIVE OR COMPLEMENTARY THERAPIES

These two terms are often used interchangeably in relation to nonmedical treatments. A variety of alternative practitioners exist, some of which belong to their own professional bodies, such as homoeopaths and herbalists, and some don't.

We use the term *complementary* in addition to *alternative* to describe potential therapies. That's an important distinction, because many of these treatments can complement those of mainstream medical practitioners. However, they shouldn't be seen as substitutes or alternatives. Treatments recommended and prescribed by doctors and other members of the healthcare team have been subjected to stringent testing and analysis to ensure their safety and effectiveness. They may have side effects, but are nonetheless safe to use and approved according to the FDA. However, everyone responds to prescription medications as well complementary treatments as individuals. Some people experience side effects and others don't. Some people find a medicine highly effective and others do not.

Gingko biloba

When it comes to complementary therapies famed for their healing properties in dementia — *gingko biloba* is probably the most lauded. It pops up so often when you search on the Internet that it can almost be considered a mainstream treatment.

This plant extract comes from the gingko or maidenhair tree. This tree is commonly called a "living fossil" because it's been a feature of the earth's landscape since the time of the dinosaurs. Gingko trees' fossilized ancestors are commonly found in rocks from the Jurassic and Cretaceous periods. Gingko trees can grow all over the world but are most commonly found in China and Japan. The oldest known specimen was 3,500 years old. Traditional Chinese medicine has used them for thousands of years. Presently, gingko is available as tablets, capsules, teas, and fortified foods.

WARNING

Don't use gingko seeds because they can be extremely toxic.

EXAMINING FREE RADICALS

Contrary to the sound of the name, *free radicals* have nothing whatsoever to do with underground resistance movements in World War II; nor are they 1960s antiwar protesters. Instead, they're atoms or groups of atoms with a spare unpaired electron (electrons are happiest hanging out in pairs) that makes them extremely unstable and reactive. Inside the human body, these free radicals go looking for another electron with which to create a pair, and they do so by bumping into other molecules and stealing electrons from them. The burgled molecule then becomes a free radical itself and, in turn, bumps into another molecule — and so on.

In the human body, these free radicals can damage the structure of cells, the components inside cells, and even the genetic material (DNA) itself. This damage stops the cells from working normally and can lead to disease. In dementia, damage to brain cells is what causes the problem.

Free radicals are naturally generated by chemical reactions that take place inside us all the time. However, environmental factors can also produce free radicals — air pollution and inhaled cigarette smoke being the main culprits.

Thankfully, our bodies produce natural antidotes to these free radicals, called *antioxidants*. These are stable molecules that can donate an electron to a free radical and then neutralize it. The body's normal metabolic processes produce antioxidants in an attempt to prevent possible damage.

Many foods also contain antioxidants, which is why you're encouraged to eat five portions of fruits and vegetables a day (and why herbal and vitamin-based therapies are advocated). To add antioxidants to your diet, put the following fruits and veggies on your weekly shopping list:

- Berries such as strawberries, blackberries, blueberries, and raspberries
- Fruits like grapes, cherries, plums, bananas, kiwis, and pineapples
- Vegetables, including kale, red cabbage, broccoli, asparagus, potatoes, and tomatoes
- Nuts such as pistachios, walnuts, pecans, and hazelnuts

Active ingredients

The leaves of the gingko tree are believed to have medicinal properties and, when analyzed scientifically, have been found to contain two main groups of active chemicals:

>> *Flavonoids* have antioxidant properties and are thought to have most protective effect on brain cells.

>> *Terpenoids* improve blood flow by dilating blood vessels and stopping platelets from sticking to each other to form blood clots within the body.

The double action of protecting brain cells and improving blood supply is thought to explain gingko's therapeutic effects. As a result, gingko is suggested to help people with both AD and vascular dementia by

>> Improving their cognitive functions, particularly memory

>> Reducing their chance of developing mood changes, especially depression

>> Improving their ability to carry out everyday tasks and to socialize with other people

Side effects

WARNING

Gingko biloba's common potential side effects include nausea, upset stomach, dizziness, restlessness, and skin rashes. However there is another major side effect to consider: gingko biloba has blood-thinning properties and decreases the ability of the blood to clot. Stop using gingko before surgery or dental work. Don't use gingko if you're on prescription blood thinners because it increases bleeding risk.

Gingko is also known to interact with a number of prescription medicines:

>> **Anticoagulants:** The similar effects of gingko can magnify the effects of all medicines used to thin the blood if the treatments are taken together. People taking warfarin (Coumadin), aspirin, clopidogrel (Plavix), or the newer blood thinners (Pradaxa, Eliquis, Savaysa, or Xarelto), should avoid gingko.

>> **Anticonvulsants:** The effectiveness of anticonvulsants, used to treat epilepsy, may be reduced by gingko, increasing the risk of seizures. Gingko decreases the effectiveness of carbamazepine (Tegretol) and valproic acid (Depakote), so don't take gingko if you're on these medications.

>> **Antidepressants:** Selective serotonin reuptake inhibitors (SSRIs — a group that includes citalopram, sertraline, fluoxetine, and paroxetine) can interact with gingko and set off *serotonin syndrome,* the symptoms of which include high blood pressure, a racing heart, excessive sweating, a tremor, muscle rigidity, increased reflexes, anxiety, agitation, and potentially coma or death. Don't use gingko with SSRI antidepressants.

>> **Antihypertensives:** Because it dilates the blood vessels, gingko can cause the blood pressure to drop for people already on medication to treat high blood pressure. This drop in blood pressure can be dangerous.

>> **Diabetes medications:** Gingko can lower blood sugar levels so don't take it with insulin or other diabetes medications.

Evidence

Gingko is marketed as a dietary supplement. Gingko has been studied as a treatment for AD, vascular dementia, and mixed dementias. And although a 20-year study published in 2013 by a team from Bordeaux, France, found that gingko reduced expected cognitive decline in healthy older people, other researchers have found that it has no actual protective benefit in reducing the occurrence of dementia. Comparisons of the effects of gingko versus those of approved dementia medicines for AD such as rivastigmine have, however, not been so positive — the pharmaceutical came out on top. However, a 2009 study found that gingko's effectiveness for AD patients wasn't statistically different from donepezil.

Some studies have found gingko to stabilize and even improve cognitive and social function of these demented patients for 6 months to a year. Other studies have shown gingko is equivalent to placebo in dementia treatment. Clearly, the jury is still out on gingko's benefit in dementia.

Gingko is thus by no means a miracle drug and no substitute for prescription medicines for dementia. However, for those dementia patients not taking any of the medicines that may interact negatively with it, gingko may have benefit.

Vitamin E

The number of people delving into Mother Nature's medicine chest to look for more organic ways to treat disease has resulted in a huge market for vitamin supplements. Never-ending combinations of vitamins are advertised as cure-alls for everything from the common cold to arthritis. In relation to dementia, vitamin E is supposed to work wonders.

Like all vitamins, vitamin E is found naturally in plant extracts, fruit, and vegetables. Ideally, you'll get all the vitamins you need from your diet rather than popping them in pill form. Natural sources of vitamin E include

>> Sunflower and olive oil

>> Almonds and hazelnuts

>> Kiwi fruit, mangoes, tomatoes

>> Pumpkins, turnips, avocados, asparagus, sweet potatoes

>> Fish and shellfish

With a list that good and wholesome, no wonder vitamin E is thought to do some good.

Vitamin E also has a role in protecting the outer layer of human cells, called the membrane, which in turn protects and maintains the normal function of cells themselves.

Active ingredient

As with gingko, antioxidants are suggested to be the active ingredient in vitamin E. (Refer to the earlier sidebar about free radicals in this chapter.)

Side effects

Unfortunately, just because something is natural and found in something as tasty as kiwi fruit doesn't mean that it can't cause unpleasant side effects when industrially concentrated into a pill. The most frequently reported problems are sickness and diarrhea, and muscle weakness.

Vitamin E can also interact with prescription medicines designed to thin the blood, such as warfarin (Coumadin) and clopidogrel (Plavix), the newer blood thinners (Pradaxa, Eliquis, Savaysa, or Xarelto) and even aspirin, increasing the risk of abnormal bleeding and bruising. Even worse, some research evidence shows that prolonged intake of high doses of vitamin E can increase your risk of death, especially in people with heart disease.

Evidence

Much of the research on the effects of vitamin E has been conducted with animals. A paper published in the *Journal of the American Medical Association (JAMA)* in early 2014 suggests, however, that the benefits accruing from vitamin E supplements may be genuine. The research team carried out a randomized controlled trial whereby 613 participants received doses of vitamin E, the dementia drug memantine, vitamin E plus memantine, or an inactive placebo. The results showed that, although none of these treatments was effective in slowing down cognitive function itself, people's ability to carry out their usual daily activities declined more slowly when they took vitamin E than if they took a placebo. Taking memantine together with vitamin E provided no extra benefit.

Unfortunately, though this finding suggests a modest but genuine benefit from taking vitamin E, uncertainty still remains regarding the safety of taking the high doses used in the study for a sustained period of time.

While the jury's out, sticking to other medicines is probably the best advice for now.

Omega-3 fatty acids

Omega-3 fatty acids are a type of polyunsaturated fatty acid found naturally in certain fatty fish (salmon, herring, sardines, lake trout, and albacore tuna), flaxseed, walnuts, soybeans, kale, spinach, and Brussels sprouts. Because the human body doesn't make omega-3 fatty acids, a person must get them from dietary sources or from over-the-counter supplements, such as fish oil or flaxseed oil. Research has shown high intake of omega-3 fatty acids can protect against stroke and heart disease.

Studies have shown that Omega-3 fatty acids may help dementia by having anti-inflammatory effects and by protecting brain cell membranes. A 2010 study had mixed results, although those patients taking the Omega-3 supplement didn't do better than those patients taking a placebo. Another study showed mild improvement on computerized memory tests in normal older adults taking Omega-3 fatty acids over those taking a placebo. Yet another study showed that women with the highest Omega-3 fatty acids in their blood had a hippocampus 2.7 percent larger and brain volume of 0.7 percent larger than those with the lowest blood levels of Omega-3 fatty acids. Clearly more research is needed. Presently, no evidence suggests use of Omega-3 fatty acid in supplement form can treat or prevent dementia including AD, although dietary sources (at least one daily) are encouraged for overall health benefits. The American Heart Association recommends eating fish containing high levels of Omega-3 fatty acids twice a week for heart benefit.

Huperzine A

Huperzine A has been around for centuries as a staple ingredient of Chinese medicine. It is a nonprescription dietary supplement used to help memory and reduce inflammation. Native to India and Southeast Asia, huperzine A is an extract from the fir clubmoss plant *Huperzia serrata*.

Active ingredient

Huperzine A is an acetylcholinesterase inhibitor like the prescription drugs donepezil (Aricept), rivastigmine (Exelon), and galantamine (Razadyne). Acetylcholinesterase is an enzyme that breaks down the nerve transmitter *acetylcholine*, which is important for many mental functions, including memory. The huperzine A sticks to the acetylcholinesterase, which prevents it from attaching to acetylcholine, so the acetylcholine doesn't break down. Therefore, the acetylcholine level rises, giving it more chance to boost brain function through improved communication between nerve cells. It also works as a NMDA receptor antagonist like memantine (Namenda).

Side effects

Huperzine A does have a few unpleasant side effects in susceptible people. The most common are

>> Chest and throat tightness

>> Slower heart rate

>> Stomach upset (pain, loose bowels, nausea, vomiting)

>> Insomnia

Huperzine A may potentially interact with prescribed medication for dementia. It shouldn't be taken with the prescription acetylcholinesterase inhibitors because they have the same type of effect and the combo can be a double whammy. Treatments for the eye disease glaucoma may work less effectively as a result of taking huperzine A, so don't use it if you're on glaucoma eye drops. Likewise Huperzine A can have additive effects with beta-blocker medications causing significant low heart rate.

Evidence

Early small-scale studies have shown some promise, with improvements in people's memory and reductions in the level of disability that their dementia causes. But so far too little evidence exists to justify huperzine A being recommended as a first-line treatment, especially because drugs are already available that not only work in the same way but have also been tested for safety.

VITACOG

VITACOG is the name given to a cocktail of B-group vitamins (B6, B12, and folic acid) developed by a team at Oxford University to see whether it could help put the brakes on the rate of cognitive decline in people with dementia. It's generated a fair amount of media coverage and excitement.

In the study, the researchers blended the ingredients, but the B vitamins used are found naturally as follows:

>> **B6:** Poultry, pork, fish, cereals, rice, eggs, milk, potatoes, soya, vegetables

>> **B12:** Meat, fish, milk, eggs, cheese, fortified breakfast cereals

>> **Folic acid:** Broccoli, Brussels sprouts, spinach, peas, chickpeas, fortified cereals, liver

Active ingredients

The vitamins themselves are the active ingredients in VITACOG. They work by reducing the levels of an amino acid called *homocysteine*. As people age, the homocysteine level in the body rises, causing damage to nerve cells in the brain and leading to their eventual death. Death of these cells causes brain shrinkage and a decline in cognitive function.

The B vitamins in VITACOG are known to reduce homocysteine levels and thus act to protect the brain from this potential damage.

Side effects

Side effects from VITACOG are minimal, but interactions with iron tablets and anticoagulant therapy are possible.

Evidence

So far, treating dementia with B vitamins shows encouraging results. The participants in the Oxford University study did demonstrate reduced brain shrinkage as a result of lowering their homocysteine levels, but it's too early to tell whether this physical improvement in brain structure improves symptoms of established dementia or actually holds off its development altogether. Research continues.

Although the VITACOG blend of B vitamins is not available in the United States, a similar B vitamin supplement named Cerefolin NAC is available and FDA-approved. It is indicated for early memory loss, vascular dementia, or AD. Most research studies have generally shown Cerefolin NAC benefits for memory loss.

Cerefolin NAC is a prescription medical dietary supplement containing the active ingredients of vitamin B12, vitamin B9 (folic acid), and methylcobalamin. Be aware that Cerefolin NAC does have drug interactions with anticonvulsants, nitrates, certain antibiotics, and other medications and shouldn't be used in people with kidney stones or liver problems.

Looking at Medical Foods

Medical foods developed to help fight dementia, and particularly AD, have received extensive media coverage. Described as "miracle milkshakes," two such products are Souvenaid and caprylidene (Axona). The two drinks contain different combinations of nutrients designed to reduce damage to brain cells and therefore improve cognitive functioning.

Souvenaid is marketed overseas to help support memory in again adults. However, it isn't available for purchase in the United States. The company that makes Souvenaid (Nutricia) lists the following among the product's ingredients:

>> Omega-3 fish oils

>> Phospholipids

>> Choline

>> Folic acid and vitamins B6, B12, C, and E

>> Selenium

This combination is designed to help nerve cells in the brains of people with AD make new connections (called *synapses*) and, as a result, repair the damage caused by the disease and thus reduce its symptoms.

Caprylidene is available in the United States, but only be prescription. In contrast to the multiple constituent ingredients in Souvenaid, it effectively has just one, caprylic triglyceride, which is derived from coconut oil. It's designed to provide the brains of people with Alzheimer's with a new form of energy when their ability to use the glucose the brain cells normally rely on for doing so is reduced.

The milkshakes both produce low-level side effects, the main symptoms being upset bowels, nausea, and a bit of gas. People with poorly controlled diabetes should be careful when using caprylidene. Because caprylidene is a triglyceride, researchers recommend that during treatment, patients undergo lipid panels including triglycerides be followed by laboratory blood work during treatment.

In terms of evidence, some small-scale studies have revealed some improvement in people with mild dementia as a result of using Souvenaid and caprylidene. Because these products are very expensive and are available only by prescription, the small potential benefit is probably outweighed by the financial cost. Due to the high cost of prescription caprylidene, caregivers of dementia patients have been using coconut oil as a source of caprylic acid, which is often available over the counter in health food stores. Although some caregivers note coconut oil has helped their loved ones with dementia, no clinical research study has ever been conducted, so no scientific evidence shows that it works. Because coconut oil is a saturated fat, avoid using it if a person has high cholesterol levels or heart disease.

Relaxing with Aromatherapy

Although the term *aromatherapy* is relatively modern, the use of aromatic oils as a treatment for illness certainly isn't. Records of the use of aromatic oils date as far back as 3000 BC. Who knows how long people used this type of therapy before they bothered recording that they were doing so? Many references are made to the use of aromatic oils in Egyptian, Greek, and Roman medicine. Today, around 400 different essential oils are in frequent use.

The oils used in aromatherapy are extracted from a wide variety of species, each one believed to have its own particular effect on the mind and body. Of the hundreds of oils available, the following are thought to help in dementia:

>> Basil

>> Chamomile

>> Coriander

>> Lavender

>> Lemon and lemon balm

>> Neroli

The following sections take a closer look at the ins and outs of aromatherapy and why some people use it to treat AD and dementia.

Applying aromatherapy

Aromatherapists work in a holistic way with their clients. First, they discuss the client's medical history and the particular symptoms causing concern, and then they decide which oil or combination of oils to use.

The aromatherapy oils can then be delivered to people's bodies in several different ways:

>> **Massage:** Applying directly to the skin.

>> **Baths:** Adding a few drops to the water, both to make direct contact with the skin and for the person to inhale the steam.

>> **Inhalations and vaporizers:** Providing the oil in the form of a smoke-like vapor, often using candles.

>> **Compresses:** Applying directly to the site of an injury or localized pain.

Considering how it works

Aromatherapists believe that oil molecules enter the body through the skin and the lining of the lungs and then work their way into the bloodstream. From there, the oil molecules travel around the body to perform their healing duties by interacting with hormones and other biochemicals.

Researchers, however, aren't yet sure about the mechanisms at work during aromatherapy. The most common theory is that the effect of the scents is achieved via the smell (*olfactory*) receptors in the nose, which are linked by nerve pathways to the areas in the brain involved in memory and emotion. Once stimulated, these areas of the brain in the limbic system (most commonly the amygdala and hippocampus) release yet more chemicals in the patient's body, leading to feelings of relaxation and calm. The theory seems to make sense.

Unfortunately, the evidence is inconclusive. However, many researchers have found small improvements in levels of agitation and distress — two of the main behavioral symptoms of dementia — as a result of aromatherapy, so it's certainly worth a try.

Tapping into Memories with Reminiscence Therapy

Chatting with friends and family about happy times shared in the past generally makes many people feel good inside. Remembering the late 1960s, 1970s, and 1980s, or even better still seeing TV clips or hearing songs from that era, can bring deep long-term memories to light even for many people with dementia.

Reminiscence therapy aims to tap into intact fond memories. The sights, sounds, tastes, and even smells of a cherished past can help to improve life for someone whose dementia makes the present day a confusing and scary place. In fact, evidence shows that this type of therapy not only improves the mood of someone with dementia but also has a positive effect on general wellbeing and maintaining relationships with caregivers, friends, and family members. And it can improve some aspects of cognitive function too.

Not all memories are happy or positive. Some prompts may remind a person of past hurt or trauma. Reminiscence therapy may bring back memories of people the person has lost, for example, and the grief she experiences may be as vivid as if the person has just died. These bad memories must be dealt with sensitively and not ignored in the hope that they'll go away on their own. Let the person with dementia talk about her feelings and have a good cry if she needs to.

Don't assume that everyone wants to spend time looking at their past. Engagement in reminiscence therapy must be voluntary if it's to be beneficial.

Reminiscence therapy holds as many possibilities as your imagination can produce. You can carry out one-to-one or group sessions, whichever seems most appropriate. Reminiscence therapy is suitable in a variety of settings, such as people's homes, daycare centers, nursing homes, and even hospitals.

You can use a whole range of media, from photos and films to books, records, and old magazines, and even favorite foods and drinks to help your loved one reminisce. Working on a scrapbook of things to refer back to time and again is a nice idea.

Here are a few suggestions for appealing to each of the senses:

>> **Sound:** Most people have a favorite song, individual piece of music, or even whole genre, such as jazz or dance hall tunes, that they like to listen to because the music takes them to a place in their heads that nothing else can reach. Maybe a particular song reminds you of a first date, the sensation of falling in love, the first dance at your wedding, or favorite film.

Reminiscing about music, playing it again, and talking about how it affects someone can be a useful part of reminiscence therapy. It can lead to discussions about the people, places, and times that made it special. (For more on music therapy, see the next section.)

>> **Touch:** Holding favorite items of jewelry or cherished ornaments can lead into some interesting conversations about where they came from and the special memories they evoke. Old clothing, like a T-shirt or fur coat, can also trigger such memories. Medals and trophies can be particularly good tools for reminiscence, although they may bring back sad as well as happy memories.

>> **Sight:** Looking at old family photo albums or home films or videos can be a good start here. Books of photographs of someone's hometown, newsreels of historic events, and favorite old films can all trigger memories.

>> **Taste and smell:** Food and drink can also be shared and used to trigger thoughts of people and places. You can involve the person with dementia in cooking a favorite meal, or set up a restaurant meal and encourage a group of participants to chat and share memories of meals abroad or with loved ones.

TIP

Quizzes and sing-alongs to old favorites can also be a great way to encourage people to communicate and connect with each other. The more fun, the better.

Trying Music Therapy

Music has the power to move people. The melody, words, or context can inspire joy or deep sorrow. Music can provide very personal experiences: Songs can both move people to tears and make them jump around the bedroom, yelling lyrics into a hairbrush or strumming the life out of an air guitar. Music can also have a powerful effect on groups of people in congregations and audiences, from the sacred connections formed while singing hymns in church to the equally spiritual experience of singing along with a band in a field at a music festival, arms raised, cigarette lighters aglow.

Music therapy, uses these emotional responses to try to improve a person's sense of wellbeing through both listening to and joining in with voices or instruments.

Looking at music and the brain

Music was probably a feature of human civilization from the very start. Music is ubiquitous; every culture has a musical tradition. It's easy to imagine early ancestors in Africa's Rift Valley singing and playing instruments while hanging out around the campfire. In fact, archaeologists have found flutes carved from animal bones and horns at sites in Germany dating back at least 35,000 years. Although not quite providing evidence all the way back to human origins, this find nonetheless demonstrates that music has been important enough to have been passed on generation after generation. Given that it has no obvious value in terms of survival, why has music become so pervasive in human society?

Neuroscientist Robert Zatorre from McGill University in Montreal, Canada, leads a research team trying to answer that question. Using modern scanning techniques, the team has shown that when people experience a spine-tingling feeling when listening to a favorite tune, a corresponding release of the chemical neurotransmitter dopamine occurs in a part of the brain called the striatum. The brain has similar responses to food and sex in this region, and some addictive drugs like cocaine also artificially stimulate it.

HOW MUSIC HELPS: MARJORIE'S STORY

Marjorie was in the advanced stages of Alzheimer's disease at age 80. She was completely dependent on others for care and didn't mix with fellow residents in the nursing home where she lived. She hadn't spoken a word to anyone for weeks. But she did let the music therapist into her room when he visited. The therapist strummed his guitar, playing a variety of different tunes that Marjorie may have known when she was younger. She opened her mouth and sang along! She wasn't singing the recognized words, and she was a few octaves out of tune, but she was making sounds in time with the music. For the first time in ages, she was communicating with another human being. Her response to the music was amazing. The music had touched her somewhere far deeper than the areas of her brain that the Alzheimer's had destroyed, and once again Marjorie had a voice. She visibly came alive when she heard that familiar music. At the end of the clip, we saw her stop singing and once again go quiet. They were the last sounds anyone heard her utter, because she died a short while later.

The effect of music on the brain is a fascinating and evolving area of research. But the fact that it leads to an emotional reward no doubt goes some way to explaining why it touches most people so profoundly. Add this to the discovery by researchers in Berlin that musical memories are stored differently than other memories and are therefore still retrievable by people with dementia, and it's easy to see how listening to music and singing along may be therapeutic.

Two main types of therapy are available:

>> **Receptive therapy:** The therapist plays and sings, and the audience simply listens.

>> **Active therapy:** People are encouraged to join in singing and playing simple instruments.

Understanding music therapy's effectiveness

The effect of music on Marjorie (refer to the nearby sidebar) and other people with dementia shows that music therapy works in ways that other treatments for dementia can't. Music clearly allowed a connection with Marjorie not otherwise seen. And a wealth of research evidence backs up anecdotal examples such as Marjorie's. And although these studies are often small scale and therefore not able to draw the hard-and-fast conclusions of large studies, plenty of evidence suggests that in moderate to severe dementia, music therapy

» Can reduce the occurrence and severity of troublesome behavioral problems

» Reduces the symptoms of anxiety and depression

» Improves communication and social functioning

» Reduces blood pressure

Music therapy is also, of course, free from side effects and doesn't interact with other forms of treatment. It's definitely worth a try.

Investigating Reality Orientation

You probably know the feeling of disorientation that occurs when waking up in a strange bed — at a friend's house, in a hotel, in a vacation cottage. You've just come out of a deep sleep and woken up in a lovely warm bed, just like your own, but the walls are a different color, the pictures are unfamiliar, and the alarm clock isn't where it should be. In fact, neither is the bedside table it should be sitting on.

Thankfully, it doesn't take long to realize where you are. The confusion dissipates, and you start to become familiar with your new surroundings. But imagine how disorientating this confusion can be for someone with dementia. You're not sure where you are or what day it is — and you may experience that sensation every morning on awakening. And throughout the day, during all activities, you may not recognize your surroundings or the person sitting next to you. As a result, you can understand why people with dementia are often very agitated and distressed.

Reality orientation aims to reduce confusion by giving a person with dementia a better sense of people, place, and time. It reinforces people's awareness of who they are, whom they're with, where they are, and the date and time.

TIP

You can reinforce someone's sense of reality by

» Displaying on a board the day, date, time of next meal, and even weather. You must remember to change it every day!

» Mounting large wall clocks in each room

» Buying daily newspapers (and putting old ones in the recycling bin)

» Putting picture signs on each door to identify the purpose of each room

>> Making sure that everyone wears name badges, if the person is in a nursing home

>> Actively discussing current events, frequently using the person's name in conversation, and referring to the day of the week as often as possible

Noting the risks and benefits

Research has shown that reality orientation can produce positive results, particularly when used alongside dementia medication. For example, a 2005 study showed improvement in memory and other cognitive test scores in participants experiencing reality orientation therapy over a 25-week period compared to those receiving pills only. And other studies have found that reality orientation also has a positive effect on people's ability to socially interact with others.

Unfortunately, the research has only been conducted with small numbers of people, meaning that definitive conclusions can't be drawn. However, a review by the Cochrane Library in 2003 suggested that sufficient positive evidence supports reality orientation therapy to encourage people to try it.

Recognizing criticisms to reality orientation

Despite the positive results that reality orientation produces, critics have suggested that repeatedly correcting a person with dementia — in terms of where she is or what day it is, for example — may actually make her worse. And taking the therapy to its extreme may mean repeatedly causing the person emotional upset. For example, a person may say she wants to go home to her husband, but is repeatedly told she can't because he died four years ago. Hearing that your spouse or parent has died when you'd forgotten about it may lead to a fresh outpouring of emotion each and every time. On a simpler level, you can easily see how being corrected about things all the time could get on your nerves and make you very irritable.

As a result of these objections to reality orientation, a few other techniques have been developed in its place:

>> **Validation therapy:** Rather than reinforcing factual information when dealing with distress in dementia, this therapy focuses on the emotional effects of such information. Thus, for example, if the person becomes distressed while waiting for her father to pick her up at the nursing home every day, rather than saying he's long dead, the caregiver's response is to say he's running late and then to provide an activity to distract the person from her worries. Although this treatment can help, insufficient evidence exists for it to be recommended as a treatment for all.

>> **Specialized Early Care for Alzheimer's (SPECAL):** Penny Garner developed this treatment while looking after her mother, who had dementia. She has since set up the Contented Dementia Trust in the United Kingdom in order to share the therapy with others. SPECAL therapy has three main rules aimed at preventing people from becoming distressed by questions their memories won't help them answer:

- Don't ask questions.

- Listen to the experts — the people with dementia — and learn from them.

- Don't contradict.

Although this method no doubt reduces distress for people with dementia — and their caregivers — critics suggest that it disempowers people with early dementia. Not being told the truth in a particular situation means people can't be involved in decision making, something that advocates of people with dementia, such as the Alzheimer's Association, believe is very important.

Whatever the rights and wrongs of these therapies, there's no doubt that they can benefit a number of people and their caregivers. Recognizing that everyone's different, regardless of illness and disability, means that trying some or all of these methods and seeing which, if any, are right for the person being cared for is a reasonable approach.

Treatments and Tests That Aren't Worth Your Time or Money

The advent of the Internet has been both a blessing and a curse for the families of AD victims. It's been a blessing because it allows families to access information about the condition and its diagnosis and treatment, as well as provide online support groups for stressed caregivers. However, the Internet is also a curse because it may not provide the latest and most accurate information. It also gives con artists an easy way to come right into your home and lure you with hope-filled emails that promise miraculous results if you send them hundreds, or maybe even thousands, of dollars.

You obviously want the very best and latest treatments available for dementia or AD to help your loved one. But how do you know what's going to help and what might hurt? In this section, we tell you about some known scams, therapies, and treatments for which promoters make outrageous claims, including the assertion that their special secret formulas cure AD. Don't fall for these scams! We also look at the self-diagnosis tests, which aren't scams but need to be utilized properly and shared with your doctor.

Nutritional supplements

Nutritional supplements may provide measurable benefits for a variety of conditions. Earlier in this chapter, we discuss how vitamin E is now being used to help patients with memory disorders. However, numerous ads blast across the Internet with claims that some nutritional supplements "cure" AD and restore patients to normal functioning. Such claims simply aren't true.

After brain cells die, no known therapy can bring them back to life. No combination of nutrients, vitamins, minerals, or secret ingredients can accomplish this miracle. The day that someone does stumble across such a miracle cure, you can be sure you'll hear about it on every news show and website, and read about it in every newspaper.

We're not trying to say that you shouldn't continue to support good general health by taking a multivitamin or some other specialized supplements with proven benefits, for example, glucosamine for joint pain. But if you see an ad for a nutritional supplement that claims to cure memory loss, particularly if the product in question seems expensive, keep your wallet closed.

Chelation therapy

In most clinical settings, *chelation therapy* is performed by slowly diffusing *chelating agents* (ethylene diamine tetraacetic acid or EDTA is most widely used) into the patient's bloodstream, where they bind the metal toxins into metal chelates that can be excreted. The average course of therapy is 20 to 30 treatments given one to three times per week.

TECHNICAL STUFF

The word "chelate" is derived from the Greek word *chele*, which means *claw*. Chelating agents "grab" toxic metal ions in the bloodstream and bind them to themselves, creating new structures known as metal chelates, which are water soluble and easily excreted in the urine.

WARNING

Some websites are now promoting rectal chelation in which the chelating agents are introduced directly into the rectum as an enema, and others advocate oral chelation. Neither of these modalities has been tested for effectiveness in the way that intravenous chelation has, so beware.

Chelation therapy is a topic that creates a lot of controversy because for more than 60 years the treatment has had an actual medical application: to increase the urinary excretion of lead when a child has been exposed to toxic levels of the metal. But even this application isn't free from controversy, because many pediatricians think that simply removing the lead from the child's environment or taking the child away from the source of the lead contamination is just as beneficial.

Relating chelation therapy to Alzheimer's disease

Given what's known about chelation — that it can reduce levels of heavy metals in the blood — it was only a matter of time before someone proposed that the therapy might be beneficial for AD patients. The belief was especially prevalent during the late 1970s and early 1980s, when some experts believed that excess concentrations of aluminum might be responsible for triggering the condition, and reared its head once again when some alternative practitioners hypothesized that high concentrations of mercury might cause the diseases.

More recently, researchers at Massachusetts General Hospital reported that a buildup of copper and zinc in the brain triggers deposits of the beta-amyloid plaques that are characteristic of the damage caused by AD. In a well-controlled study with mice, the researchers used a chelating agent known as clioquinol, which reduced the abnormal accumulation of beta-amyloid plaques by half. But clioquinol is so toxic that most experts are deeply concerned about the safety of the drug for use in humans.

Unfortunately, the poor clinical results didn't stop many alternative practitioners from claiming that chelation therapy could halt and even reverse the effects of AD. Following close on their heels came the quacks and con artists. Because chelation therapy is an FDA-approved application, consumers can easily take claims made for the therapy at face value. In an area where the science is murky and confusing, the public finds it especially difficult to make informed choices.

Figuring out whether chelation therapy really works

Here's the real scoop on chelation therapy for AD: Despite what you may read on the Internet or hear from some practitioners who claim to be able to cure AD with chelation therapy, no controlled clinical human studies have been conducted to prove the effectiveness of any particular chelation therapy in AD (at least not at the time of this publication). The practitioners answer that by saying that it's impossible to administer a double-blind chelation study, and that we should believe their claims simply because so many people improve after receiving chelation therapy. The difficulty comes in when researchers try to identify these "cured" and "vastly improved" patients, and they can't find any of them.

If someone tries to convince you that chelation therapy will cure your loved one's Alzheimer's, don't listen.

REMEMBER

Self-administered tests for AD

Although self-administered tests that are supposed to diagnose AD don't strictly fall under the heading of bogus cures, we include them in this section because of the absence to date of any single accurate test to diagnose AD.

In general, screening tests are valuable diagnostic tools that save many lives every year. They're designed to identify patients who need follow-up testing to reach a definitive diagnosis. For example, a man whose colon cancer screening reveals the presence of blood in his stool undergoes additional testing by colonoscopy that reveals the presence of a small, localized tumor that's removed surgically. The patient's doctors order these tests and then interpret the results and order any additional tests and treatment that may be required.

WARNING

Self-administered AD screening tests have the potential to cause a great deal of psychological distress and harm.

REMEMBER

AD screening tests available for use by individual consumers are offered on a self-referred basis. *Self-referred* means that the patient has decided to take the test, and the doctor didn't order it. It also means that the patient must pay for the test because few insurance companies reimburse for self-referred tests. Finally, self-referred test results are reported directly back to the consumer who bought and paid for the test. Because most consumers have little or no medical training or background, they may be unable to correctly interpret the test results and have no way of knowing if the results are accurate or if they need additional testing or treatment.

Gerocognitive Exam

The self-administered Gerocognitive Exam (SAGE) is composed of 12 questions that are based on different regions of the brain and takes 10 to 15 minutes to compete. Dr. Douglass Scharre, Director of Cognitive Neurology at the Ohio State University Wexner Medical Center designed it. The SAGE exam is available free on the Internet at `www.wexnermedical.osu.edu/patient-care/healthcare-services/brain-spine-neuro/memory-disorders/sage`. It can be downloaded, printed, competed, and scored at home, but individuals taking the test are advised to bring it their doctor to evaluate results, so if you chose to use this test (for yourself or your loved one) be sure to share results with the doctor and discuss concerns so an appropriate comprehensive medical evaluation for dementia can be provided if appropriate.

Minnesota Cognitive Acuity Screen

The *Minnesota Cognitive Acuity Screen (MCAS)* is a screening test that can be self-administered, but insurance companies use it more often. The MCAS was developed as a risk-management tool to help insurance companies avoid selling policies to patients who were likely to develop dementia. CareLink (now Univita), a firm that specializes in geriatric assessment, developed it. At one time, CareLink marketed the test fairly aggressively over the phone to a targeted audience of older people. Although it's no longer for sale to the general public, insurance companies still use it. You can find samples of the assessment questions online.

The test consists of a 15-minute telephone interview administered by a registered nurse. The test is designed to measure an individual's level of cognitive functioning by asking for her name, address, birthday, and so on, asking her to follow a series of commands and perform simple tasks such as tapping on the phone when asked, and finally asking her to respond to a question that requires executive planning, such as, "What would you do if there were a fire in your home?" People who don't achieve a certain score are considered to have "failed" the test and are identified as people who require supervision and monitoring because of their impaired cognitive status. Translated into English, they don't get the long-term care insurance policy.

When your insurance agent administers the test, he may make you think he's doing you a favor, when in reality, he's gathering information that keeps you from being able to purchase long-term care insurance if you don't pass the test.

Sniffing Out Scams: Five Warning Signs to Look For

Because new scams pop up all the time, you need to arm yourself with some good, basic information to help you determine if a particular treatment has merit or is simply a new member of the "Bogus Dementia Treatments Hall of Shame." Here are some things to look out for:

>> **Outlandish claims:** A manufacturer claims that its product or device cures "everything" or cures a wide variety of unrelated conditions, such as, "Completely reverses the debilitating effects of Alzheimer's, arthritis, diabetes, ingrown toenails, and the heartbreak of psoriasis." There's no such thing as a magic bullet. No one product can treat every condition effectively.

>> **Exaggerated language:** The advertising uses phrases such as "miracle cure" or "revolutionary breakthrough" or "the secret that doctors don't want you to know." The reason doctors don't want you to know about bogus treatments is that they're afraid that you'll waste your hard-earned dollars and valuable time pursuing treatments that have no measurable effect except the ongoing slimming of your wallet.

>> **Undocumented testimonials:** People who've supposedly tried the cure claim amazing or miraculous results, such as, "My brother had advanced Alzheimer's disease, was bedridden, bald, and hadn't recognized me as his sister for two years, but just two weeks after starting Dr. Codswallop's Amazing Herbal Alzheimer's and Baldness Cure, he's out of bed, dancing, singing, calling me Sis, performing his normal chores, and all his hair has grown back!!!" Of course, you have no way of contacting Miss T. Rosen of Los Angeles, California, so you can't check out these wondrous claims for yourself.

>> **Emphasis to buy right away:** The call for an order creates an exaggerated sense of urgency and implies that if you don't order right away, you might miss out. "Limited supply," "Reserve your supply now," or "This offer might not last" are favorite ploys. By the way, "This offer might not last" is probably as close to the truth as you'll ever get with people advertising fraudulent treatments, because if the FDA moves in to stop their scam, the offer does end — at least until they can set up a new post office box.

>> **Money-back guarantees:** A company may swear to hold your uncashed check for 30 days until you can see how miraculous its product is for yourself. Don't believe it for a minute. Your check will be cashed less than one nanosecond after they rip open the envelope.

REMEMBER

Don't get sucked in by products that are advertised as "all-natural" or that claim to be some ancient cure that's only recently come to light after archaeologists finally interpreted Hammurabi's Code correctly. Rest assured that when a truly effective treatment or real cure for Alzheimer's disease is found, the news will blare from every website, television, newspaper, and radio station in the world. Unless you're living in a sensory deprivation tank, you'll hear about it.

3

Providing Care for Your Loved One

Chapter 10

Managing Your Loved One's Care and Day-to-Day Life

Not everyone is born to be a caregiver for someone else, particularly other adults. Yet the wedding vows people say to their spouses usually include the proclamation that they'll love them in sickness and in health. The same applies to caregiving. When sickness such as dementia strikes a loved one, it seems only right that family and close friends step up to the plate, roll up their sleeves, and get on with the job of caring. As sons or daughters who were looked after by parents as children, not lovingly reversing that role when parents are unable to care for themselves seems cruel and unfair.

But being a caregiver isn't easy, and the cognitive and behavioral changes that accompany dementia can make caring for someone you love even more difficult. And that's not to mention the potential problems created by incontinence and other debilities.

While at some point it may be necessary to employ professional caregivers, if the person with dementia or Alzheimer's disease (AD) is your spouse, parent, other family member, or close friend, you may still be involved in looking after him to one degree or another. This chapter provides hints and tips about how to best handle that role while pointing out some of the common errors and pitfalls that can make life harder.

Being a caregiver isn't easy, but it doesn't have to be impossible and can actually be extremely rewarding.

Caring for Dementia and AD Patients

You're about to enter a new world. The parent or spouse or sibling you've known all your life has been diagnosed with dementia or AD and is changing before your eyes — perhaps even changing into someone you don't understand or feel as close to as you would like.

REMEMBER

Remember that your loved one has no more control over these changes than you do over the rising and setting of the sun. If you keep that in mind as you interact with him, you may find it easier to be truly compassionate, patient, and caring in your treatment of him. Simply maintaining a calm and upbeat approach can help keep a patient with a memory disorder content and happy and, therefore, easier to manage.

TIP

If you're having trouble handling your loved one or find yourself becoming frustrated by his behavior, consider that your response may be triggering some undesirable behaviors or making the behavior worse. If you feel overwhelmed and out of control, you may not be getting the breaks you need. Remember to schedule regular respite care so you have time for yourself. In addition, it may help to give yourself some visual cues.

For example, get a large marker and some index cards and write one of the following words on each card: patience, tolerance, compassion, love, acceptance, gratitude, flexibility, and any other keyword you think may help you remember your mission — which is to provide the best possible care for your loved one. Now tape the cards in prominent places around your house where they can remind you of your daily caregiving goals and keep you focused on the task at hand and away from negative thinking.

Even with the best possible care, your loved one's condition will progress and his symptoms and problem behaviors will increase. This isn't a reflection of anything you have or haven't done. Blaming yourself and feeling like you're a failure as a caregiver can create more problems. Seek help immediately if you start to experience these negative feelings.

All the things you take for granted in the course of your day — taking care of your personal needs like bathing, going to the bathroom, preparing and eating a meal, doing a load of laundry — can become monumental challenges for a dementia patient as the disease progresses. Devise ways to help your loved one take care of his needs without demeaning him or triggering conflicts between the two of you.

You'll need an extra dose of patience as your loved one's skills erode. Try to focus on the positive; as long as you're caring for him and trying to help him with the activities of daily living, you have an opportunity to continue your relationship with your loved one, even if it's very different from the relationship you had in the past. Remember . . . patience.

Designing a Daily Routine That Works

Sticking to regular daily routines and schedules makes life much less confusing for the person with dementia and also allows you, as a caregiver, to know what you're supposed to be doing, when, and on which days. In theory, a set schedule is a win-win situation all round.

Generally, it's easier when your days are planned. It can make some people anxious when things go awry. However, no off-the-cuff, ready-to-wear daily routine exists for everyone with dementia or AD because no two people are exactly the same. Everyone has different likes, dislikes, and physical needs. So telling you to take your loved one out for a walk every day would be useless advice if he's bedbound. Likewise, if someone hates singing and always has, pushing him to go to a music therapy session will really upset him. The plan has to be tailor-made to fit the individual.

Clearly, a daily plan has to work for you as the caregiver too. Thus, if you need to pick up your children from school at 3:30 p.m., signing the pair of you up for a session at a memory-enhancement program at the same time is pointless.

Before working out a suitable routine for the person with dementia, consider the following:

>> His previous routine

>> His interests, strengths, weaknesses, and physical abilities

>> His best times of the day, both physically and mentally

>> How long necessities like washing, dressing, and eating meals take

>> His bedtime routine

>> The timing and location of clubs or activities

>> Your own daily needs

>> Flexibility for unexpected opportunities, interruptions, and visits from others

Taking these considerations into account, you can then establish a routine for each day of the week.

TIP

Review the routine after a trial period to see what works and what doesn't, which times of the week are perhaps too busy, and which leave you and the person you're caring for twiddling your thumbs. You'll have to tweak the routine as the dementia progresses. Alterations to accommodate the person's changing needs and abilities are inevitable as time goes on. However, no matter what happens, a routine is still a good idea.

TIP

Create a simple chart detailing the events of each day and place it on the wall in an obvious place so both of you know what's going on. Also keeping a write-on/wipe-off board to write more temporary notes and reminders can be helpful.

Simplifying Washing, Dressing, and Grooming

Bathing, dressing, brushing your teeth, and combing your hair are simple routine things most people can do with their eyes closed in a matter of minutes. But to perform them quickly and appropriately requires

>> Awareness that they need doing

>> Ability to plan in which order to do what, from the need to take off pajamas before putting on clean clothes, to knowing that it's best to bathe before getting dressed rather than after in order to have more of the body available to clean

>> Awareness of the risks of drawing a bath too full of hot water or stepping into too hot a shower

>> Realization that it's important to put on clean clothes daily and put dirty ones in the laundry

>> An appreciation of which are the appropriate clothes to wear for the weather conditions

>> Physical dexterity and balance, which can obviously restrict a person's ability to perform these tasks on his own

Washing and dressing are also activities that can provoke embarrassment because they have always been done independently in private. However, with increasing dependency, this basic self-care now may involve undressing and being naked in front of someone else. Remember that your loved one has always washed and dressed himself since childhood, but now he needs help with such seemingly simple tasks, which can be tough for him to swallow.

And finally, remember that jumping in to help, often due to the frustration of watching your loved one struggling to do tasks, isn't necessarily the best approach to take. People can quickly become lazy and deskilled, losing what independence they had left. Remember the adage "use it or lose it"? Help your loved one to maintain his function as long as feasible by encouraging him to do as much as possible for himself, even if it takes longer.

Ensuring dignity and independence

"Do unto others as you would have them do unto you" is appropriate advice for a caregiver. If the roles were reversed, you'd probably have pretty strong feelings about how certain intimate tasks should and shouldn't be performed on you. For example, if someone unceremoniously pulled your clothes off, leaving you naked, you'd probably be a little bit disgruntled. If that person then escorted you into a lukewarm shower and scrubbed you with a sponge on a stick, you'd no doubt lose your mind.

Unfortunately, well-meaning family members and caregivers have been known to wash and bathe people in this way. Don't even begin to think, "Well, it doesn't matter because he won't remember anyway." Actually, neuropsychological research suggests that the emotional memory of people with dementia and AD remains intact. As a result, they can remember when they've been cruelly treated (the nearby sidebar "Emotional memory" has the details).

REMEMBER

Everyone deserves to be treated with dignity and respect.

Not wanting to dwell on the negative implications of the way in which you help someone you're caring for to wash and dress (and do pretty much anything for that matter), consider something you can do to have a positive impact on him: encourage independence.

EMOTIONAL MEMORY

Experiments in 1911 by Swiss neurologist Édouard Claparède provided the first inkling that even people with memory loss retain emotional memories. One of the neurologist's patients was a woman with severe amnesia. Her memory was so bad that every time Claparède met her on the ward, which could be many times during the day, he had to reintroduce himself because she'd forgotten who he was.

One day when he shook her hand to say hello, he was holding a small, sharp tack, which pricked and hurt her. The next time she saw him, even though she couldn't remember ever having seen him before and couldn't explain why, she refused to shake his hand.

Since then many more experiments using brain-scanning techniques have discovered the different nerve pathways involved in emotional memories that are preserved in dementia, particularly AD. And other research has shown that, despite significant memory loss, people with dementia retain memories of hurt, sadness, and pain. They're therefore likely to behave in an agitated or frightened manner when circumstances they can remember from the past repeat themselves. This is particularly true about the ways in which others have treated them.

The flip side of this, though, is that scientists have also suggested that people with AD can better retain memories for events if they're associated with positive emotions at the time they occur.

Doing things for yourself, the way you want to, feels good. It's an empowering experience, especially when you're doing things for the first time. People with dementia may see their previous capabilities slipping away from them. It can be empowering for them to know they can still do some things for themselves and that you still value their efforts.

You can't leave the person with dementia or AD completely to his own devices when washing or dressing, a situation that will become increasingly obvious as the condition progresses. However, by the two of you sharing tasks, he'll certainly feel he has an important part to play.

Doing it together

Here we give some tips about how to work collaboratively when helping the person with dementia or AD wash and dress. And we throw in a few other bits of advice for good measure. Some of them may strike you as obvious, but others involve putting yourself in the shoes of the person and seeing things from his perspective.

REMEMBER

Washing and dressing are important elements of helping people to feel calm, relaxed, and good about themselves. Don't turn these activities into a chore or, worse still, a battle. These experiences can set the tone for the day. It can be a lengthy process, though, so patience is needed.

Washing routines

To encourage independence and ensure that the process goes smoothly and safely:

>> Offer the choice of either bath or shower, and go with whichever option he prefers (unless getting in and out of the bathtub is unsafe).

>> Let your loved one choose the soap, shampoo, conditioner, bubble bath, toothpaste, and other toiletries he wants to use from a couple of options so he can have some control.

>> Be kind and not irritated when offering tips about which step comes next in the process; holding out the soap or towel at the appropriate moment can be helpful.

>> Try to make bathing a relaxing and enjoyable experience with nice fragrances and time to relax and chat, rather than a rush that suggests you have better things to do. Make it something the person looks forward to rather than dreads.

>> Make sure everything you need is nearby to avoid a kerfuffle at a crucial moment; for example, towels, pajamas, shampoo, a hairbrush, and perhaps soothing moisturizer for afterward.

>> Always make sure the floor isn't slippery, that the water temperature is just right (for the other person, not you), that he can't get locked in the bathroom, that you're available to help without distractions and interruptions, and that cleaning products aren't around to be mistaken for shower gel.

>> Be flexible about the number of showers or baths your loved one must take. Even if you're from a family whose members bathe every day, it isn't necessary to force your loved one to take a full bath daily. Full bathing a couple of times a week is enough (and usually what is provided for residents at an assisted living or nursing home facility). You can get by with sponge baths on the other days of the week as long as the genital and rectal areas are kept clean.

DEALING WITH FEAR OR STUBBORNNESS AT BATH TIME

If you're having trouble convincing your loved one to bathe, don't turn it into a battle. Try to distract her with another activity and then try the bath again 20 minutes later. Be willing to do sponge baths for a few days until she settles down or try associating the bath with a reward to make the idea more appealing. For example, if your loved one enjoys a foot massage, get some nice lotion and tell her, "Let's take a bath and then I'll give you a foot massage." Hopefully, she will begin to associate the reward with the bath and be more willing to bathe.

If you're dealing with someone who wants to "do it all herself," use simple, one-step commands to get her started. For example, "Here is the soap. Wash your arms." Take your time and be patient; don't overload your loved one with too many products or too much to do at once.

If your loved one is still adamant about not wanting a bath, you can try giving her sponge baths for a few days until she gets over her objections. Or you might try one of the pre-packaged personal bath cloths that are widely available at discount and drug stores. You can gently warm these bath clothes in the microwave; they contain an emollient, skin-soothing formula. They make a good substitute for those days when your loved one just won't allow you to bathe him in a tub or shower.

Dressing routines

Everyone has their favorite types, styles, and colors of clothes, which all contribute to their sense of self. Being told what to wear can stifle independence. To encourage people with dementia to dress themselves:

>> Make sure the room is warm and privacy respected as much as possible. Close the curtains. If the person needs help, try to provide a caregiver of the same gender if at all possible.

>> Lay out clothes in the order in which they should be put on, so trousers don't precede underwear and shoes aren't put on before socks. Doing so makes the job simpler and much less likely to cause anger, frustration, or embarrassment.

>> Choose clothing with simple fasteners — Velcro straps on shoes rather than laces and zippers not buttons.

>> Avoid anything that slides on over the head. It's hard for a dementia or AD patient to coordinate the complex movements required to get a pullover on properly.

>> Put out a choice of clothes to allow the person to choose what he wears. Don't get irritated if he puts patterns or colors that you don't think work or don't think are appropriate.

>> Change what's in the wardrobe according to the seasons so the person's attire is appropriate for the weather.

>> Choose rubber-soled shoes and slippers to help prevent slips and falls.

>> Allow time for dressing so the process isn't a stressful rush for either of you.

REMEMBER

AD and dementia patients have trouble with buttons, zippers, and fussy clothing that's hard to get into. This can become a source of frustration and may contribute to incontinence if they can't get out of their clothing in time when they have to go to the bathroom. Opt in favor of comfortable fabrics like cotton knits and easy styles like pull-on pants with elastic waists and knit tops that close in the front.

Oral hygiene

Taking care of your loved one's teeth is not only difficult; it can be downright dangerous. Even if you've persuaded him to open wide and allow you to put a toothbrush in his mouth, he can change his mind and clamp down at any moment, giving you a painful bite.

But you have to persist; oral hygiene is every bit as important to your loved one's health and overall wellbeing as regular bathing is. AD and dementia patients have many nutritional challenges, and teeth that hurt or ill-fitting dentures can be a big part of what's keeping your loved one from eating properly. For more on this issue, take a look at the "Managing Diet and Eating Difficulties" section later in the chapter.

WARNING

Pain is one of the major triggers of agitation and violent outbursts in dementia patients. Pain can result from cavities or gum infections that your loved one can't really tell you about. So be sure to maintain a regular schedule of daily oral hygiene along with annual trips to the dentist to check for hidden problems. Notify your dentist in advance that your loved one has AD or dementia so she can make any adjustments necessary to ensure a good visit. You should sit in the room with your loved one during the examination to help keep him calm and ask the dentist to play soft music and speak in a calm voice as she explains each step of what she is doing to the patient.

Try brushing your teeth together. Seeing you put a toothbrush in your own mouth can relieve some of the fear of the unknown a dementia patient may feel when confronted with a toothbrush, particularly if you make brushing an enjoyable game. If your loved one will allow you to floss between his teeth, that's good, but it may well be too dangerous to floss if he's unhappy about it.

What about using an electric toothbrush? Although electric toothbrushes certainly help you get your loved one's teeth cleaner faster, some AD patients may be frightened by the sound of the motor. You'll have to experiment to see what reaction your loved one has to an electric toothbrush. If he tolerates it well, it can make your job easier.

You can buy sponge-tipped swabs pre-loaded with toothpaste; swabbing may be easier than brushing.

If your loved one wears dentures, they must be cleaned every day. Check your loved one's gums for any signs of irritation; if you find reddened areas or sores, the dentures don't fit as well as they should. If necessary, arrange to bring your loved one to the dentist for denture adjustment. Ill-fitting dentures can have an adverse effect on a patient's nutrition because they make it harder for her to eat.

Schedule an appointment for a regular check-up and cleaning with the dentist at least once each year, or more frequently if oral hygiene becomes a chronic problem.

Grooming

A caregiver can easily become frazzled over grooming issues, but be aware that your loved one may not understand what you're asking him to do. Dementia and AD patients may forget the norms and routines for proper grooming, refusing to comb their hair or bathe, mixing and matching awful combinations of clothing, refusing to wear shoes, insisting they have on clean clothes when you're looking at a tattered, stained, stinky outfit.

Keep hair and nails neatly trimmed and the hair preferably in an easy-to-maintain style that doesn't require a lot of fuss. Depending on whether your loved one's scalp is oily or dry, you may have to wash his hair several times a week to keep him looking fresh or just once a week.

Shaving can be tricky, particularly with traditional razors. Try to switch over to an electric razor to avoid the possibility of cuts. If shaving becomes a battle, just skip it. An older woman doesn't need to have her legs or underarms clean-shaven, and an older man can easily sport a mustache and/or a beard.

Pay attention to your loved one's nails, particularly his toenails. Both fingernails and toenails should be trimmed twice a month. While you're trimming the toenails, check for signs of corns, bunions, ingrown nails, or foot sores. If you find anything that might be hampering your loved one's mobility, visit a podiatrist. Pedicures may be scheduled if your loved one enjoys them.

Grooming can be a struggle, but if you stick to the basics and try not to get too upset or embarrassed if things don't go exactly the way you planned, you should be able to accomplish most grooming chores with minimal hassle.

Handy gadgets

As time goes on, both bathing and dressing can become distinctly tricky procedures for someone with dementia. As a result, they can be tricky procedures for caregivers to facilitate too.

Thankfully, a variety of gadgets designed to help with these activities is available online and in shops specializing in disability aids. The person's physician can also refer you to an occupational therapist who will undertake an assessment, offer advice on suitable aids, and possibly supply some of them.

Washing aids

Loads of aids are available to help with bathing and showering, such as

>> Inflatable bath pillows to allow someone to lie back comfortably as he soaks

>> Anti-slip bath or shower mats to prevent falls getting in and out of the bathtub or shower

>> Bath seats to allow those who can't get right in and sit on the bottom to bathe, albeit in shallower water

>> Tap turners for people with weak hands or problems with coordination

>> Steps to help people get in and out of the bathtub without having to step over the side in one try

>> A walk-in shower can be useful for those with compromised mobility or those who needed assistance

>> Bath and shower toilet grab rails

>> Shower seats

>> Long-handled back brushes

>> Mobile shower chairs with wheels that can be wheeled in and out of an accessible shower, therefore preventing the need to stand or walk on wet surfaces

MODESTY ISSUES

TIP

A big reason dementia and AD patients may refuse to bathe is embarrassment over being seen naked. A daughter who had to care for her ailing mother came up with a modesty garment called Honor Guard that can be used to cover private areas during dressing and bathing. This product gets high marks from both patients and caregivers and reduces or eliminates bath time troubles related to modesty issues. At $49.95 for the women's style, which has a top and a bottom, and $39.95 for the men's style, it's very affordable. Visit www.dignityrc.org for more information.

Dressing aids

These aids are designed to help with more difficult dressing tasks, and thereby increase independence:

» Non-tie shoelaces, which are made of elastic, don't need tying or untying, and aren't long enough to trip over

» Sock and stocking aids, which have long cotton tapes attached, allowing footwear to be pulled up easily

» Button hooks, which are pretty self-explanatory and allow small buttons to be pulled through buttonholes easily

» Long-handled shoehorns, which prevent the need to bend when putting on shoes

Dealing with urinary incontinence

Perhaps no problem causes families more distress than dealing with ongoing incontinence. Dementia patients may not even be aware they have an incontinence problem. Or they may do their business in inappropriate places like closets because they confuse it with the bathroom, a fact you may only discover when you try to track down that awful smell that's been lingering in the air for the past week or so.

Patients with advanced disease may become incontinent for two reasons:

» They suffer from weakened pelvic muscles that cause them to lose urine when they laugh or cough.

>> They may not have any physical problems that cause incontinence directly, but are wetting and soiling themselves because they can't find a bathroom, can't get to a bathroom in time, can't get their clothes off in time, or have forgotten the proper process altogether.

Don't ever scold your loved one for having a toileting accident. He may already be embarrassed and upset as it is. If he can no longer tell you when he needs to use the bathroom, watch for visual signs such as restlessness or tugging at the genitals. Schedule regular toileting times into your daily routine. Generally, every two hours is a good interval for a bathroom break to avoid incontinence.

WARNING

Don't withhold water from your loved one in an attempt to manage incontinence. He may become dehydrated, which can lead to a urinary tract infection, which in turns exacerbates the incontinence. However, limiting caffeinated beverages can be helpful because caffeine stimulates the bladder.

Ruling out a UTI

Patients with any stage of dementia may become incontinent at any time if an underlying medical condition like an urinary tract infection (UTI) is present. A doctor should evaluate the cause of any new onset incontinence. Get to know the symptoms of UTI and monitor your loved one for them. Symptoms include

>> A strong urge to urinate that can't be delayed

>> Pain or a burning sensation when urinating

>> Scant urine

>> Urine tinged with blood

>> Complaints of pain or soreness in the back, sides, or lower abdomen

>> Chills, fever, nausea, vomiting, or lethargy if infection isn't caught and treated early

UTIs are easily diagnosed with a urine sample, so don't hesitate to take your loved one to a doctor if you suspect a UTI.

Trying a few tricks

Caregivers have several proven options for managing incontinence; although no one technique is foolproof, the following strategies do help to reduce or eliminate episodes of incontinence:

>> **Scheduled toileting:** The number one intervention to reduce incontinence is to establish a toileting schedule. A prompted trip to the toilet every two hours will significantly reduce the frequency of incontinence episodes or eliminate them altogether.

>> **Prompted voiding:** Check to see if your loved one is wet or dry. Ask, "Do you want to use the toilet?" Help him to the toilet if he needs to use it. Praise him for being dry and trying to use the toilet. Tell him when you will come back to take him to the toilet again.

>> **Habit training:** Habit training takes advantage of the fact that most people have a fairly regular natural schedule of toileting. Watch your loved one to find what times he urinates. Take him to the bathroom at those times every day. Praise him for being dry and using the toilet.

It may help to tape a picture of a toilet on the door of the bathroom to remind the patient what that room is used for or keep a light on in the bathroom to guide him. Also, keep clothing simple; avoid complicated things like buttons; opt instead for pull-on pants that are easy to slide off in a hurry.

Be patient. Toileting treatments take time to work. Treat the person with dementia as an adult with dignity. He may feel bad about being wet, and your inappropriate anger may only serve to make the problem worse or trigger an emotional outburst from your loved one.

Purchasing some incontinence supplies

A number of excellent supplies are available for dealing with incontinence, including disposable underpants, adult diapers, panty liners, and bed pads. You will have to help with wiping and flushing. Therefore, you may want to use one of the soft, pre-moistened cleansing wet napkins so you can do a thorough job of wiping with less discomfort, particularly after a bowel movement. If you use disposable underpants or adult diapers for your loved one, be sure to check them regularly, and change them as quickly as possible when they're wet or soiled to avoid skin irritation.

Addressing bowel incontinence

In advanced dementia or AD, bowel incontinence develops in addition to urinary incontinence. It occurs because patients lose the ability to interpret defecation and urination body signals and no longer can process how to properly use the toilet. The most important issue at this point is to change disposable underwear or adult diapers promptly after soiling to avoid skin irritation that can lead to rashes or bedsores. Good cleaning with each change using disposable wipes and/or a soft washcloth is essential after each episode of bowel incontinence.

Preventing bedsores

As people age, skin cells tend to flatten and lose their protective barrier of fat and collagen, and oil-producing glands become less active, making skin thinner, drier, and more sensitive to damage. In addition, as AD or dementia advances, your loved one may become less mobile. When you add aging skin to immobility, that's a recipe for a bedsore. A bedsore is a skin ulcer that may develop when the blood supply to the skin is cut off for more than two to three hours.

Bedsores occur most frequently on people who are bedridden or confined to a wheelchair, but anyone who's sedentary and stays in the same position for long hours can develop a bedsore. They tend to form on areas of the skin that are under pressure for prolonged periods of time, such as the buttocks or the heels of the feet.

If your loved one is sedentary, bedridden, or spends long hours in a wheelchair, you should regularly inspect his skin for bedsores. The first sign is a red, painful area that eventually turns purple. If you don't intervene and treat the bedsore at this point, the skin can break open and make an ulcer that can become infected. These infections can be dangerous. After these ulcers become deeper and work their way into underlying tissue like muscle, healing can be very slow.

If you pay good attention to the condition of your loved one's skin and take care to move them regularly, you can prevent most bedsores. Here are some tips to keep bedsores from forming:

>> Turn or reposition your loved one frequently to keep pressure from building up in any one spot on the skin.

>> Buy a special mattress overlay (available at medical supply stores) designed to reduce pressure points across the body of a bedridden person.

>> Add soft padding like soft pillows to any spot in your loved one's bed, wheelchair, or favorite chair that seems to be putting pressure on his body.

>> Buy a commercial pressure relief seat cushion at your local medical supply store or on the Internet to put in your loved one's wheelchair or favorite chair.

>> Keep your loved one's skin clean and dry and inspect it regularly for any signs of redness or breakdown.

Even with the most diligent care, people with a memory disorder can still develop bedsores, particularly as the disease advances and they become more sedentary. Here are some pointers for treating bedsores, but remember that your loved one's doctor should promptly evaluate any bedsore. The doctor can prescribe appropriate treatments based on the severity and location of the bedsore. The doctor may even be able to arrange a visiting nurse to treat the bedsore at home.

>> Eliminate all pressure on the affected area.

>> If the bedsore is open, protect it with a wound dressing or medicated gauze.

>> Keep the bedsore clean to prevent infection — especially if it's in an area affected by urinary or bowel incontinence.

If all else fails and a bedsore develops dark *necrotic* (dead) or pus-filled tissue, it won't heal until the tissue is removed. In that situation, the doctor will refer your loved one to a surgeon to remove this tissue in a procedure called *debridement*.

Managing Diet and Eating Difficulties

Food isn't just a basic human necessity; it also provides opportunities for enjoyment and socializing. In fact, the act of preparing and eating food can also be a source of stimulating physical and mental activity.

Although nutrition and energy are essential for human survival, regardless of whether you have dementia, preparing meals and sharing them with others are important and therapeutic even for a dementia or AD patient. These sections explain some issues you may encounter with your loved one with diet and eating and how you can deal with them.

Getting plenty of fruits and veggies

However much a person may enjoy coffee and doughnuts, they aren't sustainable. People need a mixed and balanced diet of protein, limited but adequate carbohydrates, good fats, vitamins and minerals, fiber, and water. A healthful diet is particularly important for people with dementia to help them maintain their independence by keeping up their strength and remaining fit for as long as possible. Poor nourishment increases the risk of illness, infection, and falls.

A vital part of a balanced diet is adequate portions of fruit and vegetables every day. These foods not only provide a rich source of vitamins, minerals, and disease-preventing antioxidants, but also contain plenty of fiber to produce firm stools and keep the bowels moving, thus reducing the risk of bowel incontinence.

Here's a quick list to help you get five servings of fruit and vegetables into your loved one daily. How much constitutes a serving varies and nowadays is often printed on the side of the can or box:

>> Fresh fruit and vegetables — a medium-sized piece of each counts as one portion; for melons and grapefruits, a quarter suffices

>> Beans — a cup counts as one portion no matter which type you eat

>> Frozen fruit and vegetables

>> Canned fruit and vegetables

>> Dried fruit

>> Vegetables in microwave-ready meals (although beware the unhealthy levels of fat and salt in most such meals)

>> Vegetable soups

>> Fruit juices and smoothies

A very wide variety of fruits and vegetables is available and can suit most tastes and budgets. Providing an adequate amount of these, in whatever form, is what's important.

Encouraging a balanced diet

Of course, fruits and vegetables are only one part of a truly balanced diet. Every-one also needs a selection of the following:

>> **Protein:** Protein helps build strength by maintaining muscle bulk and is found in milk, yogurt, eggs, seafood, nuts, meat, fish, beans, and soy products, meaning that both vegetarians and meat eaters can get their fair share.

>> **Carbohydrates:** Recent research suggests that excess carbohydrates may not be helpful in people with dementia. However, an adequate amount of carbohydrates helps provide energy. Rice, pasta, potatoes, whole grain bread, and breakfast cereals are all good sources.

>> **Fats:** Although a low-fat diet generally was thought to be healthy in the past, researchers have discovered that good fats are needed to keep bodies ticking. Healthy sources of fat are oily fish, olive oil, coconut oil, and some level of milk and cheeses, with the caveat of being cautious about lactose intolerance.

>> **Fiber:** This is the stuff that keeps bowels regular. Fiber can be particularly important for people with dementia because relative inactivity can predis-pose them to constipation. Foods high in fiber include whole grain break-fast cereals and breads, brown rice, potatoes with their skins on, fruits, veggies, beans, and lentils.

>> **Calcium:** This mineral is found in milk, cheese, and most other dairy products. It's important for keeping bones strong and reducing the risk of broken bones from falls.

Including some of each of these food groups in the diet of someone with AD or dementia is vital if he's to remain as healthy as possible for as long as possible. In early stages of dementia, you may be able to have your loved one accompany you to the supermarket to choose food items, which can be an activity you share together.

WARNING

Avoid foods that may cause choking (see the list in the "Choking" section, later in the chapter). Also avoid foods that are hard to chew, like tough cuts of meat or hard snacks, like pretzels or taco chips.

TIP

If the person with dementia lives alone or is left alone for long periods during the day, he may either forget to eat or simply forget where the food is. Placing a bowl of fruit and accessible finger foods in easy sight and reach can be helpful. The visual prompt helps him know when to eat or question whether he's hungry. Remember not to put out individually packaged items as snacks if your loved one has difficulty opening the packages. You want these snacks to be easily eaten.

Ingesting fluids

Keeping track of fluid intake is important to ensure your loved one doesn't get dehydrated. Dehydration can cause confusion in its own right as well as contribute to urinary tract infections, which can also cause confusion. Leaving a glass of water or juice in near reach or plain sight can give someone a visual reminder to have a drink. Other ways of increasing fluid intake without pushing drinks are to have soup, popsicles, ice cream, and gelatin. Anything with a high fluid content can help.

Using Meals on Wheels

For those without family nearby, or who live alone and aren't safe or able to prepare their own meals, healthy, balanced foods can be delivered directly to them. Most local communities around the country have a Meals on Wheels service or a private company that offer these services.

Local community Meals on Wheels programs

Arrangements no doubt vary around the country, but as a guide to the sort of service provided, here's the way it usually works:

>> Anyone can apply to be part of Meals on Wheels without the need for a referral from his physician or social services.

>> You can set up the service for yourself, a relative, friend, or neighbor.

>> Hot meals are delivered to the person's home. They're ready to eat and can be provided up to seven days a week if needed.

>> A sandwich or cold salad can also be delivered at the same time for use later in the day.

>> A wide choice of foods is available, catering for all tastes and special dietary requirements, including kosher and diabetic meals.

>> The person delivering the meals can assist the client with getting started with her food, if needed, by getting silverware, opening cartons, and removing lids. The delivery person also checks that clients are okay and will call a relative or doctor if he has concerns.

This great service, run by volunteers, provides not only good food but also reassurance that the person with dementia is checked on every day. You can contact your local senior service organization for details of the services near you. Meals on Wheels charges vary across the country, but are in the range of $10 per day for a hot meal. Most organizations charge based on a sliding scale so no one is turned away. Go to www.mealsonwheelsamerica.org/signup/find-programs to find your nearest provider.

Private companies

Home food delivery services have sprung up around the country and can be found on the Internet. Like local senior service organizations, many provide daily hot meals, but some companies also deliver frozen meals that can be heated later when needed. This service provides the flexibility of being able to have meals out or with family without wasting a hot delivered meal or getting in a pickle about canceling a delivery. It also means that people have more choice about what they want on a particular day. Of course, this service is only suitable for people who are still fully able to operate a microwave or conventional oven safely and able to check that food is heated through thoroughly before eating it. Otherwise, they need a caregiver to do these tasks for them.

An extensive array of foods is available, and all dietary and religious needs are catered for. The cost of individual meals varies, but delivery is often free. Check company websites for details. Individual meals are useful because families can easily check on whether they are being eaten regularly by how many are left at the end of the week.

Monitoring weight changes

Many dementia and AD patients lose weight because they forget to eat or just don't eat enough. Their sense of taste and ability to smell may be diminished and that takes away two of the prime biological appetite boosters. A routine family dinner may be too chaotic for dementia or AD patients. They may have problems selecting the food from the serving platter or bowl or in using utensils.

Despite your best efforts, your loved one may lose weight. If this happens, consult your doctor about adding a calorie- and nutrient-rich beverage supplement to the diet. A number of brands are available at most supermarkets and drugstores, but they're expensive and you have to be careful of high-sodium content. Because these products are liquid and taste good, they're usually easy to get down, but be aware that even with liquids, choking is always a possibility with a dementia patient.

TIP

Even if your loved one is losing weight, try to stick to a regular meal schedule. If your loved one forgets that you served a meal just 15 minutes before and expresses an interest in food or tells you she's hungry, put out a plate of nutritious snacks like cheese cubes, soft fruit, or scrambled eggs cut into small squares, rather than preparing an entire meal again or denying him the opportunity to eat.

As your loved one progresses through the stages of dementia, you may find it more and more difficult to get her to eat. She may lose interest in food entirely and refuse to open her mouth when offered food. This is just part of the disease process. Be sure to keep the doctor informed of any changes in nutrition and weight, and ask for suggestions to encourage better eating habits in your loved one. (Meeting with other caregivers at a local support group or online can provide opportunities for you to ask what works for them; refer to Chapter 17 for more information.)

For other patients, memory problems may cause them to think they haven't eaten even though they've just completed a meal. They may demand another meal and gain weight as a result. If you're thinking, "How can my mom be hungry? She just ate!" remember that AD wreaks havoc with the senses and the sense of *satiety*, that lovely feeling that tells you when you're full and have had enough to eat, diminishes in AD patients along with the other senses. So do monitor the amount of food you give to make sure your loved one isn't eating too little or too much.

Trying other strategies to boost nutrition

The basics of eating involve selecting some food, preparing it, and getting it into your digestive system. However, for someone with a memory disorder, everything that surrounds these fundamentals can get in the way of successfully completing this process. In addition to the strategies outlined in the preceding sections, here are other tactics you can try to help boost nutrition:

>> Schedule meals for the same time every day and make sure mealtime is a calm and pleasant event. Don't let the dinner table become a battlefield over eating; both you and your loved one lose if you constantly fight over meals.

>> Keep the surface of the table clean and uncluttered. Don't use tablecloths or table linens like place mats and napkins; these can be a source of distraction for the patient.

>> Keep knives and other sharp utensils out of reach in a locked drawer or cabinet. Serve food already cut up and ready to eat.

>> Serve five or six small meals instead of three large meals. Dementia patients are easily distracted, and you may have a hard time getting your loved one to sit still long enough to consume a large meal. Smaller meals composed of just one or two tasty, nutritious foods are easily managed often bring better results.

>> Meals don't have to be served in the dining room or kitchen. If your loved one has a new favorite room or special nook in the house, serve snacks and small meals there.

>> Don't serve junk food. Avoid snacks and meals that are either too highly salted or loaded with sugar or artificial ingredients.

>> Watch the food's temperature to make sure it isn't too hot or too cold.

>> Don't rush. Allow plenty of time for your loved one to chew and swallow each bite before presenting the next one. If you try to hurry her, she may run the risk of a choking episode.

>> Lock medicine and cleaning supplies away, or better still, remove them from the bathroom and kitchen so they aren't mistaken as food or drink to avoid poisoning.

Helping when eating becomes tough

You can have the most appetizing-looking meals created by the finest chefs delivered directly to your plate, but as the mechanics of physically eating erode, getting any nourishment from the food can be very difficult. Sadly, as dementia progresses, not only do people lose their appetite, but they also begin to struggle to eat and swallow. The physical dexterity necessary for using silverware also begins to fail, meaning the whole process becomes a struggle.

As a rule, Alzheimer's and dementia patients have an easier time swallowing thicker liquids like milkshakes and soups. They also seem to prefer soft foods and sweet foods, but make sure the sweets you serve are natural. Don't load them up with too many artificial sweeteners or too much refined sugar.

Stimulating an appetite

Bland, boring food is a turnoff for most people, hence the age-old jokes and moans about school lunches and hospital food. Nothing's worse than being served the same food day after day or food that you don't like.

TIP

Try these ideas for keeping people with dementia interested in their food:

>> Encourage them to eat small portions often.

>> Give them a choice and involve them in preparation if able to do so.

>> Use strong flavors and good seasoning that you know they like.

>> Offer sweet, tasty desserts.

>> Provide softer foods if chewing is a problem.

>> Try finger foods, milkshakes, and smoothies, which can be easier to get down while still providing plenty of nutrients.

>> Turn off the TV and cut down on other distractions and noise so they can focus on what they're eating.

>> Make mealtimes relaxed and sociable occasions rather than battlegrounds for disputes about nourishment.

>> Ensure that no obvious physical obstructions to enjoying food exist, such as ill-fitting dentures or teeth problems, by taking them for regular dental check-ups.

>> Check that they're wearing their glasses, if they have them; they may not fancy eating simply because they can't see what you're offering.

Dealing with problems getting hand to mouth

Coordination fails as dementia progresses. Therefore, getting started eating a meal, let alone finishing it, can be difficult and embarrassing. The fear of tipping things over, spilling drinks, dropping food on the table or floor, and having a face covered in sauce like a toddler can be very stressful for a dementia patient, never mind a loss of dignity.

Being aware of coordination difficulties is important because they can stifle the person's desire to eat for fear of looking foolish. Thankfully, this problem can be worked around very easily:

>> Chop food up to make it easier to get onto a fork or spoon and into the mouth.

>> Encourage the person to use a spoon if a knife and fork is proving too difficult.

>> Provide finger foods such as cocktail sausages and soft fruit or vegetable pies for lunch and snacks rather than thick sandwiches or messy soups.

>> Invest in specially designed silverware, cups, and tableware aimed at helping people who have difficulty gripping or difficulty with coordination to maintain

independence. You can buy silverware with easy-grip handles or angled heads, nonspill cups (sippy cups), partitioned bowls and plates, angled bowls, and plate surrounds to make scooping easier.

Aiding with chewing and swallowing

Even when food has been successfully brought from the plate to the person's mouth, the eating process still isn't complete. Chewing and swallowing are necessary to get the food from the mouth to the stomach. Sadly, people with dementia may forget to chew or experience physical difficulty chewing and swallowing, especially as the disease progresses.

TIP

The Alzheimer's Association offers these tips to stimulate chewing and swallowing in dementia and Alzheimer's patients who are having difficulty eating:

>> Use rough-textured foods, such as toast or sandwiches made on toasted bread, to stimulate the person's tongue and encourage chewing and swallowing (if he is able to chew effectively).

>> The person with a memory disorder sometimes has little sensation of food in the mouth. By gently moving the person's chin, you can get him to chew.

>> Stimulate chewing by touching the person's tongue with a fork or spoon. By lightly stroking his throat, you can remind him to swallow.

If your loved one is having trouble swallowing, cut his food into very small pieces or mash or puree it. Alternate bites of food with a sip of a beverage to help him swallow and clear his throat between bites.

TIP

A speech and language therapist can provide advice on eating and swallowing difficulties. If the preceding tips don't help, ask the person's primary care physician for a referral to a speech therapist.

Finally, if things reach the stage where independent feeding is neither possible nor safe, you can feed the person yourself, but be sure not to put too much in his mouth at one time. You can make homemade milkshakes or buy prepared, nutrient-rich drinks to ensure the person makes up the deficit resulting from smaller meals. If your loved one has diabetes or kidney disease, special preparations are available. Ask your loved one's doctor or pharmacist for suggestions.

Choking

Chewing and swallowing become less and less coordinated as dementia progresses, making it difficult for your loved one to take in proper nourishment. Another problem that results from this loss of coordination is choking.

A number of things can minimize choking episodes. The first is to limit foods that are prone to trigger choking. Here are some examples:

>> Hard candy

>> Taffy

>> Hot dogs

>> Nuts

>> Crunchy foods like chips or crackers

>> Peanut butter

>> Chewing gum

>> Grapes or cherries

>> Thin liquids if given too rapidly

Give liquids in a cup with a sipper lid or use straws to help regulate the flow of the liquid and prevent choking.

Choking can also happen when patients with a memory disorder eat inappropriate things like dirt, glue, or pieces of fabric. You should try to keep the environment around your loved one as clean and clutter-free as possible to minimize the chances for this sort of behavior.

If your loved one does choke, don't slap her on the back because this could worsen the problem. The safest way to rescue someone who is choking is to perform the Heimlich maneuver. For illustrated instructions, go to www2.sptimes.com/pdfs/heimlich.pdf.

You should review these instructions now so you'll know what to do should the need arise. Remember that an older adult is frailer, so be careful about the amount of force you use in performing the Heimlich maneuver, or you could inadvertently crack a rib.

Preventing Boredom

Boredom's a killer. Nothing's worse than having to spend day after day staring at the same four walls with no hope of change in environment or circumstances. It's isolating, lonely, and depressing. But getting fresh air, a change of scenery, and some gentle exercise is invigorating and stimulating, and provides a boost to people's moods and emotions. This applies whether you're 9 or 90, with or without dementia. If a person has dementia, however, getting out and about can be a vital way of staying fit and mentally and physically active for longer. Make sure the Alzheimer's or dementia patient is supervised to prevent wandering or getting lost.

If you develop a series of quiet and enjoyable activities for your loved one, you gain a few minutes of respite in your busy day. Patients with a memory disorder like things that keep them occupied and respond favorably to activities that stimulate their senses in a gentle way. The following sections offer a few suggestions to avoid boredom.

WARNING

Over the course of caring for your loved one, you'll have to drive her around in your car to transport her to a doctor's office or accompany her while doing errands like picking up a prescription or going to the grocery store. *Never* under any circumstances whatsoever leave your loved one in a parked car, not even for a minute. She could get out and get lost, or, if it's a hot day, she could actually suffocate or have a heat stroke and die. *Always* take your loved one with you into a store or an office to run an errand. Or do these things while your loved one enjoys spending time with another responsible person at home or when she's at an adult day-care program.

Providing fresh air and exercise

Everyone should try to get at least half an hour's exercise five days a week to stay fit and healthy. Exercise keeps the heart ticking, strengthens bones, helps prevent insomnia, and keeps the body supple. And evidence suggests that exercise can reduce the rate of cognitive decline in people with dementia too.

As people age, exercising can become more difficult as osteoarthritis makes joints stiff and painful, balance falters, and energy levels aren't what they used to be. Certain types of dementia, such as Lewy body disease and vascular dementia, can exacerbate these difficulties, whereby disease processes in the brain can affect mobility.

Not everyone with dementia is old or physically incapacitated, however, and exercise and activity outside the home or in the garden can help maintain mobility and independence for longer. Getting out and about also increases opportunities to have a change of scenery, which makes life generally more interesting.

If you're worried that the person you're caring for is out of shape or has other medical conditions that may be adversely affected by exercise, by all means ask his doctor to check him over and provide advice on what exercise he should and shouldn't do. But given that exercise helps most conditions, the person is more than likely to be given the thumbs-up for gentle activity.

Exercise need not mean training for marathons or squeezing into workout clothes and heading to the gym. Fantastic ways for people with dementia to keep fit include swimming, walking, dancing, and stretching exercises.

If the person is up to it physically and has the mental ability to coordinate movements, be creative to find what works best for him. Exercise needn't stop in the later stages of dementia, although it will obviously have to be adapted. People can still be encouraged to do simple stretches and upper-body exercises if their legs have gone on strike. People who are wheelchair-bound also benefit immensely from getting outside regularly for fresh air and a change of scenery. They can also benefit from regular range of motion exercises of their arms and legs to prevent them from getting stuck in a flexed position called a contracture, which can be painful.

If your loved one wants to swim and it's safe to do so, fit her with a life jacket and jump in the pool with her. You can find creative ways to incorporate exercise into a dementia patient's life.

REMEMBER

Researchers at the Mayo Foundation for Medical Education and Research have found that exercising four times a week improves both the emotional and physical health of women who are caring for a relative with dementia. Study participants slept better, felt less stressed and depressed, and experienced a drop in their blood pressure, leading researchers to conclude that physical activity is beneficial for both the caregiver and the person he or she cares for.

Adult daycare centers may offer exercise programs for seniors; check with your local providers — some may even offer exercise classes separate from their daycare program. The YMCA also offers a broad range of classes for older adults and the one in your area may offer a special class for patients with a memory disorder.

Start slowly and don't try to push your loved one to do too much to start. Ten to fifteen minutes is plenty to begin with. You're just trying to help your loved one stay as healthy as possible for as long as possible.

WARNING

If at any time during the exercise session, your loved one complains of dizziness, shortness of breath, or any sort of pain anywhere in his body, especially chest pain, stop exercising immediately and call 911 for medical assistance.

Offering social opportunities and entertaining activities

Socializing with others is another great way to try to prevent boredom and promote mental stimulation. For those to whom exercise is a burden, meeting others at a club or coffee shop can be an excuse to get them out of the house and walking about too.

The Alzheimer's Association or other local support groups may run programs particularly set up so people with dementia and their caregivers can enjoy a cup of coffee and take part in stimulating activities such as quizzes, reminiscence work, and music therapy. Go to www.alz.org to access information about local programs.

REMEMBER

When you plan activities for your loved one, be sure to keep his current level of ability and his natural interests in mind. Choose entertaining activities that provide gentle stimulation. Avoid anything that's too complex because that will only lead to frustration.

Here are some ideas for planning activities:

>> If you have a well-trained pet that your loved one cares for, let the dog or cat spend a few minutes with her at around the same time each day. Some animals have an uncanny sense around ill humans and seem to know just how to conduct themselves to provide the most comfort. If your cat climbs onto your loved one's lap, curls up, and starts purring, watch to see the reaction. If she accepts the animal and even starts petting it or talking to it, then you've found a pleasant way to help your loved one occupy her time for a portion of each day. If, on the other hand, the animal's presence upsets or frightens your loved one, then this isn't a good idea.

>> Some patients respond favorably to stuffed animals or dolls, particularly female patients. Sometimes simply holding a doll or stuffed bear can be calming.

>> Other patients respond favorably to photos of family members. Let him help you select the photos he likes and assemble them into a 4 x 6 album he can carry around and look at whenever he likes.

>> Another good idea is to make a memory box. Cover a shoebox with bright contact paper and put in five or six of your loved one's favorite keepsakes from his past. For example, you may include a prom photo or baby pictures or a souvenir postcard from a favorite vacation, even a soft piece of cloth cut from one of his children's baby blankets. Include anything that you know has special meaning for your loved one, but don't include any sharp or breakable objects. Then, whenever he wishes, he can sit down and go through the box and enjoy the fond memories the objects bring back.

WARNING

You may be baffled when, without warning, an activity that your loved one has enjoyed for many weeks or months is suddenly refused. Remember that dementia is a progressive illness, so something that worked yesterday may not work today because your loved one may not have the same abilities, memories, and knowledge today that he had yesterday. Don't let it upset you. Just devise some simpler activities to take the place of the one being rejected.

Preparing for Bed

It would be wonderful if, at the end of a long and busy day, you could simply tuck your loved one into bed, say a prayer, turn out the light, and then go to sleep yourself. Unfortunately, that's rarely the case with dementia and AD patients because many of them have trouble sleeping through the night.

WARNING

Physical restraints to keep a patient with a memory disorder in bed at night and prevent wandering should never be used. They can increase episodes of agitation as the person tries to free himself. Restraints are dangerous because they make it difficult to evacuate the patient in case of an emergency, like a fire. They can also cause injury including suffocation.

David Harper, a research psychologist affiliated with Harvard Medical School found that caregivers cite sleep disturbances as one of the main reasons why they decide to place dementia patients in residential facilities. Take a look at the following list for a few steps you can take to help make bedtime easier and give your loved one a better chance of getting a full night's rest. Instead of making bedtime into a combat zone, try to make it as pleasant an experience as possible.

>> **Restrict caffeine intake after noon.** Caffeine takes a long time to pass through the body and can keep your loved one up and buzzing around for a full six hours or more after one little cup of coffee. Also, try to not let your loved one nap excessively because that can lead to additional difficulties in falling asleep at bedtime.

>> **As often as possible, put your loved one to bed at the same time each evening.** Depending upon her needs, start the before-bed routine about a half hour to a full hour before bed. Help her into her nightclothes and with her grooming and toileting. Speak in a soft and pleasant voice. When you have her dressed for bed, take her to her bedroom and help her into bed. Sit and talk with her for a few minutes until she begins to feel sleepy. Play soft music, turn on a nightlight, and use aromatherapy to help your loved one associate bedtime with pleasant feelings. Offer an incentive if she settles down quickly, like a foot massage with her favorite lotion, or read her a story.

>> **You can't stay up all night long just to watch your loved one.** If she has a habit of wandering at night, try installing motion alarms to alert you and high locks on the door to lessen risk of wandering outside.

Remember that sleep problems are part of dementia and AD. You must be patient with your loved one and try to understand that she isn't waking you up in the middle of the night with any malicious intent. When she awakens in a darkened room, she doesn't know where she is. No wonder she becomes frightened and disoriented.

Making the House Safer

Patients with memory disorders function best in a calm and well-structured environment. That means eliminating potential sources of trouble as much as you can.

Most of us take our homes and familiar surroundings for granted. If you've lived somewhere for ten years and you've completely adjusted to the little half step up into the kitchen where a tile has cracked and shifted, you probably don't think too much about it. Your foot just automatically hitches up that extra half inch every time you go into the kitchen.

WARNING

According to the National Center for Injury Prevention, falls are the leading cause of injury deaths in adults aged 65 and older. One in every three older adults falls at least once each year. One out of every five falls causes a serious injury such as a broken bone or head injury. Every 13 seconds, an older adult is treated in the emergency room for a fall; every 20 minutes, an older adult dies from a fall. Among people aged 65 to 69, one out of every 200 falls results in a hip fracture; that increases to 1 out of every 10 falls for those age 85 and older. In 2013, the total cost of fall injuries in the United States was $34 billion and is expected to increase to $67 billion by 2020.

So remember: For a dementia patient, that half-inch step into the kitchen could be disastrous, leading to a serious fall and maybe even hospitalization. In this section, we talk about making the house safe for your loved one.

TIP

To help you patient proof your home, download a free copy of the document or read it online at www.nia.nih.gov/alzheimers/publication/home-safety-people-alzheimers-disease.

Patient proofing your home

In addition to locking up knives and other sharp objects in the kitchen, you should lock up matches and lighters. You should also put a kill switch on your stove or remove the knobs so your loved one can't accidentally start a fire. Put childproof latches on all your cabinets, and if you have any throw or area rugs in the kitchen, remove them. Throw rugs are tripping hazards, even if you have them secured to the floor with carpet tape. Remove any electrical wires that run across open spaces to prevent tripping, and put childproof plugs in all your electrical outlets.

Walk around your house and look at each room with a critical eye. If you see something that looks like it could cause a problem for your loved one, remove it or secure it so it no longer presents a hazard. Then you can rest assured that you have done your best to patient proof your home. Even with all reasonable precautions taken, accidents can still happen. Don't blame yourself. Seek treatment for whatever injuries your loved one may have and move forward.

Here are some more specific tips:

>> If your loved one wanders, you need to secure the entire house and yard to keep him from getting lost. Install locks on top of entrance doors to keep your loved one from getting outside unsupervised. Install locks on windows and use childproof doorknobs to make it more difficult for him to escape. Put locks on your garden gates, and if your yard isn't fenced, consider putting in a high fence as soon as possible so you can keep your loved one secure at home while allowing him to engage in normal, healthy outdoor activity. But remember, no fence is tall enough and no gate is secure enough to substitute for your supervision!

>> Disengage the garage door opener. Install alarms at the exits to let you know if someone is trying to get out. You also can use alarm mats that sound if someone steps on them. If you can't afford alarms, hang a bell on the door to alert you if someone is leaving (although this may not be enough to wake you from a sound sleep).

>> Let your neighbors know about your loved one's condition so they can alert you if he manages to sneak out despite all your precautions. You may even want to take your loved one on a nice walk around the neighborhood to introduce him to your neighbors, but remember, discuss your concerns with

neighbors, either before or after this visit. As you might imagine, patients don't like to be discussed as if they weren't standing right there.

>> If you have a flight of stairs in your home, you must put gates at both the top and the bottom to keep your loved one from trying to go up and down unassisted. Mark the first step, top and bottom, with a wide, brightly colored tape so they'll be aware of where it is. Make sure a handrail is securely fastened to the wall on both sides of the stairs and will support the weight of a falling person. If the handrails are flimsy, have them replaced.

>> Use technology to help. Cameras, coined as Grannie-cams, can allow monitoring over the Internet, and baby monitors can provide audio monitoring from another room in the house. Alert-button necklaces or bracelets also allow someone to push for help in the event of a fall or other emergency. Realize that such alert buttons require the wearer to understand and remember to push the button when needed for them to be effective, which may be impossible for a dementia or AD patient. (Refer to the nearby sidebar for more about alert buttons.)

>> Install smoke alarms and don't use portable space heaters because they're a huge fire risk. Cover the fireplace and put cushioned corner bumpers on sharp edges of furniture to prevent injury in case of a fall.

Keeping track of an Alzheimer's patient

No one knows exactly why Alzheimer's patients wander, but the reality is that a certain number of them do. If your loved one wanders, it probably scares you to death. To help make sure the wandering isn't a tragic experience, a number of programs are available to help find your loved one and return him home.

Use iron-on labels with your loved one's name, address, and phone number imprinted on all his clothing, even his socks. This could make a big difference between a speedy return or a lot of red tape if your loved one gets lost.

The Alzheimer's Association and MedicAlert Foundation sponsor a program called Safe Return. For a registration fee of $55, you receive an ID bracelet or necklace with the organization's 24-hour toll-free emergency crisis line. In addition, when you report your loved one missing, Safe Return sends his picture and information to local law enforcement agencies. If someone finds your loved one, she calls the number and you can be reunited. Finally, membership in the program provides important medical information that doctors or paramedics might need in the event of an emergency. Call 800-432-5378 for complete information or visit www.medicalert.org/safereturn to register.

Getting clutter out of the way

Something you may live with every day and not pay too much attention to is clutter, but clutter can be dangerous for your loved one.

You may love your stacks of magazines and newspapers and laugh when you open a cabinet and 20 plastic containers come tumbling down. But what seems cozy to you may present a real danger for your loved one. In his weakened condition with diminished ambulatory skills and impaired balance, it may be almost impossible for him to navigate around your treasures.

If you just can't bear to part with all your treasures or simply don't have time to deal with cleanup at the moment, gather your stuff in boxes and cart it to a mini storage. But be careful about reorganizing your loved one's familiar environment too quickly and too drastically. Familiar spaces and old routines are the dementia patient's friend; changing too much too quickly can trigger undesirable behavior or cause anxiety or paranoia. These clutter tips are for you, not for your loved one.

Considering remodeling

When you walk through and assess your house, you may come to the conclusion that certain areas simply aren't going to work, no matter how much reorganizing you do. At that point, you may consider remodeling part of the house to accommodate your loved one's needs.

Talk to local contractors. It may be more economical to build a small addition with a bedroom and accessible bath than to tear out an existing bath and walls to remodel. Whether you remodel depends on your financial situation and your loved one's needs. Perhaps by combining two households, you can find the capital to make the needed structural changes in your own home.

Addressing Driving and Mobility

Driving safety is an increasingly important public health issue with the growing population of aging drivers who may have impairments in vision, hearing, movement, and cognition. Driving is a privilege, not a right. In the case of a person with dementia, driving becomes more dangerous as the disease progresses. Don't take the decision to stop someone from driving lightly because the ability to drive is often equated with independence and freedom. However, families and doctors must consider not only the impact to the person with dementia, but also to others whose safety may be compromised by the impaired driver's actions.

If your loved one's doctor decides that it's time for him to stop getting behind the wheel, then it's time to hang up the keys. The reporting requirements vary depending on the state you live in. Your loved one's doctor will know the state requirements. In many states, the doctor is required to report to the Department of Motor Vehicles (DMV) that the patient is no longer safe to drive. In Pennsylvania (and other states), the required physician's report triggers an evaluation process that may include a test of current driving ability and ultimately lead to recall of the patient's driver's license. Failure of the physician to report cognitively impaired drivers can lead to the physician being held responsible for accidents the impaired driver may cause and even criminal penalties. Hence, physicians recognize the importance of this issue.

TIP

If possible, talk to your loved one about driving concerns, if he is capable of such a discussion, soon after diagnosis and develop a strategy together. Discuss the issues — liability, safety, and peace of mind — that are important to both of you. It may be necessary to obtain a driving examination to evaluate his driving ability. If the person administering the evaluation says your loved one can no longer drive safely, then take the keys. If your loved one passes the evaluation, repeat it every three to six months or sooner if needed to stay informed about his actual level of driving skill.

When and how to intervene regarding driving without risking demoralization of your loved one is a tough call. The Alzheimer's Association (www.alz.org) lists the following signs of unsafe driving that indicate it is time for your loved one to give up the keys and also offers other tips related to driving.

TAKING A DRIVING TEST

If you're not sure whether your loved one is fit to continue driving, he can take a driving test. Of course, if the DMV requests it (after required physician reporting), your loved one has no choice but to undergo this test. He must demonstrate that he knows the rules of the road and can apply them when behind the wheel of a car. He must also prove that he can drive safely in different road and traffic conditions.

The Automobile Club of America offers professional driving assessments. For more information, you can check out http://seniordriving.aaa.com/evaluate-your-driving-ability/professional-assessment.

(continued)

(continued)

The AAA's driving assessments fall into two categories: driving skills evaluations and clinical driving assessments. A driving skills evaluation includes an in-car evaluation of your loved one's driving abilities and a recommendation regarding the need for additional specialized drivers' training. Clinical driving assessments identify underlying medical causes of any driving performance deficits and offer ways to address them so driving remains a safe option.

State-licensed and trained driving instructors conduct the in-car driving skills evaluations. The evaluations can provide a relatively quick and inexpensive checkup. Results may

- Show that your loved one's driving skills are adequate and current with no need for specialized drivers' training.

- Reveal deficits that could be addressed with specialized drivers' training (not a realistic option for a person with dementia).

- Lead to a recommendation for a clinical driving assessment by an occupational therapist driving rehabilitation specialist (OT-DRS).

Clinical assessments by trained specialists are the best way to fully evaluate someone's driving capabilities. In some cases, getting a clinical driving assessment can help decide whether your loved one should continue to drive and if so, under which conditions. Results may

- Show he is perfectly fit to drive without restrictions.

- Indicate he would benefit from extra training (which may not be able to be absorbed by a person with dementia) or need special adaptive vehicle equipment (this is more likely the case with a physical disability like an amputated leg than a cognitive disability like dementia).

- Reveal that he is no longer safe to operate a motor vehicle.

Get an evaluation if you're concerned that your loved one's driving skills have diminished; were recommended to take a driving skills evaluation by a physician, occupational therapist, or family member; or may benefit from supplemental in-car training.

Giving up a driver's license

Your loved one has driven for many years, and maybe he is the only driver in the household. Surrendering his license for good can be quite upsetting. However, the last thing you want to do is put other drivers or pedestrians at unnecessary risk by not addressing your loved one's driving impairments. And the money saved by not having to pay for gasoline, car insurance, maintenance, and repairs due to owning a car can be spent on using other forms of transportation such as buses, subways, and taxis. Clearly, a person with a memory disorder needs assistance to use public transportation to avoid getting confused and lost.

REMEMBER

When weighing the loss of independence for your loved one to the danger of him driving, remember the injuries a motor vehicle accident can cause to himself, his passengers, and those around him. You must pick safety for all concerned over his independence.

TIP

If you're the caregiver and are having trouble convincing your loved one that he should no longer drive, enlist the help of your doctor. You can also check out the Alzheimer's Association Dementia and Driving Resource Center at `www.alz.org/care/alzheimers-dementia-and-driving.asp`.

The Hartford Insurance Company has excellent advice, guidelines, and tips for addressing the issues of memory disorders and driving. You can read it at `www.thehartford.com/alzheimers`.

Finally, if you're still having trouble facing this issue, ask yourself: "Would I want my child or grandchild to ride with my loved one at the wheel?" The answer will tell you what you need to do.

Making arrangements for others to drive

When the day comes that a dementia or AD patient has to give up his driver's license, the caregiver faces a big decision: Who's going to provide transportation? At the same time you discuss when to end driving privileges, start recruiting volunteers to help you with transportation. Call your local Administration on Aging to see what sort of transportation services are available in your area, and check with senior centers and daycare centers to see if they provide round-trip transportation as part of their service.

REMEMBER

Don't try to do it all yourself. Ask other people for help in driving; if you're the primary caregiver, your plate is already full enough without taking on all the transportation duties for your loved one as well. The key is to not miss a beat. Have a plan in place so your loved one's schedule and social activities can continue without interruption.

Another solution is to consider hiring a private driver or paid companion who can also serve as a driver. Don't assume that your loved one will fight you on this; even though he may be loathe to give up driving, his real fear is giving up his freedom. If you provide another way for your loved to get to his appointments and activities, he should be agreeable to the new arrangement. He may be particularly happy to have the companionship of the new driver.

Using handicap placards

Many disabled people and their families around the United States benefit from a handicap parking placard, which allows them to use specially allotted parking spaces near their destinations. The person with the disability need only be a passenger in the car for it to qualify for a placard. Strict criteria govern who is and isn't eligible for a handicap placard. Currently, people typically qualify if they

>> Have significant lung disease

>> Have disabilities limiting the ability to walk

>> Have cardiovascular disease

>> Have significant limitation in the use of the lower extremities

>> Have a "permanent and substantial" disability that makes walking very difficult or means they can't walk at all

REMEMBER

Handicap placards aren't automatically issued to everyone with dementia — only those people who also have a physical disability or a type of dementia that causes problems with walking, particularly vascular dementia or Lewy body disease. Physicians must issue a prescription for a handicap placard to be attached to the application with the appropriate (usually nominal) fee and submitted to the DMV. Ask your loved one's physician if a handicap placard is appropriate.

Staying on Top of Healthcare Issues

In the United States, most people older than 65 have access to the Medicare program. In other parts of the world, people with dementia who can't afford to pay for their healthcare can become unnecessarily disabled as a result.

Making good and sensible use of what is available is thus important. People with a memory disorder obviously need help specifically for whatever disease is producing their symptoms. But they may also have other medical conditions such as heart disease, diabetes, high blood pressure, asthma, thyroid disease, or arthritis that also need treatment and monitoring. The following sections point out how you can help your loved one with all types of healthcare issues.

REMEMBER

People with chronic diseases such as diabetes, high blood pressure, and heart disease should regularly be seen by their physician. Keeping these appointments is vital.

Visiting doctors, dentists, podiatrists, and opticians

Looking after the person's teeth, feet, and eyes is important. Make sure they're checked at least annually, if not every six months. Prevention is always better than cure.

Bear in mind that people with dementia and AD may feel anxious about visiting the dentist or being in an unknown, potentially busy, environment. Behavioral problems and agitation may result. Try to keep stress levels to a minimum by

>> Attending appointments with your loved one to offer support and give him confidence

>> Trying to attend the same clinics and see the same clinicians each time so your loved one gets used to the surroundings and personnel

>> Letting the professional know that the person you are with has dementia, and giving him useful tips for minimizing the potential stress of the situation for all concerned

>> Taking along a written list of points you want to cover with the clinician, including any concerns voiced by your loved one

>> Allowing the person with dementia to talk for himself if he is able and not irritating him by talking over him

>> Not covering too much in one visit and making the experience exhausting

REMEMBER

Don't let a previously stressful visit or the person's declining dementia keep you from taking him to appointments again. His physical health is vital to him.

Coping with pills and medicines

Prescription medicines often have ridiculous names that make them hard to pronounce and remember, even for caregivers, let alone people with a memory disorder. Pills for different conditions can also have extremely similar names, which can lead to confusion. Penicillin, for example, has a very close namesake — penicillamine — that's no help at all in treating infections because it's designed to modify the symptoms of rheumatoid arthritis. And if that's not enough, drugs often go by both their generic and brand names. A common capsule to treat the symptoms of reflux and heartburn is known by its brand name, Prilosec, and its generic name, omeprazole. For all these reasons, mixing up pills is very easily done.

WARNING

A person on multiple drugs for lots of different conditions could be made very ill as a result of confusing different medicines. Mixing up medications also involves the risk of under- or overdosing.

Checking what's what with the doctor

The person's primary care physician's nursing staff should be happy to sit down and take you through each medicine the person you're caring for is taking and what it's treating. Try to arrange such a meeting as early as possible when you begin caregiving so you have a clear understanding of what's going on. You can then explain the pills to the person you're caring for, and repeat as necessary each time he asks. Knowing the purpose of each medication also means you can stress the importance of taking each one and when it should be taken.

Using pill boxes and blister packs

Some pharmacies dispense the person's medication in a blister pack for a charge. This involves grouping together pills in a packet to be taken at a particular time of day for each day of the week. Automatic pill dispensers provide another way to ensure medication is taken safely. These dispensers give access only to the pills needed at that time of day and have the added advantage of an alarm to remind the person when to take his tablets. They may even be able to close after a period of time even if the person hasn't taken the pills to avoid them from being taken to close to the next dose. And having the pills safely locked in the automatic dispenser until the allotted time minimizes the chances of overdose. You can buy these dispensers online. They have to be filled by family or caregivers.

TIP

The most common method of tracking medication use is to set them out in weekly pillboxes where the pills for each day are put in that day's slot identified as S/M/T/W/TH/F/S. As caregiver, you have to fill these pillboxes appropriately (with the help of your loved one if he is capable). Then you can leave out only that week's pills and make sure your loved one takes only the appropriate daily dose.

Dealing with the Patient's Emotions

Throughout the process of caring for your loved one, you're going to be dealing with a lot of emotions — yours, his, and those of your other family members and friends. Dementia patients are particularly subject to frustration because it's so difficult for them to navigate their days, always looking for something, trying to remember something, worrying about something. It's a huge burden for any one person to bear.

A great deal of the successful management of a patient with a memory disorder rests with the way the caregiver treats him. If you always try to respect the person's dignity, let him know you love him, and treat him with courtesy, patience, and compassion, you can minimize outbursts. But even if you're so good and thoughtful and caring that you're about to be nominated for sainthood, the day may come when your loved one pitches a tantrum or sinks into a spell of the blues. It's not a failure on your part — it's the disease advancing. Seek counseling for yourself and take your loved one to his doctor for a checkup; if the change in his behavior is sudden, the reason might be a medical one.

Managing mood swings

Wild mood swings can actually be one of the early signs of dementia, but as the condition progresses, you may start to see more persistent tantrums or depression in your loved one (although the apathy of some AD patients is frequently misdiagnosed as depression). Other families have to contend with a loved one who always seems to be in a bad mood for no discernible reason. It's tough to deal with someone who is always finding fault and picking at you, but try to remember why this is happening and separate the event from your feelings for your family member. He isn't being difficult on purpose.

Caregivers and healthcare providers should look for possible underlying causes for these behavioral problems, including pain, psychosis (paranoia), medical conditions, and side effects of medications.

Doctors are reluctant to treat psychiatric symptoms pharmacologically in AD and dementia patients because many psychiatric drugs, particularly the antipsychotic medications, have undesirable side effects in older adults. These drugs can cause fogginess, disorientation, and sleepiness that can contribute to a fall and can even increase mortality when used to treat dementia-related psychosis. See Chapter 8 for details on antipsychotic medications.

So what can you do if medications aren't appropriate? A good therapy for mood swings in an older adult is to get her out of the house and into some enjoyable and appropriate activity. Many families have found that enrolling their loved one in an adult daycare center, even for a half day, two or three times a week, can greatly improve dispositions all around.

Recognizing depression

If your loved one is not sleeping or eating well and seems sad all the time, or expresses negative feelings, she may be clinically depressed. In the early stages of dementia, your loved one's depression may result from her diagnosis and the realization that she will gradually lose her capacity to function.

Regular exercise can help an older adult feel better, both physically and mentally. Talk to your doctor about other treatments. If nothing you do seems to lift your loved one's spirits, you should schedule an appointment for an evaluation to determine if your loved one needs medication to treat depression. Antidepressant medications may be helpful and are generally well tolerated. In addition, your loved one may benefit from counseling or participation in a support group designed especially for people with mild dementia if she is capable of talking about her worries.

Chapter 11

Making Medical Decisions

A lzheimer's disease (AD) and other dementias are complex diseases that aren't entirely understood — not even by doctors and scientists working on the forefront of memory disorder research. It would be nice if, like treating a cold, your loved one could have some chicken soup, rest a few days, and then feel better. But memory disorders are progressive conditions, and the medical decisions that you and your loved one make become more and more critical with the passing of time.

The first and, perhaps, most important decision is choosing the healthcare providers who'll be your partners throughout the journey you're embarking on. Having a sympathetic and knowledgeable healthcare team that's willing to take the time to listen to your concerns and dispense thoughtful advice will prove immensely helpful. In Chapter 5 we outline the process of selecting healthcare professionals to assist you and your loved one as you navigate the many twists and turns of the road ahead.

After you have a good healthcare team in place, you'll have to make dozens of other decisions, including end-of-life care and whether a *Do Not Resuscitate (DNR)* order is appropriate. You'll need to consider funeral and burial planning. You also may want to consider brain donation for ongoing research projects that have already yielded valuable clues in the fight against dementia and AD. However, this decision needs to be made in advance of death.

In this chapter, you find practical advice and information to guide you as you try to make the best possible medical decisions for yourself and your loved one.

REMEMBER

According to the Alzheimer's Association, a person with AD lives an average of 8 years from the onset of symptoms, but may live as long as 20 years. That's one reason why finding healthcare providers that you like and trust to serve as your partners during this journey is so very important.

Building a Team

In Chapter 5, we talk about the different kinds of specialists who may see a dementia or AD patient. We also tell you that your family doctor is a good place to start and, in many cases, can provide the majority of the care your loved one requires. Your primary care physician (PCP) can refer you to specialists, if needed, and other sorts of healthcare providers, such as visiting nurses and therapists, who may be available to help your family provide proper medical care for your loved one.

Working with a primary care physician

In many ways, though, continuity of care with the patient's PCP who knows the person best may be ideal. This doctor knows the patient's background and is therefore better placed to observe any changes than is a physician who has just become involved. The existing PCP can also continue to monitor other, more long-standing conditions the patient may have.

To ensure you get the most from working with the PCP:

>> Try to see the person's usual PCP and ask for a double appointment. Most appointments are only around 10 to 15 minutes long, which won't be enough.

>> Think about what you want to get from each appointment before you go.

>> Write down a list of questions so you don't forget anything.

>> List any symptoms that are causing concern so they can be addressed.

>> If tests are suggested, ask what they involve, what the test results can show, how long they'll take, and how soon the results will be available.

>> Ask whether referral to a specialist memory clinic is available or appropriate.

>> See what local services are available, such as organizations and support groups for caregivers.

>> Discuss what you can do to keep yourself healthy.

>> Find out about how to get in touch with social services and what they can provide in terms of support and home adaptations.

Keep in mind that not every person with a memory disorder needs to see a specialist. Many PCPs can do a fine job, particularly if they're familiar with the patient and his or her family. In addition, finding and regularly visiting a specialist is unrealistic for many families because of finances or geography.

REMEMBER

Although your PCP may be aware that you or someone you love has dementia, he's not psychic and doesn't automatically know when things aren't going well or new symptoms have developed. Let him know of problems as they arise so that he can offer help as soon as it's needed.

Adding other health professionals for regular checkups

Focusing on caring for a person with a chronic condition like dementia can mean a caregiver forgets to also consider that person's general health. Patients with memory disorder are unable to attend to their own health issues and medical needs. People with dementia develop arthritis, cataracts, and poor hearing, just like everyone else, and leaving these problems untreated can dramatically add to their disability.

Ear, teeth, and eye specialists

People with dementia may experience problems with their hearing, teeth, and eyesight. And with memory disorders in particular, it's important that people can make full use of their senses. It's easy to think someone isn't remembering when he simply didn't hear what was said. Dealing with these issues will improve someone's general wellbeing.

Here are some of the specialists who can help:

>> **Audiologists:** Poor hearing is disabling enough on its own, but when combined with the symptoms of memory loss, it can lead to increasing confusion and isolation. Hearing checks are vital, but may need to be preceded by a trip to the doctor's office to ensure that a buildup of wax isn't the culprit. Hearing

aids are recommended if needed. But after they're obtained, keep hearing aids tied to a necklace to prevent loss because they're expensive.

>> **Dentists:** These professionals aren't everyone's favorite, and a visit to the dentist can become increasingly difficult as dementia or AD and their associated confusion progresses. However, it's a good idea for people with dementia to have regular check-ups with a dentist they already know to help maintain healthy teeth and gums.

>> **Opticians/optometrists:** As people get older, a multitude of eye conditions, from cataracts to macular degeneration, can affect the eyesight. As with hearing difficulties, the sensory deprivation resulting from poor eyesight can worsen symptoms of confusion, so regular eye checkup and treatment for problems (including eye glasses) are vital.

Mobility specialists

Mobility is often an issue for elderly people, whether or not they have dementia. Maintaining muscle strength and flexibility is vital for staying mobile, and taking care of your loved one's feet can make a big difference to the quality of life of a patient with dementia. The two specialists you're likely to encounter are

>> **Physical therapists:** Physical therapists work in hospitals, nursing facilities, and in private practice. They can treat pain and immobility resulting from arthritis, help mobilize someone after a fracture or joint surgery, and provide exercises to help improve stability and prevent falls. Although they work in hospitals, many physical therapists also treat people in outpatient settings, and some even do home visits.

>> **Podiatrists:** These foot specialists play a vital role in keeping feet healthy and pain free. They can treat a wide variety of problems from simple corns and ingrown toenails to bunions. They also can provide toenail-trimming services for very thick nails.

Bringing in specialists as needed

Other factors may influence the number and type of professionals included in your loved one's medical team. For example, if your loved one has diabetes in addition to memory loss, your medical team might include a diabetes specialist, such as an endocrinologist, or dietitian — experts who typically wouldn't be required for the day-to-day care of an AD or dementia patient but who can provide essential expertise when needed. If your loved one has cardiovascular disease, your team might include a cardiologist, and you may seek out a rheumatologist if your loved one has arthritis. In other words, the makeup of your particular medical care team is dictated by your loved one's medical needs. If a memory disorder is the only diagnosis and your loved one is healthy otherwise, you may do very well with a small team consisting of your family doctor, a specialist in memory loss, if needed.

As the disease progresses, you should be alert for changes in your loved one's condition that may require the addition of a new doctor or other healthcare professional to your team. For example, if your loved one develops hearing difficulty you may need an audiologist or if foot problems occur you may need a podiatrist.

WARNING

Sometimes families get so used to the day-to-day routines of caring for a loved one with memory loss that they're unsure how to react when a medical crisis not related to memory loss presents itself. If your loved one shows any signs of unusual pain, persistent heartburn and/or indigestion, dizziness or fainting, bleeding, or any other symptom that would indicate a significant medical problem, you should have him evaluated as quickly as possible by the family doctor. If the condition seems critical or life threatening, call 911 or immediately transport your loved one to the nearest hospital emergency room for treatment.

Keeping Good Records

Now is a good time to prepare a filing system to keep track of the many medical documents you'll receive over the course of your loved one's treatment for his memory disorder. You don't need anything fancy to store your files; a simple cardboard filing box is fine. If you want to get a little more elaborate, purchase a filing cabinet. Whatever you choose, the important thing is that this place is where every single piece of paper relating to your loved one's memory disorder will go. Try to get in the habit of filing the papers as soon as you get home from a doctor's appointment. If this isn't feasible, keep one manila folder in the front of the filing cabinet where you stick all the medical records until you have time to file them properly.

TIP

Keeping medical records straight will be much easier if you establish a good filing system to begin with. Get a box of manila folders and give each one a specific label, such as "Prescriptions," "Medicare Documents," "Hospital Bills," "Dr. John Doe," and so on. You'll be surprised how much time you save by keeping your loved one's medical records in one easy-to-access place. It beats digging frantically through piles of papers and junk mail any day.

If you don't have time to file the documents yourself, consider paying another family member (perhaps a teenage son or daughter who always seems to be asking for money?) or a neighbor you know and trust to help you. All these little pieces of paper may not seem important now, but down the road, you may need to correlate information on two different medical records to make a more informed medical decision. If your loved one is seeing several doctors, keeping them informed of what medications the other doctors are prescribing will help prevent an accidental conflict in prescriptions. By keeping all this information at hand, you'll always be ready to answer any questions your healthcare providers may have, and you'll also have exact times and dates available.

TIP

To keep track of medications more easily, make up a list of medications (including any vitamins or other supplements) your loved one takes and place it in your wallet, and make a copy for your loved one's wallet as well as copies for various healthcare providers. Be sure to update the card each time a medication is added or stopped, or the dosage is changed.

Before each appointment with a doctor, or other member of your loved one's care team, make a list of concerns you want to share at the visit. Having the info written down on your list can help you remember to discuss any questions you have or important issues that have come up since the last visit.

REMEMBER

Always bring copies of medical records or advanced directives rather than the original documents. If you were to lose the originals along the way, they'd be difficult to replace. If obtaining copies is difficult, ask the physician's office to copy the originals or directly scan them into the electronic health record while you're there and then return them to you before you leave.

Using Alternative Therapies

More information is available than ever before, and it's coming 24/7 from a dozen different directions. To say the least, trying to decipher whether the information is good or bogus is difficult.

Nowhere is separating good info from bad more confusing than in the world of alternative therapies. If you believe half of what you read on the Internet, you'd think that doctors had already cured AD. (But if that were really true, don't you think the mainstream press would have reported that breaking news by now?)

On the other hand, don't assume that just because a treatment isn't mainstream medicine doesn't mean it has no therapeutic value. For more info on alternative therapies that work, see Chapter 9.

REMEMBER

If you decide that you want to investigate alternative therapies for your loved one, just be sure that you don't use them in place of proven medical care. And please keep your doctor informed of everything you're doing, so she can advise you of any potential conflicts or problem areas.

Deciding on End-of-Life Care Options

Talking about end-of-life care options may seem a bit disheartening, especially because the end may still be many years away. But now, as soon as possible after diagnosis, is the time to discuss your loved one's wishes for her end-of-life care. You're going to have to make more decisions than you might think, so you want to start early.

If a patient is in the early stages of a memory disorder, she should be asked her wishes and make her own decisions (as much as she is able). Her caregivers should then carry out her wishes. Depending on the severity of your loved one's dementia at the time of diagnosis, she may still be capable of participating in the decision-making process in a meaningful way. You can consult an attorney to have any necessary documents drawn up for signature, if your loved one is still mentally competent to sign.

GETTING AHOLD OF THE CODE STATUS LINGO

REMEMBER

Code status refers to the formal physician's order defining whether to attempt resuscitation in the event her heart stops beating or she stops breathing. *Resuscitation* means administering *cardiopulmonary resuscitation* (doing CPR), *defibrillating* (shocking) the heart, *intubating* (inserting a breathing tube), and administering emergency medications. Code status becomes most important when a person is admitted to an assisted living facility, nursing home, or hospital so staff members have guidelines of to how to handle emergency situations in accordance with the patient and family wishes.

Code status is defined differently in different states, but in general two opposite options are available:

- **Full code:** *Full code* means everything will be done to try to resuscitate the person. Realize that making a choice for a full code means that doctors will attempt resuscitation, but there is no guarantee that it will be successful.

- **Do Not Resuscitate (DNR):** Also known as no code, this status means that if a person's heartbeat or breathing stops, then there will be no attempt at resuscitation. Generally DNR or no code is chosen if the person wants to let nature take its course.

TIP

To make sure that the patient's choices for end-of-life care are carried out according to her wishes, *advance directives* are necessary documents. (For more information on advance directives and how they work, see Chapter 12.) When a patient hasn't prepared an advance directive and is no longer capable of making such choices, the family caregiver must make these decisions for the patient.

Many patients succumb to physical ailments other than dementia or AD, such as heart attack, stroke, or complications of diabetes. In fact, most people with a memory disorder don't die from the dementia but rather from a complication of the disease, such as aspiration pneumonia or urinary tract infections. No matter how excellent their care has been, as their disease progresses, dementia and AD patients are unable to make decisions for themselves. That's why you should discuss these issues as much as possible while your loved one can still make her wishes known.

When your loved one is in advanced stages of dementia or AD, she may experience a life-threatening medical crisis, such as pneumonia, and you must decide what sort of care will be provided. In this sort of situation, you have three major choices available: letting nature take its course, palliative care, or aggressive care. Read on for an explanation of each option.

Letting nature take its course

When you've lived with a patient with a memory disorder for many years, as you near the end of the road, you may decide that you'll ride out whatever happens and let nature prevail. If you choose this course (based on your knowledge of your loved one's wishes), you absolutely must make these wishes known to your healthcare provider by signing a DNR (Do Not Resuscitate) order. All this order means is that when your loved one is dying, the medical care facility and its staff will allow that natural process to proceed without interfering.

Only doctors can complete DNR forms, but only competent patients or their power of attorney (POA) can request them. If you do ask for a DNR, the doctor will sign and ask the patient (if she is capable) or whoever is legally empowered to represent the patient to sign the document as well. Different states have different options for DNR orders, so ask your doctor what these are where you live. The DNR, which is a binding, legal document, is then put into the patient's medical record so anyone who provides care knows what to do if the patient experiences a life-threatening crisis. (Chapter 12 has more details about DNRs.) However, realize that this DNR form usually will need to be re-created each time your loved one is admitted to a hospital or nursing home.

Maybe your loved one signed an advance directive called a living will while she was still mentally capable of making end-of-life decisions. Living wills specify the exact types of medical treatment and interventions that patients do and don't want performed if they're in a crisis situation. For more information on living wills and where to find forms for your state, refer to Chapter 12.

You may be thinking, "Well, of course if a dementia or AD patient is dying, doctors are just going to let them go." That's not always the case, though. Even when a patient's quality of life isn't good, some healthcare providers are determined to prolong her life no matter what. They may aggressively resuscitate a dying patient, inserting ventilator tubes and performing other invasive procedures to restore life. But if your loved one has had the foresight to sign a living will and you have made sure there is a DNR, then the attending doctors and the medical facility must honor that request.

Palliative care

Palliative care means that your loved one will be fed and kept comfortable and free from pain. It also means that appropriate care and medications will be given to alleviate any distressing symptoms the patient may display. For example, if a patient is running a fever and is uncomfortable, the doctor may administer acetaminophen to bring down the fever. But no aggressive or invasive measures will be taken to artificially extend the patient's life.

TECHNICAL STUFF

The verb *palliate* derives from the Latin, *palliatus,* which means "to conceal." Palliative care does just that; it "conceals" the intensity of an illness through moderation of its effects with appropriate care and medications. However, it doesn't change the course of the illness. It is a way of letting nature take its course but at the same time treating pain and other distressing symptoms.

REMEMBER

Palliative care often goes hand in hand with a DNR order. It's a way for family members to let healthcare providers know that they want to ensure their loved one's comfort and safety without taking any extraordinary or aggressive steps to save that person's life if she experiences a potentially fatal health crisis. This helps prevent unwanted medical intervention at the end of life.

TIP

One way to provide palliative care is to enroll the person with dementia or AD in hospice. Unless your loved one has another terminal condition (like advanced cancer or heart failure), in order to qualify for hospice using dementia or AD as the terminal diagnosis, certain requirements must be met. The patient with dementia of AD must be at Stage 7c on the Functional Assessment or FAST SCALE, which we explain in detail in Chapter 7. This stage requires that your loved one is unable to walk without significant assistance and the ability to speak is essentially gone. In addition, she must have had at least one of the following conditions in the last 12 months:

>> Aspiration pneumonia

>> Kidney infection

>> Multiple severe bedsores

>> Recurrent fever

>> Weight loss of at least 10 percent of body weight

Medicare pays for hospice and requires your loved one's physician to certify that life expectancy is six months or less. To stay on hospice during that time, the patient must continue to show decline. Hospice can be provided at home if a caregiver is present 24/7 to care for and monitor the patient and provide medications for comfort as needed. It can also be provided in an assisted living facility or nursing home. Some larger cities have an inpatient hospice center where patients can be admitted. For details of what hospice covers, refer to the Medicare website for latest information at www.medicare.gov/what-medicare-covers/part-a/part-a-coverage-hospice.html.

Aggressive care

Some families just can't accept the idea of letting go of a beloved family member, no matter how far advanced her illness. These families may choose to opt for aggressive end-of-life care, authorizing their physicians to employ whatever means necessary to prolong their loved one's life, including the use of ventilation equipment to maintain breathing and oxygenation and defibrillators to restart the heart.

Although end-of-life care is an extremely personal choice, choose carefully if you're considering an aggressive approach. Aggressive care is appropriate and understandable in situations where someone has suffered a traumatic injury or is in a critical stage of an illness that could be treated. If these patients can be helped through their crises, they may recover fully and go on to enjoy many more years of a good quality of life. Other times, it can be the beginning of a long road on life support, promoting quantity of life over quality of life.

You need to remember your loved one's dementia or AD is a progressive disabling condition. Even if you "save" your loved one, ask yourself: "What am I saving her for?" You have to determine to what degree your loved one has quality of life. You and your loved one have already been through a lot simply dealing with a memory disorder. If there is no quality of life, there's absolutely nothing wrong with choosing to let life end naturally.

FUNERAL AND BURIAL PLANNING

Because the death of a loved one is a stressful enough situation in itself, have funeral and burial plans in place before they're needed. Planning the details ahead of time can alleviate significant stress at this difficult time.

Pre-paid burial plans are available in which all the details of a funeral can be selected and paid for in advance of death.

Ask your loved one his wishes if he's still able to discuss his desires. If the dementia or AD is too far advanced to allow your loved one's participation in these decisions, then you make the necessary decisions based on your knowledge of your loved one's values and beliefs. Questions to answer include the following:

- Does your loved one want to be buried or cremated? If he wants to be cremated, what are his wishes for his ashes?

- Has a cemetery plot already been selected and purchased or if not, does your loved one want to buried in a specific cemetery?

- Does your loved one prefer a religious-based funeral service in a house of worship or a memorial service in a funeral home?

- Does your loved one desire specific speakers, music, or flowers that would be important to your loved one to have at that service?

Considering Brain Autopsy and Brain Donation

Many advances in scientists' understanding of AD and its effects upon the brain have come from the study of brains donated by the families of deceased Alzheimer's patients. In addition, some families find closure when they choose to donate their loved one's brain, because a post-mortem brain autopsy is still the only way to confirm a diagnosis of AD with absolute certainty. Brain autopsy may involve cost, and special arrangements must be made prior to your loved one's death.

If you decide to donate your loved one's brain after her death, you need to start the process now. Through brain donation, you help researchers as they look for answers to prevent dementia and AD as well as define future treatments. However, because brain tissue is only viable for 24 hours after a person dies, arrangements must be made well in advance of your loved one's death. Contact a research center, brain bank, or university to make brain donations arrangements.

For more information on brain donation, contact your local Alzheimer's Association or check these websites:

>> www.alzforum.org/brain-banks

>> www.bu.edu/alzresearch/education-resources/brain

>> www.alzprevention.org/prevention-research.php (Click at the bottom of this page to be directed to the PDF document about brain donation.)

Chapter 12

Addressing Legal Issues

A diagnosis of dementia or Alzheimer's disease (AD) gives you a chance to plan for your loved one's future. So although you may be overwhelmed by the fact that your loved one has dementia, it's important to make practical plans to avoid problems later with future care or financial decisions. Make plans now while your loved one may still be able to make his wishes known.

Legal decisions in these situations can be emotionally wrenching; in many states, you must first have your loved one declared mentally incompetent before you can activate a previously prepared power of attorney (POA) or begin guardianship proceedings. Families may be understandably reluctant to do this. But in order to protect your loved one's assets and get your family through the next few years in the best possible shape, everyone involved must sit down together as soon as possible and make these important decisions.

In this chapter, we explain the ins and outs of many legal issues that can affect patients and their families. We also explain why getting your legal ducks in a row as soon as possible after your loved one's diagnosis is so essential. Legally, only the person with the memory disorder can make these decisions. If you wait too long, your loved one becomes incompetent in the eyes of the law and then your family will have to go to the trouble and expense of seeking guardianship in order to manage your loved one's affairs.

REMEMBER

The information provided in this chapter is in no way intended as a substitute for professional legal advice. If you have a specific legal question, your best bet is to consult an attorney who understands your state and local statutes and the laws that apply to your particular situation.

Getting Started

Before you pick up the phone and call an attorney, take the time to do a bit of organizing. You'll save yourself a lot of time and money down the road.

First, get a sturdy manila accordion file or similar file to hold documents in an organized fashion. Because you're going to be dealing with a lot of paper over the coming years, you may want to invest in a hanging folder system that helps keep your files together and your paperwork in good condition.

TIP

If space is tight in your home and you don't want a giant, ugly metal filing cabinet cluttering things up, consider using a cardboard banker's box to store your loved one's documents. They come in packs of three or six and are ideal for storing either letter- or legal-size documents, or you may have access to empty copy boxes with lids at work that can serve as file boxes. Use one box for medical records, one for legal records, and a third for financial records.

Get a packet of manila file folders and label them. For example, in a folder marked "Will," you might have a copy of your loved one's will and written documentation stating where the original, legally binding copy of the will is stored. If you have more than one attorney, such as one that deals with elder law issues and another that deals with financial issues, make a separate folder for each one. Proceed in this fashion until you have folders for every legal issue you're dealing with.

Ultimately, although all this labeling and preparation may seem like a lot of work, doing so will help you stay organized and ultimately it saves you so much time in the long run that you'll be happy you prepared your filing system properly. And don't make the mistake of thinking that you have to do all this work by yourself. Your loved one or your children and grandchildren may be happy to help with this important paperwork.

THE PAPER CHASE: WHAT SHOULD YOU FILE?

Over the next few years, you'll more than likely handle hundreds of pieces of paper for your loved one. So how do you decide what to keep and what to throw away? Well, your legal advisor is the best person to ask, but we recommend that you keep the following info handy:

- Contact information for your attorney or your loved one's attorney

- A copy of your will or your loved one's will, along with precise information about where the original will is stored

- Copies of any trusts that have been executed, along with info stating where originals are kept

- Copies of other pertinent legal documents, such as advanced directives, including Do Not Resuscitate forms, living wills, durable power of attorney (POA), documents for healthcare POA, and POA for finance

- Include the title to the cemetery plot where your loved one has chosen to be buried

- The name and contact information for the individuals who have the financial POA and medical POA for you or your loved one, as well as copies of each and location of originals

- The name and contact information for the person appointed to carry out the will, also known as an *executor* or *personal representative*

Setting Up an Advance Directive

An *advance directive* is a written statement of a person's wishes indicating the types of medical treatment he does and doesn't want under certain circumstances in the future if he is unable to make these decisions for himself or to communicate it to others.

An advance directive can take the form of a written living will, which a person defines instructions for medical treatment or a healthcare POA or healthcare proxy in which the person appoints a person to serve as his agent to make healthcare decisions when he is no longer able to do so. We recommend both documents.

In legal parlance, an advance directive allows your wishes to be respected if at any time you "lack capacity." Decisions about competency and capacity in the United States are based on federal Supreme Court decisions as well as state laws. This can be a complex and confusing issue. The following sections focus on advance directives and what you need to know about them.

Looking at the UK's Mental Capacity Act to understand the concept of capacity

In order to understand the approach that one may take to determine capacity, looking at the approach the United Kingdom has taken is worthwhile. Practitioners in the UK presently base their approach on the Mental Capacity Act of 2005.

The Mental Capacity Act aims to empower and protect all vulnerable people when they're no longer able to make important decisions for themselves. Its underlying principle, according to the UK's Ministry of Justice, is "to ensure that those who lack capacity are empowered to make as many decisions for themselves as possible and that any decision made, or action taken, on their behalf is made in their best interests."

In order to try to achieve this outcome for vulnerable people, the act has five key principles (sourced from www.justice.gov.uk):

>> Every adult has the right to make his own decisions and must be assumed to have capacity to make them unless it's proved otherwise. Therefore the onus is on the assessor to prove the individual lacks capacity, not the individual to prove he has it.

>> A person must be given all practicable help before anyone treats him as not being able to make his own decisions.

>> Just because an individual makes what may be seen as an unwise decision, he should not be treated as lacking capacity to make that decision.

>> Anything done or any decision made on behalf of a person who lacks capacity must be done in his best interests.

>> Anything done for or on behalf of a person who lacks capacity should be the least restrictive of his basic rights and freedoms.

This law is intended to protect people in the UK with a range of different underlying medical problems, such as brain tumors, strokes, severe depression, schizophrenia, or learning disabilities as well as people with dementia. You may be thinking that's interesting about capacity as defined in British law, but what about in the United States?

Defining capacity

The law deems that for people to have capacity, they must be able to do the following:

>> Understand information given to them

>> Retain information long enough to be able to make a decision

>> Weigh the information available to make a decision

>> Communicate their decision

REMEMBER

Assessment of capacity is decision specific. In other words, not all decisions require the same level of mental functioning — some are much more basic than others. An assessment has to be made on a case-by-case basis, looking at one particular issue at one specific time only. This situation exists because a person with dementia, for example, may not be capable of making decisions about managing his money, but may be able to very clearly state that he'd like his appendix removed when he's in severe pain as a result of appendicitis.

Assessing capacity and competency

A person's doctor usually makes an assessment of cognitive function through mental status testing and in consultation with the person's family and main caregivers. During the assessment, the doctor does his best to communicate the issues at stake to give the person the best chance of coming to grips with the situation and its ramifications. The doctor then tries to establish whether, on the balance of probabilities, the person lacks the ability to make the particular decision because he's unable to understand, retain, and weigh the information he's just been given and then effectively communicate it.

Recognizing what an advance directive can cover

An advance directive helps your loved one to be one step ahead of the game in relation to losing capacity, because it enables your loved one to decide what will or won't be in his best interests if certain important decisions need to be made. These decisions will therefore be made by the patient and not for the patient.

Examples of such decisions include your loved one's wishes regarding life-saving treatment such as

>> Antibiotics and intravenous fluids

>> Blood transfusions

>> Cardiopulmonary resuscitation

>> Dialysis (artificial kidney machine)

>> Intensive care treatment

>> Intubation (insertion of breathing tube)

>> Mechanical ventilation (breathing machine)

Your loved one's decisions expressed in an advance directive are legally binding, thus any doctors involved in care have to uphold them.

REMEMBER

While your loved one still has capacity, his word overrides anything written in an advance directive.

Completing the paperwork

Some organizations working with people with dementia, such as the Alzheimer's Association, or with terminal illnesses, provide downloadable example advance directive forms on their websites. But you don't need to complete an official document. If you're preparing an advance directive for yourself, you must include the following details:

>> Your name, date of birth, and address

>> The name, address, and phone number of your physician, and whether he has a copy of your advance directive document

>> A statement making clear that this advance directive document should be used if you ever lack capacity to make decisions

>> A statement regarding which treatment(s) you will refuse, and the circumstances in which your decision will apply

>> The date you created your advance directive

>> Your signature

>> A dated signature of at least one witness

If you're writing an advance directive to refuse medical treatment that will keep you alive, it must also include the statement, "I refuse this treatment even if my life is at risk as a result."

TIP

Talking through possible scenarios with your physician as you draw up your document and before putting pen to paper and signing it is always best. Your doctor can help you understand what you may face in certain circumstances, and what refusal of treatment will mean in terms of the symptoms you may therefore suffer and the effect on your life expectancy.

Examples of statements covering scenarios you may want to include after this discussion are

>> "I refuse artificial feeding and rehydrating fluids, even if my life is at risk as a result, if I have terminal cancer and become unconscious and unable to eat or drink without assistance."

>> "If I have a condition from which I'm expected to die in a matter of days or weeks, I only want treatment to help manage discomfort and distress and not to prolong my life, even if my life is at risk as a result."

Many people say that they don't want to be a vegetable, which is slang for long-term dependence on life support and machines. But even those individuals may be willing to accept temporary life support (like breathing machines) if they'll likely recover to their previous function. One way to express this is to say "no aggressive treatment if poor quality of life is expected."

As a caregiver, if your loved one is still able to do so, then you should help her review her advance directive with her family and doctor at regular intervals, because it can be rescinded or altered at any time while they still have the mental capacity to do so in the light of changing circumstances.

Identifying which professionals to involve

If she still has capacity, your loved one can still complete advance directives. However, unless she really wants to, she doesn't have to involve an attorney in drawing up an advance directive, which will definitely keep the cost down. Forms are available on the Internet that are state-specific and can be downloaded and completed. However, to be sure all the latest legal jargon is used, have an attorney involved — even if it is just to check over the forms. After her advance directives are signed, ensure that all those looking after your loved one have copies for their records.

This list of people may include your

>> Next of kin

>> Family or paid caregivers

>> Assisted living facility or nursing home staff (if that is where your loved one resides)

>> Primary care physician (or geriatrician)

>> Neurologist

>> Case manager

>> Social worker

And, of course, she can give her lawyer a copy for safekeeping too.

Looking into a Durable POA

Recognize that a person must prepare and sign advance directives while he still has the capacity do so. After he has lost significant cognitive function and can no longer speak for himself, he can't complete an advance directive and you can't do it for him. We can't stress the importance of this enough.

REMEMBER

A *durable power of attorney* (POA) is a legal document that authorizes a person to make caregiving, financial, and/or medical treatment decisions on behalf of a patient who's become incapable of making her own decisions. In most states a distinct medical POA exists for a person to appoint someone to make healthcare decisions for him. In other states, a general POA is sufficient. The person who receives the AD patient's legal authority is called an *attorney in fact,* but you may also hear this person called an *agent* or a *proxy.* The person granting the POA is called the *principal.* A durable POA can be granted only if the patient transferring the authority is still considered mentally competent.

When dealing with a health situation where a person may become increasingly incapacitated, you need a durable POA. This instrument that transfers broad legal decision-making authority to the designated person designed for future unknown circumstances. A POA allows dementia and Alzheimer's patients to exercise their authority and choose someone trustworthy to handle future decisions while they're still able to make informed decisions. After the POA is designated, the person with memory loss should discuss his future wishes with that person to make sure he's understood.

Two types of POA exist:

>> Health and medical

>> Property and financial affairs

You can choose to make one type or both.

WARNING

If your loved one is diagnosed with dementia or already holds a POA for another family member such as his spouse or child, you should arrange to transfer that authority as soon as possible. Discuss the situation with the person who gave him the POA so that person can appoint an alternate person to serve that role if he hasn't already determined an alternate in the original document.

Healthcare/medical durable POA

This document allows your loved on to choose someone to make decisions for him when he can no longer make those decisions for himself concerning issues such as

>> Medical care to receive

>> Medications

>> Surgical operations

>> Diagnostic testing

>> Life-sustaining treatment and resuscitation

>> Moving from his home into a long-term care facility or an assisted-living facility

The person serving as POA can only make these decisions if the person who completed the document has lost the capacity to do so. Certain decisions, however, can already be written into his living will or other advance directive to guide the POA in making these decisions the way he would have made them for himself. The attorney can't overrule decisions in advance directives unless explicitly given permission to do so in the directive.

General or financial durable POA

This document allows a person to choose one or more people to make decisions about money and property on his behalf. The POA or agent can pay bills, collect benefits, or sell property, among many other responsibilities.

Taking a look at the benefits offered by a durable POA

As any Boy or Girl Scout will tell you, it's best to be prepared. Setting up a durable POA document while your loved one is still capable to do so means he can define who will make decisions for him when he is no longer able to do so, which allows him to cover all potential eventualities. This can put his mind at ease that a trusted person will be looking out for his interests.

A durable POA also means that everyone who cares for your loved one is aware at an early stage of his dementia of his future wishes. This is particularly important if he lives alone or has a family where different members don't get along and may have their own conflicting ideas about what will be best for him.

Sorting out a durable POA also makes sense from a financial point of view, because if your loved one loses capacity to make decisions without a durable POA, you or your family will have to go through the court system to manage his affairs. This legal process is costly in both time and money and adds unnecessary stress at a time when life may already be difficult for all of you.

And finally, by putting agents in place, your loved one avoids the risk of either a stranger or someone he may have known but didn't trust making decisions for him.

Figuring out how many agents are needed

The number of agents appointed depends on the particular situation and the abilities of the individual agents. The only person who can make these appointments is the person who is still capable of stating who he wants to manage his medical decisions and business affairs when he is no longer able to do so. For example, if your father has AD and doesn't appoint an agent before becoming incompetent, you can't appoint an agent for him. Hence, the following discussion assumes that your loved one still has the capacity to make that decision.

Each family can tailor its POA to fit its needs. For example, if a woman has two children, one a nurse and the other an accountant, she may choose to draw up two powers of attorney, giving the nurse the right to make medical decisions and the accountant the right to make financial and legal decisions for her when she can no longer make these decisions for herself. When appointing more than one agent, to avoid conflict, you should appoint people who get along well together and who'll work together to protect your interests.

Another consideration is proximity. Typically, a family must deal with caring for a loved one with dementia or AD over a long period of time. Hence, it's most practical if the agent lives relatively nearby. A woman in New York City who has the best relationship with her eldest daughter who lives in Seattle, Washington, and trusts her the most out of all her children may want her to be POA. It may be difficult for that daughter to be onsite to handle affairs. However, many of the responsibilities of a POA especially (in regard to medical decision making) can be done by telephone between visits so don't let distance be the only factor in POA or guardian appointment. Ultimately, your loved one has to be comfortable that the person appointed will do the best to make decisions in her best interest.

TIP

When your loved one is selecting an agent, help her identify someone she loves and trusts who can be forceful if required. As caregiver, it can be convenient if it's you. However, sometimes a family member other than the caregiver has already been appointed in the past. Then you have to work with this person to do the best for your loved one. If no one in the immediate family is able to take on this responsibility, POA can be given to a close friend or significant other. But your loved one must be sure that person is willing to accept the responsibility before proceeding and must also make sure the person is someone trusted implicitly to do the job because that person is about to get a lot of power.

Your loved one can grant her agent as much or as little power as she wishes. Most durable POA forms actually have checklists of powers that may be granted — for example, real estate transactions and banking. If your loved one wishes the agent to have a particular power, she leaves it on the list, but if your loved one wants a specific power to be excluded from the agent's authority, she crosses that off the POA document.

TIP

Appointing several alternate agents in order of preference is wise because if, for some reason, the first choice of agent is unable to carry out his responsibilities, backup agents are named.

Your loved one may be happy with just one agent, but most attorneys say that appointing alternate agents is a good idea.

REMEMBER

Handling the legal, financial, and medical affairs of another person is a lot of work, so don't beat yourself up if it's something you'd rather not do. Perhaps the responsibility can be split between several family members so the entire burden of care doesn't fall on one person.

Choosing the correct type of POA

Durable POA can be handled in two ways:

>> If your loved one's health is deteriorating rapidly, the durable POA can take effect immediately upon the signing of the legal documents. That means that from the moment your loved one lifts the pen from the signature line and the form is notarized, the designated proxy (agent) will be handling all of his affairs.

>> If your loved one is still able to manage his affairs and prefers to do so for as long as possible, he can sign what's known as a *springing durable POA.*

This type of POA automatically springs into effect after your loved one meets the definition of incapacity set out in the document and his attending physician has certified that incapacity. In other words, with a springing durable POA, your loved one won't give up legal authority until and unless he becomes incapacitated.

Although springing POA may seem like an attractive alternative, in actual practice they can be problematic because there is nothing concrete on the face of the document that states the document is now in effect. As a result, third parties such as banks and insurance companies are frequently reluctant to honor them, even after the necessary certifications have been obtained. Consult your attorney to see what POA is right for your loved one.

WARNING

In all states, a patient must still be demonstrably competent and capable of making informed decisions when he signs a durable POA. That's why setting up a durable POA as soon as possible after a diagnosis of a memory disorder is so essential. If you wait until after your loved one has lost significant mental capacity, the courts will no longer allow you to obtain your loved one's POA because he's no longer capable of giving informed consent to the arrangement.

Recognizing the kind of "powers" a POA bestows

You may feel confused about what a person can or can't do with a POA. Though specific authority varies from state to state, generally speaking, agents acting on behalf of an incapacitated individual (also known as a *principal*) may

>> Collect by whatever means are necessary any money or valuables that are owed to the principal

>> Save, invest, or disburse money, or use them on behalf of the principal for the purposes intended

>> Sign new contracts or modify existing contracts on behalf of the principal, on terms agreeable to the POA

>> Buy, sell, or lease property on behalf of the principal

>> Settle claims or court cases in favor of or against the principal

>> Hire and fire attorneys, accountants, or any other personnel necessary to attend to the principal's business and legal affairs

And that list is just the short one. In plain English, an agent may handle real estate and personal property transactions, stocks and bonds, commodities and bonds, banking, business operations, insurance, annuities, estates, trusts, claims and litigation, personal and family issues, Social Security, Medicare, Medicaid, pensions from private corporations or from civil or military service, retirement plan transactions and income, and personal and property taxes.

REMEMBER

In addition to the things an agent may do, there are also some things that she must do to satisfy the requirements of the law. Agents must

>> Always act in the best interests of the principal and not engage in any act that furthers his own interests rather than those of the principal

>> Keep appropriate records of each transaction, including a complete accounting of receipts for expenditures and disbursements

>> Manage the principal's legal and financial affairs in an honest and competent manner

WARNING

A POA gives the agent an enormous amount of authority. Some unscrupulous people will try to force someone to sign a POA in order to gain legal authority over that person's assets. If someone in your family, a friend, or an acquaintance is trying to force your loved one to inappropriately give him POA, don't let it happen! Contact the police or your local elder abuse hotline immediately for guidance and information about how to handle the situation. In some states, trying to force someone to sign a POA through threats and abuse is considered extortion, so if you feel that your loved one is unsafe, don't hesitate to call the authorities for help in removing and dealing with the person who's threatening your loved one.

Changing your mind

If your loved one is unhappy with the appointed agent's conduct, the POA can be revoked at any time, as long as the person who granted the authority in the first place is still considered competent to make decisions. Your loved one must inform the agent in writing that the POA is revoked and must also inform the lawyer, bank, and other financial institutions that the agent no longer has the authority to manage your affairs. You may need to assist your loved one with these notifications.

TIP

After your loved one becomes incompetent, you should keep watch over his affairs even if you're not the agent to make sure the person granted the POA is behaving responsibly. If you're not the agent but you feel that the agent is abusing the POA, you should file a complaint with local law enforcement authorities or pursue guardianship yourself. Because the person with the memory disorder is no longer competent to make his own decisions, the court must intervene to investigate any instances of misconduct. Only the court has the authority to dissolve a POA in situations where the principal is no longer competent and the existing agent isn't performing his duties responsibly. But the court doesn't have the authority to grant a new POA; that's why appointing several agents at the time the POA is granted is a good idea. If one doesn't work out, another can step up and take over the job. If the principal names only one agent and his authority is revoked or he is no longer able to do the job due to illness, his own incapacity, or death), then the family must apply for a guardianship to gain legal authority to manage the affairs of the person with AD.

If your jurisdiction required the POA to be filed with the local clerk of court, the lawyer must file a copy of the revocation with the clerk to make things official. At the same time, if your loved one still has the mental capacity to select a new agent, then you need to help him consult with his attorney about appointing a new agent through the creation of a new durable POA. If you put this off and don't select a new agent in a timely fashion while your loved one still is able to do so, then your family will be required to go to the expense and burdensome process of getting a conservatorship or guardianship approved by the court.

Considering cost

A POA is a relatively inexpensive legal procedure. If your loved one's situation is straightforward, you can obtain the form by downloading it from `http://powerofattorney.com/durable/` or picking one up from your local bank.

However, if your loved one's situation is more complex, then the best bet is probably to hire an attorney who's experienced in elder law to help, especially if his legal, financial, and/or family situation is complex and requires sorting out.

TIP

To find an elder law specialist in your area, call the state Bar Association or the local Alzheimer's Association or your area Office on Aging for suggestions. You can also talk to other families dealing with dementia or AD to see if they can suggest a good lawyer. If you want to use an Internet search engine, enter the phrase "elder law" and then the name of your town or city. The results should give you contact information for any attorneys specializing in elder law in your area.

REMEMBER

In addition to attorneys' fees, your loved one should be aware that it's reasonable for an agent to ask for a monthly stipend to cover the expenses that she may incur while managing the affairs of the person with the memory disorder. The agent may have to give up her job to care for your loved one, or change from full-time to part-time work, so she may suffer a real loss of income as a result of agreeing to be the agent. Even if the agent keeps working full time or already doesn't work at all, she could still incur considerable expenses, such as gas, postage, phone, legal bills, and other professional fees. The amount of this stipend can vary dramatically, depending on the number and value of the assets to be managed, the relationship between the agent and the principal, and prevailing rates in your area. Ask your attorney what amount is customary.

Families tend to prefer durable powers of attorney because they transfer broad authority to manage their loved one's assets without the hassle and expense of constant court interference required by guardianship. However, if your loved one's diagnosis of dementia or AD is made well after she has become incompetent, you'll be required to seek a conservatorship or guardianship in order to make legal decisions for her. We discuss other valid reasons why some people choose to seek a guardianship instead of a durable POA in the next section. So read on if you aren't sure which route to take.

Looking At Guardianships or Conservatorships

Depending on where you're located, the next level of legal oversight and decision-making authority may be called either a *guardianship* or a *conservatorship.* Simply put, a *guardian* or *conservator* is charged with guarding the assets and interests of his ward and making decisions based solely upon that person's best interests. The court oversees and supervises all decisions that the guardian makes.

REMEMBER

For the purposes of a guardianship, a *ward* is defined as a person who, by reason of incapacity, is under the protection of a court either directly or through a guardian appointed by the court.

When a dementia or AD patient has already passed the point of being able to make competent decisions in his own best interest, guardianships can be used to give a family member the ability to manage the affairs of the patient. Guardianships are also a good idea if there are disagreements between the patient and family members or among various family members about how the situation should be handled and who should get the POA. In the case of family squabbles, a guardianship with court oversight is a good way to guarantee that the best interests of the person with the memory disorder are maintained.

If your loved one set up the guardianship while he was still considered to be competent, then your loved one was able to set out the exact terms and conditions he wanted, including selecting his own guardian. If the guardianship was set up by the court after your loved one was already considered incapacitated, the court appoints the guardian, and a family may not have as much say-so in that appointment as they'd like. There may be disagreement among family members who are vying for the appointment, and if the judge so chooses, he may appoint a guardian that is not even a member of the family. (Yet another argument for settling legal matters long before your loved one loses his legal status as a competent person.)

Understanding a guardian's duties

When a guardian's appointed, the first thing that she must do is deposit a court-determined amount of money called a *bond* to ensure that she will honestly manage the protected person's assets. Sometimes, however, the court won't require this bond, especially if the assets of the estate are limited.

A guardian must provide for the basic needs of

>> Food

>> Shelter

>> Medical care

In addition, the guardian must manage the ward's assets in a skillful and prudent manner and pay the wards' bills in a timely fashion, using the ward's assets whenever possible. Finally, the guardian must prepare an annual report for the court describing all transactions made on behalf of the ward.

Grasping how guardianships are awarded

If your loved one has set up a guardianship in advance, its provisions will kick in as soon as the court is satisfied that your loved one has reached a point of incapacitation. If your family hasn't made any legal plans in advance and your loved one is now incapable of caring for himself, you may now determine that a guardianship is right for your family (at this point, a durable POA is no longer an option). In either case, the first thing you must do is petition the court:

>> If the guardianship has been set up in advance, with you as appointed guardian, then you simply have to prove to the court that your loved one is no longer capable of caring for himself. In this case, courts usually accept a written report from the attending doctor as proof, but in some instances, they may require the doctor to appear and testify in person.

>> If your family hasn't planned for a guardianship in advance, you (or whoever's up to the task) must ask the court for the right to be named your loved one's guardian. Before the court appoints you, you must prove that your loved one

is incapacitated by providing valid medical documentation. Sometimes, when the presiding judge isn't happy with the way the family's conducting itself, she may decide to appoint the court itself or a court representative as the guardian. This may also happen when the ward doesn't have any immediate family members available to act as guardian. To ensure the best outcome, hiring an attorney to represent you at these proceedings is imperative.

Choosing a guardianship or not

Sometimes, people who are still competent choose a guardianship over a durable POA. In the following situations, this is a wise move:

>> **The individual has no one to look after her.** If an individual doesn't have anyone to look after her, setting up a guardianship while she's still competent allows her to choose how her assets are managed and also have a say in her medical care, living arrangements, and end-of-life care options. Because the court manages the guardianship, your loved one has a way of making sure her wishes are carried out.

>> **The individual's family members don't get along.** When family members either don't get along or engage in out-and-out warfare, a guardianship outlines what must be done on behalf of a dementia or Alzheimer's patient. Even though the family members may still fight, they must follow the guidelines of the guardianship exactly and have no authority to change them or go against the wishes the principal or the court have set out in the guardianship documents.

REMEMBER

Guardians must operate within very narrow parameters set out by statute in their jurisdictions. If they mismanage an estate or commit acts not in the best interest of the protected person or engage in outright fraud, they may face severe civil and criminal penalties, including fines or even a jail sentence.

Court supervision of all transactions under guardianships makes it almost impossible for a guardian to pull any kind of stunts with the principal's assets. So if your loved one is worried that certain family members may not be trustworthy when handling her assets, she can sidestep the entire issue by setting up a guardianship.

REMEMBER

On the downside, guardianships make it much more difficult for family members to conduct business or make decisions for their loved one because every single thing they do has to be approved by the court prior to doing it. And each time the family's involved with the court, fees must be paid; papers must be signed, notarized, and filed; and a dozen other little details must be dealt with in order to satisfy the dictates of the court. So overall, guardianships are more expensive to set up and manage than durable powers of attorney.

Comparing durable POA versus guardianship

Your loved one's lawyer can review the relative benefits and drawbacks of both types of asset management and help her decide which is best for your loved one. We offer a quick comparison of the two in Table 12-1.

TABLE 12-1 **Durable POA Versus Guardianship**

Type of Instrument	Advantages	Disadvantages
Durable POA or Springing Durable POA	Gives a patient the ability to plan his own future and make sure someone he trusts carries out his wishes. Can be tailored to meet the family's situation; authority may be split between several people. Provides for broad range of authority along with the freedom and flexibility to make decisions for the principal without court oversight. Relatively inexpensive.	Gives broad powers to the appointed agent; lack of monitoring makes it possible for an unscrupulous agent to steal assets. May make patient feel left out or overlooked unless springing form is used.
Guardianship or Conservatorship	Has the built-in safeguard of court supervision of the agent's activities on the person's behalf, which helps to prevent fraud and abuse. Can serve to settle arguments when family members don't get along or disagree on how the principal's assets should be managed.	Much more expensive compared to a durable POA, generally costing several thousand dollars at least. More difficult to make decisions because everything must first be approved by the court. Crowded court dockets in most areas mean that months or even years may pass before a court renders its decision. Cuts patient out of the decision-making process and deprives him of many rights. Principal must be declared incompetent in an open court before guardian can be appointed.

Examining the Ins and Outs of Living Trusts

Living trusts take effect as soon as they're executed and can be an excellent tool to manage assets during the grantor's life. Trusts can take one of two forms:

>> Trusts can be either *revocable,* which means that the person creating the trust can change the terms or cancel it entirely even after it's put in place, as long as he is still competent to do so.

>> Trusts can be *irrevocable,* which means that the trust can't be changed or revoked.

REMEMBER

The person who creates and funds a trust is called the *grantor.* The person who manages the trust is called the *trustee.* In most cases, the grantor and the trustee are the same person. Property and assets are placed in the trust and managed by the trustee for the benefit of the grantor in accordance with the terms of the trust. However, a *successor trustee* is usually designated. This successor trustee assumes his responsibilities upon the death or disability of the trustee. These documents provide an extraordinary amount of flexibility in the management of assets.

Your loved one transfers property ownership to the trust, and then after he dies, the trust transfers the property to the people he selected, effectively avoiding probate. *Probate* is the process a court goes through to establish the validity of a will and to distribute an individual's assets. Probate can take anywhere from 12 to 18 months or longer, playing havoc with a family's finances. Because living trusts don't require court validation, they save a huge amount of time and trouble for families.

The following sections examine the pros of a living trust and how your loved one can transfer property into a living trust.

The advantages of a living trust

Living trusts bypass the probate courts, so they save more of your loved one's assets for distribution to her heirs because they won't have to pay court costs, attorneys' fees, and executor's commissions. They also help to reduce estate taxes. In addition, living trusts can help shield a family's privacy because your family's business isn't being aired out in open court.

Transferring property into a living trust

How your loved one transfers property into a living trust depends on the kind of property and whether or not she has an ownership document, such as a deed, for the property. For things that have deeds, like cars, boats, land, and houses, your loved one must actually transfer ownership of the property to her trust by re-registering the property in the name of the trust so the trust then hold the deed. This action effectively makes the trust the legal owner of the property. If your loved one doesn't take this step while she is alive, the person she appoints as her trustee won't be able to transfer this sort of property after she dies.

REMEMBER

Even though your loved one transfers ownership of her property and possessions to her trust, she still retains full control and use of the property during her life-time as long as she is mentally capable of doing so.

REMEMBER

Property that doesn't have an ownership document, such as household furnish-ings and personal possessions, can be transferred easily to your loved one's trust by simply listing them on what's known as the *trust schedule*, which is just an inventory of the property that's owned by the trust.

Making Decisions about Resuscitation (DNR)

Advance directives can stipulate which medical treatments your loved one wants withheld and when, including resuscitation. Your loved one's physician can sign *do not resuscitate (DNR)* orders to dictate your loved one's wishes regarding resuscitation in the event he has a cardiac or respiratory arrest.

Your loved one needs to have considered this very important scenario ahead of time, because if an ambulance is called, without a DNR form to hand to the para-medics, they will be duty bound to begin resuscitation and transport him to a hospital. If your loved one doesn't want an ambulance crew jumping up and down on his chest and inserting needles into his veins, while zapping him with 360 joules of electricity to try to jump-start his ticker when he is on his death bed, then make sure a DNR is completed and available.

Checking out the forms

Depending on where you live in the United States, you'll have to fill in a DNR form specific to your state. This form features the following information:

>> Your loved one's name, address, date of birth

>> The name, address, and contact number of his physician

>> The level of care he desires in the event of a cardiac or respiratory arrest (including the decision for no intervention and what interventions are acceptable)

>> Signature line for the physician and your loved one (if able) or his representative (POA)

Different states have different forms with different choices. Some states have tiers of resuscitation to be selected. Copies of your state forms can be found online or requested from your loved one's physician.

REMEMBER

"Do not resuscitate" doesn't mean "do not treat." If doctors or paramedics are given this form, they do all they can to ensure that your symptoms are managed as well as possible and that you're made comfortable. They won't take you to a hospital and they won't start CPR if your heart stops or you stop breathing, but they will take very good care of you and do everything else necessary.

DO NOT RESUSCITATE

In 2011 an 81-year-old woman from Norfolk, Virginia, took the unusual step of getting a tattoo, the first she'd ever had, so ambulance crews and doctors would be in absolutely no doubt about her resuscitation wishes should her heart or breathing stop.

Inked across her chest she had "DO NOT RESUSCITATE," and, hedging her bets in case she was discovered lying face down, "PTO" (please turn over) was tattooed across her back. Despite having an advance directive in place for 30 years, she told the national press at the time that the tattoo was to ensure that there was "no excuse for not knowing what I think."

As experts in medical ethics pointed out to the media, despite her novel way of getting her message across, it would hold no weight legally, and without her advance directive, paramedics would be duty bound to start CPR.

Telling the necessary people

If your loved one's physician competed this form for him, then it will be in that doctor's records. However, if an emergency department or hospital physician completed this form, we suggest that you make sure a copy gets to his primary care physician for inclusion in his record. All your loved one's friends and family should also be aware of the existence of this form and his wishes. In a panic situation, and without an understanding of what he wants, dialing 911 will be second nature, and with no form to hand the paramedics, he'll be treated or taken to an emergency department even if that wasn't his choice.

Taking a Peek at Another Mechanism

Many states have worked to improve the mechanism for patients to document and share their advance directives and provide healthcare treatment instructions for when they're seriously ill and nearing death. This initiative is called POLST, also referred to as MOLST, which stands for *Physician Orders for Life Sustaining Treatment* or *Medical Orders for Life Sustaining Treatment.* Sometimes these documents are referred to as *Physician Orders for Scope of Treatment (POST), Medical Orders for Scope of Treatment (MOST),* or *Transportable Physician Orders for Patient Preferences (TPOPP).*

A national organization and its website, www.polst.org, gives more information. On this site you can see if your state has a means for using the POLST or similar form. If you have completed one of these documents, any healthcare provider and at any location including emergency personnel should recognize them.

The POLST (and these other forms) not only lists one's resuscitation status, but also identifies one's wishes regarding end-of-life care in general. Included is language regarding choices about comfort measures, including the desire whether to be hospitalized or whether to receive antibiotics in the case of an acute infection. A pragmatic rule for completing a POLST is when the doctor wouldn't be surprised if the patient were to die in the next year. The form should only be completed for seriously ill or frail patients. POLST is a standardized short (often one page) summary of physician orders. It documents a discussion between the physician and the patient and/or the surrogate decision maker (healthcare POA) and must be signed by the doctor and in some states by the patient or POA.

WARNING

These forms don't take the place of a living will or healthcare POA document. They are actual physician orders that complement these other advance directives but don't replace them.

Drawing Up a Will

Generally speaking, anyone who's an adult over the age of 18 and sound of mind and body is legally able to make a will. A person who makes a will is called a *testator*.

As with all other legal issues, making a will is much easier to do while your loved one is still considered competent and capable of making informed decisions. If you wait until after she's incapacitated, the courts will oversee the writing of the will and the distribution of the estate, and it'll be a lot harder on your family and cost a lot more money than if you take care of it while she is still able to decide on a will and sign for herself.

WARNING

Never throw an original will haphazardly into a drawer or file box or bury it in a stack of unrelated papers. A will is a valuable legal document that helps an executor or the courts settle your loved one's estate according to her wishes. The original copy of the will should be stored in a fireproof box, and notarized copies should be kept with the attorney who drew up the will. By taking these precautions, in the unlikely event of a fire, flood, or natural disaster, your loved one's wishes can still be carried out. Please note that a safety deposit box in a bank is not a good place to store a will. In many states it may be necessary to open the estate before anyone can gain access to the safe deposit box of the person who has died.

Understanding the benefits of a will

Wills allow people to control how they want their assets to be distributed after death. They help people transfer their assets to their surviving spouse, children, friends, or charitable organizations in a way that eases the tax burden and also satisfies the desires of the person making the will as to how those assets will be divided among the heirs. A will also serves as a road map for the court that lets the court clearly understand the wishes of the person who's died.

A will does many things besides the obvious. Along with allocating your loved one's estate in the way he wants, a will can also do the following:

» Leave more assets for heirs by minimizing estate taxes and other expenses that would be incurred in a court-managed distribution of your loved one's estate

» Provide for the most economical distribution of assets

» Ensure that assets are distributed to heirs without undue delay

REMEMBER

The property a person leaves behind after he dies is called his *estate.* An estate includes all property and cash assets owned at the time of death, including bank accounts, the family home, other real estate and buildings, land, furniture, cars, jewelry, royalty income, stocks and bonds, and proceeds from investments, along with proceeds from life insurance policies and pension plan policies that are payable to the estate.

Deciding if you need an attorney to make a will

Like any other legal documents, wills can be simple and straightforward, or they can be complex and hard to understand. If your loved one has a small estate and just one or two heirs, you and your loved one can certainly write out the will yourselves, have it witnessed and notarized, and file it with the court. Doing so is fast, and it's economical. Many websites provide forms for simple wills valid in your state at little or no expense.

If your loved one has a larger or complex estate and a number of heirs, trying to write the will yourself can be a mistake that costs your family thousands of dollars in unnecessary taxes, not to mention court and attorneys' fees. Lawyers can often make money-saving suggestions that more than cover the cost of their fees.

When making a will, your loved one needs to take several things into consideration. For instance:

>> Does she own the bulk of the property with her spouse?

>> Does your state have forced heir laws that require a certain percentage of her assets go to her children?

>> Does she want to leave a bequest to a favorite charitable organization or research institute, or make sure that her son with the 12 nose rings and orange hair gets nothing until he reaches a certain age?

Attorneys experienced in probate, estate planning, and the laws of your state can help your loved one make her way through the conflicting information and also help her make good decisions about how to distribute her estate.

Dying without a will

If you or your loved one dies without a will (referred to as dying *intestate*), your family may be thrown into a maelstrom of trouble. Heirs may fight over the distribution of the assets; the spouse can be left destitute. All sorts of undesirable things can happen. And worst of all, the state will step in and tell your family how they have to distribute the assets, and they'll take a bigger chunk of your loved one's property as taxes than they would've if an attorney experienced in estate planning and probate had been hired to draw up a will.

More than half of Americans don't have a will. The legislature of your state has already determined how to distribute the assets of people who die intestate and you may not like some of their ideas very much. For example, if your wife dies without a will in Louisiana, all her estate automatically goes to your surviving children, leaving you, the spouse, high and dry. So if your wife wants to be the one who decides how her estate is divided and who gets what, she needs to make her will while she is still mentally capable to do so.

Making a will for an incompetent person

In order to write a legal will for a person who's been declared incompetent, you must be appointed as his guardian. Along with the other powers granted by the court, you have the power to write a will for your loved one and determine, with the court's guidance, how his assets should be distributed following death.

Writing a will can get tricky because guardians aren't supposed to do anything in furtherance of their own self-interests, but if you're appointed guardian for one of your parents, it's reasonable to expect to inherit a portion of the assets remaining after their medical and burial expenses have been paid. You should consult an attorney to familiarize yourself with the statutes that govern the making of a will for an incapacitated person because they vary widely from state to state.

If family members disagree as to how assets should be distributed or who should be named as your loved one's guardian, consider visiting a mediator to work through your disagreement and reach an equitable compromise. Your family is going through a difficult time and everyone is going to have his own opinions about how things should be handled. Try not to let this be the cause of a permanent rift.

Despite what you see in the movies, recorded wills aren't acceptable because all wills must be in a written form and signed in order to be valid and legally binding.

Chapter 13

Working through Financial Issues on Behalf of Your Loved One

Taking care of a loved one who has dementia or Alzheimer's disease (AD) for an extended period of time can leave a family financially devastated. You must figure out not only how to pay for your loved one's normal expenses, such as food, clothing, and shelter, but also how to cover all of his medical expenses — without bankrupting either your loved one or your family. It can be a daunting task to say the least.

A long bout with severe memory loss can wreck even the most careful financial planning. Money put aside to pay for a carefree retirement must be diverted to pay for long-term care. Families without health insurance face even more dire circumstances, sometimes falling into poverty in order to maintain a good standard of care for their loved one.

If your loved one is still gainfully employed, you must help him determine when to stop working and how to deal with the loss of his job and his income. If he is retirement age, pension money and Social Security payments may provide needed money for care. When it becomes apparent that he can no longer manage his own finances, you have to decide who in the family can step in and take over or find a trustworthy professional to handle financial issues. You have to evaluate your loved one's health insurance coverage and formulate a plan to cover gaps in coverage.

In this chapter, we guide you through the complexities of the many financial issues that families and patients may face. We offer some savvy tips for making the most of what resources you do have and point you in the direction of community resources and local organizations that can help you cope with your situation.

Reviewing Financial Needs and Resources

Yes, the cost of dementia or AD is an 800-pound gorilla, and you have to wrestle with it whether you want to or not. But don't be afraid to face the financial situation head-on. Having accurate financial information can empower you to make better choices.

TIP

You should have only one unknown variable in your financial equation: how long you'll have to provide care for your loved one. That's the one thing you can't be sure about. However, a good bet is to plan for rising costs as your loved one's disease progresses and additional care is required.

Before you worry yourself into a tizzy, take some time to sit down and review your loved one's current and projected financial needs, and also take a look at his resources. Doing so gives you a reasonable idea about whether your loved one's available resources are sufficient to cover his needs. If not, then you at least have an idea of how much the projected shortfall may be. After you have this information in hand, you can use it to chart a financial course and figure out if you need to develop additional resources to cover the cost of care.

Comparing resources to needs

Make two columns on a sheet of paper and label one "Resources" and the other "Needs." Under "Resources" list the following:

» Your loved one's cash on hand and in savings, checking, and money market accounts

» Any recurring monies due from:

- Salaries
- Social security
- Rents
- Trusts
- Pensions
- Royalties
- Stock dividends
- Outstanding loans
- Any other source of steady, recurring income

» Any payments due your loved one from:

- Insurance settlements
- Retirement packages
- Any other type of investment including individual retirement accounts (IRA)

» Real property assets, such as the family home, car, land, jewelry, artwork, collections, and so on

Under "Needs" list current monthly bills and a projected amount that will be required to maintain your loved one as memory loss progresses. Depending on whether you provide care in the home as a family member, hire an outside caregiver, or place your loved one in a residential care facility, your medical costs can range anywhere from about $1,000 a month to more than $6,000 a month. Most families find that costs increase as needs increase and require more hands-on care.

Projecting future costs

Although not every patient ends up in a nursing home or other residential setting, those patients who do usually stay an average of two-and-a-half years. Sometimes, families admit patients to a hospice for their last few months of care, particularly if the patient has other serious health problems, such as diabetes, cancer, or heart disease.

In order to qualify for hospice, the patient must meet specific disease criteria and be certified by a physician to have only six months or less to live. Clearly, doctors aren't all-knowing and can't predict exactly when a patient will die; however, with experience, doctors can make reasonable estimates of life expectancy for hospice purposes. Many assisted living facilities and nursing homes can provide hospice services without the patient having to move to a formal hospice center. Hospice programs work with the staff of these facilities to provide end-of-life care. Medicare pays for the majority of hospice costs; call 800-633-4227 for complete information or download a free hospice care booklet at www.medicare. gov/Pubs/pdf/02154.pdf.

Nursing home and hospice costs vary widely from region to region, so call local care facilities and get an average cost for residential care in your area. Then determine the average number of doctor visits per year, the cost of prescriptions, and so on, and add to your estimated costs for providing care, and you have a reasonable estimate of how much you'll have to pay each month to care for your loved one.

Compare available resources with needs to see whether sufficient resources are available to care for your loved one. Knowing what is available helps you determine how to manage your situation and whether you need to liquidate some of your loved one's investments to generate additional cash. Be sure to have a contingency plan in place if your planning indicates that your loved one's needs outstrip his ability to pay for his care.

You may find that your loved one has enough resources to cover his care, but those resources are in the wrong form. For example, your loved one may have stocks or bonds that must be liquidated to provide cash to pay bills. Or he may have some property that he was holding as an investment in the hope that it would appreciate. Even if you don't net as much as you may want, selling the property and investing the money in a liquid fund may be a good idea so it will be available to pay bills as needed.

TIP

Before you make any financial decisions that you may regret later, consult an expert for advice. Many banks offer financial counseling services to their customers; you may also seek financial advice from an accountant, attorney, broker, or an independent financial adviser such as a Certified Financial Planner (CFP).

What if the worst happens, and you find out that your loved one doesn't have a penny saved and can't contribute to his own care at all? Although this news may not be exactly what you wanted to hear, finding it out now so you can figure out what to do about it is far better than finding out when it's too late to do anything. We give you some tips for dealing with this situation later in this chapter.

Managing paperwork

When you do take over your loved one's finances, you must establish a well-organized filing system right from the get-go, not only for tax purposes but also for legal and insurance reasons.

TIP

Consider using a cardboard box or buying a small, inexpensive filing cabinet so you can store your loved one's paperwork separately from your own. If you don't keep up with the paperwork, you may have to pay dearly.

Although filing may just seem like extra work in an already overburdened schedule, it'll save you lots of time and energy in the long run when you realize that you can always put your hands on whatever papers you need simply by opening a drawer or lifting the lid from a box.

Reviewing your own financial needs and resources

In the midst of taking care of all your loved one's business, don't let yourself lose sight of your own finances. You absolutely must review your own needs and resources, just as you did for your loved one (see "Comparing resources to needs" earlier in this chapter), and come up with a financial plan for yourself. This is especially important — particularly if you're planning to be at least partially responsible for your loved one's expenses. If handling both sets of financial records is too big a job for you, ask your spouse or an adult child to help. Or consider hiring a financial professional to do it for you.

Letting your own bills slide is all too easy when you're caring for a loved one with AD or dementia, but you don't want to wreck your own credit while protecting your loved one's interests. Try to achieve a balance by setting aside an hour or so each week to review your own finances and pay any bills that are due. Then set aside a separate hour to deal with your loved one's finances. After you get organized, you'll probably find that you can manage more easily and quickly.

Taking Over the Financial Reins

As the fog of dementia or Alzheimer's begins to cloud your loved one's mind, her ability to handle even the simplest financial transactions becomes impaired. Early on, she may have problems calculating tips, writing checks, or using a credit card. She may lose money, forget to pay bills, or pay the same bill twice. She may hide money and then accuse someone else of stealing it when she forgets where she hid it. When these things happen, it becomes clear that she's no longer capable of handling her money independently.

You don't want health insurance or long-term care insurance policies to be canceled for nonpayment of premiums, which is important especially because your loved one can't get long-term insurance back after being diagnosed with AD or another form of dementia. Likewise, not having health insurance in effect during an emergency illness can cause bankruptcy due to huge medical bills.

TIP

Begin discussing financial issues when your loved one is first diagnosed with AD or dementia. Perhaps another family member can serve as a financial manager to take this pressure off the primary caregiver. Transfer of the day-to-day management of money to this financial manager can be done in steps if need be. For example, the patient with early dementia can sit with the financial manager and open bill envelopes. The financial manager then writes the check to pay the bill, and the patient signs the check. This enables the patient to feel involved until she is no longer able to understand sufficiently to properly participate.

Ideally, you have already arranged for durable power of attorney (POA). Then soon after your loved one's diagnosis (unless she arranged it previously), all you have to do when you reach this point is have the family doctor declare your loved one incapable of handling her own affairs, and the POA put in place then springs into effect. This gives you the authority to manage your loved one's finances with very little hassle. We discuss obtaining a power of attorney, as well as other legal issues, in Chapter 12.

WARNING

If you wait until a crisis occurs to figure out how to manage your loved one's finances, it may be too late. After your loved one is incapacitated, your options are much more limited and much more costly than if you'd planned ahead and put a POA in place while your loved one was still mentally competent. Planning ahead gives you the chance to protect your loved one's assets from fraud or mismanagement by others and also minimizes the bite that court costs, attorneys' fees, and taxes will take if you have to apply for guardianship.

If you didn't put a POA in place, you may have a fight on your hands. A frequent characteristic of memory disorders is episodes of suspicion, in which the patient believes that family members or others are stealing from her. This atmosphere isn't exactly conducive to finding a way to transfer control of your loved one's finances into your hands. That scenario plays right into a patient's suspicions that everyone is out to rob her blind.

Remember that as the disease progresses and ultimately your loved one is no longer mentally able to declare her wishes, you may have problems obtaining a POA because your loved one may not grant it. The person granting the POA must be of sound mind when granting it. If your loved one's condition is advanced, you'll have to seek guardianship through the courts in order to gain authority to manage your loved one's finances. And with today's crowded court dockets, getting guardianship can be a lengthy and expensive process.

If you need to apply for guardianship, in the meantime, do what you can to make sure that bills are paid on time and that there is sufficient money to buy groceries, gas, and other everyday necessities.

PROTECTING YOUR LOVED ONE FROM FRAUD

Congress estimates that telemarketing fraud involving sweepstakes and prizes costs Americans about $40 billion a year. According to AARP, more than half those victims are 50 years of age or older. The sad but true fact is that millions of elderly Americans become victims of fraud every year. This is particularly true for people who have a memory disorder. Older people are vulnerable to scams for lots of reasons, including the simple fact that they were raised in a time when it was considered rude to hang up on a caller, even a dishonest one. Con artists know this and use it to help their schemes succeed.

Create a plan for a checks-and-balances system to monitor your loved one's finances for signs of fraudulent activity that might indicate that she has fallen prey to a dishonest scheme. If you do suspect fraud, try to gather as much evidence as you can and contact the appropriate authorities. Then change your loved one's phone number immediately to get her out of the clutches of the con artists because they don't stop until they've wrung every possible penny out of their victims. Some con artists have even convinced some of their older victims to sell their homes and send them all the proceeds.

You should also report the problem to the fraud divisions of your loved one's bank and credit card companies. Ask them for guidance in canceling existing accounts; they can flag the accounts to monitor them for fraudulent activity. In the meantime, you're protecting your loved one. You may have to spend some time and effort recovering lost assets and seeking reimbursement. Attach doctors' statements of the dementia diagnosis (such as a note written on a prescription pad) to the letters you write when attempting to have charges waived.

In 1995, the National Consumer's League launched a project to help determine those factors that make older people more vulnerable to fraud. The organization created a document called "They Can't Hang Up" that includes tips to help seniors recognize and avoid fraudulent schemes. Check out www.fraud.org/learn/older-adult-fraud/they-can-t-hang-up.

If you don't get control of your loved one's finances before she becomes incapable of managing her money on her own, she'll be an easy target as a potential victim for scammers and con artists. And even if the person with AD or dementia doesn't fall victim to a fraud, multiple subscriptions to the same magazine and series of books can still be damaging and costly.

Understanding Changes in Tax Status

Along with all the other changes dementia and Alzheimer's disease brings to your life, it also changes your loved one's tax status and gives you another chore that you must manage — handling their taxes as well as your own — all while trying to figure out which deductions you can take to compensate for the cost of your loved one's care.

If you're going to take even one deduction, take as many as you qualify for because only the person who's filing a return that itemizes deductions can claim many of the following benefits. Generally speaking, a caregiver can only deduct his loved one's medical expenses if the caregiver pays for them and they total more than 7.5 percent of adjusted gross income. If you're filing as a head of household and are claiming your loved one as a dependent, the amount to be deducted can include the total medical expenses for you and all the members of your immediate family as well as all the medical expenses you paid for the patient. This helps you reach the 7.5 percent figure.

Where you deduct the expenses depends on your situation. If your loved one is living with you and you're claiming him as a dependent, you'd make the deduction on your 1040. If your loved one is still living independently, you may deduct qualified medical expenses on your loved one's tax return. They include necessary improvements to your home or your loved one's home, in order to better provide care, including ramps, stair chair lifts, or shower grab bars that qualify as medical expense.

REMEMBER

If you're claiming your loved one as a dependent, because she has dementia and is dependent on you for care, she must be certified as meeting the requirements of a chronically ill person. A licensed healthcare professional should do this certification "within the preceding 12-month period," which implies an annual certification (Internal Revenue Code 7702B).

Deciding Whether You Need a Financial Adviser

If you have a trusted financial adviser who can help you and your loved one look at resources and formulate a plan to pay for ongoing expenses, you're ahead of the game. But you don't have to have a financial adviser to survive, particularly if you're fairly knowledgeable about how money works and feel confident making financial decisions. But like legal issues, financial management can be complex. Unless you have a thorough understanding of money and long-term financial planning, for your own peace of mind, you should consult an accountant, attorney, financial adviser, or other expert.

People with early-onset AD or dementia especially require thoughtful financial planning because their young age means that they don't qualify for some programs and benefits available to older adults. Also, 20 to 30 percent of people with dementia and AD live alone. Family members or trusted friends should accompany them to the financial counseling appointments to help them understand and implement the advice they are given.

REMEMBER

Before you can formally start managing your loved one's finances, you must first have written legal authorization to do so, either in the form of power of attorney or guardianship. See Chapter 12 for complete information.

TIP

Financial adviser fees vary widely, so be sure to get a quote in writing. Check out the person's credentials and find out whether he has any complaints on file with the Better Business Bureau (BBB), the Certified Financial Planner Board (CFP), National Association of Securities Dealers (NASD), or the Securities and Exchange Commission (SEC). A good financial adviser can save you the cost of his fees many times over, but a bad one can cost you money, or worse yet, engage in dishonest, commission-producing practices that eventually drain your entire account.

Knowing what to look out for in an adviser

Just because someone is the parent of one of your children doesn't mean you should automatically make him your financial adviser. You should take several steps to ensure that the person you select to help you with your finances is honest and knowledgeable, and he doesn't have any potential conflicts of interest.

What kind of conflicts of interest? For example, if the financial adviser is encouraging purchase of a particular security over another, more highly rated security, you may discover that he receives a commission on sales of the less desirable product. When advisers recommend products that they also earn commissions on, that represents a potential conflict of interest. However, just because the potential for a conflict exists doesn't automatically mean that the adviser is up to no good. As long as he fully explains his relationship to the recommended product and that he earns commissions from its sale, he's satisfied the requirements of full disclosure and provided everything needed to make an informed investment decision. Remember, it's your loved one's money. The adviser is just that — an adviser. Final decisions rest with you if you are your loved one's POA or guardian. You need to make sure that all decisions regarding these resources are made for the best benefit of your loved one.

WARNING

If you give the adviser too much autonomy in handling your loved one's money, he may be tempted to churn the account to make extra money. Always maintain a hands-on involvement in your loved one's finances to provide an extra measure of security and oversight.

REMEMBER

Churning has a very different meaning in the world of finance than it does in the world of dairies and cows. In financial circles, it means that your adviser is turning your money over again and again, investing first in one stock or bond and then in another to earn more commissions. Before this type of fraud came to light, many people had their entire investment accounts drained by unscrupulous investors who churned their way right down to the bottom of their clients' capital, producing not butter, but gravy for themselves.

Recognizing the types of financial advisers

Many different types of financial advisers are available, and they all must be licensed, which means that you can check their backgrounds and performance histories. Although honesty is certainly an important characteristic to look for, you also want someone who's compassionate and caring, who understands your loved one's needs, and who can assess her resources and advise you on the best way to make those resources stretch to cover the cost of her care.

In recent years, *Certified Financial Planners* (CFPs) have emerged as leaders in the field of financial advice because they have a broad range of knowledge and experience and can help people put together comprehensive financial plans tailored to their individual requirements and tastes. However, several other types of financial advisers may meet your needs just as well. Check out your options in the following list:

>> **Certified Financial Planner (CFP):** CFPs have studied and passed a rigorous examination administered by the Certified Financial Planner Board of Standards. CFPs commit to uphold high ethical standards and voluntarily submit to the regulatory authority of the CFP Board. CFPs must stay current in their skills by passing a new certification test every other year.

>> **Certified Public Accountant (CPA):** CPAs have completed extensive education and supervised work experience before taking a national examination to receive certification. Although the majority of accountants are concerned with tax returns, financial statements, and audits, in recent years, many CPAs have expanded into the area of financial planning.

>> **Attorney:** Attorneys who specialize in estate planning may sometimes diversify into financial planning as well, particularly when their practice concentrates on elder law and the preparation of documents, such as wills and trusts, that enable families to take over the management of their loved one's assets.

>> **Stockbrokers:** Stockbrokers are licensed, certified, and regulated by the National Association of Securities Dealers (NASD). Stockbrokers recommend securities, such as stocks and bonds, for investment purposes and earn commissions on those transactions that their clients execute.

>> **Investment advisers:** Investment advisers provide advice regarding the purchase of securities in exchange for a fee. Depending on the breadth of their practice, any professionals who perform this service must either register with the Securities and Exchange Commission (SEC) or the local state securities agency.

>> **Money or asset managers or portfolio managers:** Money managers manage their clients' investment portfolios. Depending on training and experience, money managers may either design the investment portfolio themselves or use a design provided by a CFP or some other sort of financial adviser. The manager's fees are usually a percentage of the value of the portfolio.

When looking for an adviser, ask your friends for the names of financial advisers they've worked with and trust and then check up on those advisers and interview them before you make a selection. The local chapter of your Alzheimer's Association may also have names of financial planners who are familiar with the specific needs of people with memory disorders.

Grasping cost issues

How much a financial adviser costs you depends on how his charges are structured. For starters, you should know how the adviser gets paid, whether by commission or by fee. This seemingly small fact can make a world of difference in how much you're charged and in whether the recommendations you're given are unbiased or based upon the adviser's desire to sell financial and investment products he represents in order to earn additional commissions.

WARNING

Never hire a financial adviser who won't fully disclose, in writing, how he's paid and how much he's going to charge you.

Financial advisers usually base their charges on one of the following five models:

>> **Fee only:** Your adviser charges you a fee for each service he renders. In the case of attorneys or accountants, you usually pay an hourly fee.

>> **Fee based:** Your adviser charges fees plus commissions. The fees are for assessing your financial situation, and the commissions are earned on the sale of investment products he recommends.

>> **Percentage fee:** The fee is based on a percentage, typically 1 to 2 percent, of the value of the assets the adviser's managing for you.

>> **Commission only:** Your adviser's earnings come strictly from commissions on investment products he sells; insurance agents and stockbrokers generally use a commission-only fee structure.

>> **Salary:** Employees of banks and credit unions who provide financial advice generally are paid a salary, but they may receive performance bonuses.

TOP FIVE SIGNS YOUR FINANCIAL ADVISER MAY BE GETTING READY TO MOVE TO ACAPULCO

Okay, so maybe we didn't really mean the Acapulco thing, but there are distinct ways to tell whether a financial adviser has your best interests at heart or is working toward her own financial goals. Think about switching to another adviser if the one you're working with exhibits any of the following behaviors:

- Starts recommending various financial products within minutes of meeting you, long before she knows anything about your loved one's personal financial situation, needs, or problems

- Baffles you with a rapid-fire presentation of dense technical lingo and then tells you not to worry; she'll take care of everything

- Asks you for permission to manage your funds independently and make trades and purchases without first getting your permission for each transaction

- Fails to disclose that she's been disciplined for dishonest practices in the past

- Fails to deliver promised documentation or contracts

Ask what sort of records the adviser keeps and what access you have to those records. Check to find out whether the adviser's records are regularly audited and by whom.

In addition, try to find out if your potential financial adviser has any conflicts of interest, has been prohibited from taking part in the management of a company for reasons of fraud, has had any criminal convictions within the past five years, or has declared bankruptcy. Some of this information may be available with an Internet search.

Quitting Work

By the time most people are diagnosed with dementia or AD, they've already retired from their careers. However, improvements in the diagnostic procedure mean that doctors are diagnosing the disease earlier in the course of the illness. Consequently, more people receiving a diagnosis of a memory disorder are still employed. These people must decide when to quit their jobs and when and how to tell their bosses and coworkers about their diagnosis.

Your loved one's decisions in this regard depend on the type of work he does and how much on-the-job authority he has. Obviously, the lead designer for a revolutionary new fighter jet has a lot more riding on the accuracy of his work than a person who performs a less challenging job or who works in a support position. Even if they don't specifically know that they have dementia or AD, people often understand early that something is wrong because they are having difficulty with tasks required by their jobs.

These sections discuss some important topics that you may have to consider with employment if your loved one has been diagnosed with a memory disorder.

Properly timing the departure

Sometimes, patients deny that anything's wrong, and a boss or compassionate coworker must tell them that their performance is lagging. If your loved one hasn't yet been diagnosed and the coworker is unaware that cognitive impairment is the cause of the problems, this confrontation can be particularly difficult. The drop-off in performance produced by early AD or dementia can baffle fellow workers, particularly if it comes from a valued long-term employee who's always been a reliable producer in the past.

When your loved one can no longer perform his job effectively and/or without undue stress, the time has come for him to quit working. If you wait too long to talk to your loved one about quitting, you may have to deal with him being let go or laid off, which may negatively affect insurance coverage. Assist your loved one in talking to the benefits counselor in the human resources department to determine the best way to quit or retire if eligible.

Your loved one may be able to use accumulated sick time or take a medical leave of absence, which may cover health insurance expenses for a period of time. Or maybe he can use a disability benefit that will pay him a portion of his salary for a period of time, as well as allow him to keep health insurance coverage. Finally, allowing the company to terminate your loved one so he's eligible for COBRA health insurance coverage may work out best. Other companies, particularly smaller ones, may not have such a variety of options available. Assist your loved one to explore the best options with his employer. Because the problem is a memory disorder, don't expect your loved one to be able to address these issues alone and remember what he needs to do or the advice given.

REMEMBER

COBRA stands for the *Consolidated Omnibus Budget Reconciliation Act* of 1985 that requires employers who offer group health plans to give their employees the opportunity to continue their group health coverage for a period of time even if they're terminated, laid off, or experience some other change in employment status. Individual companies handle COBRA insurance in different ways, so be sure to accompany your loved one when he speaks to the HR benefits counselor to determine the best way to handle leaving.

If your loved one is forced to stop working and is too young to retire with a pension or receive Social Security benefits, and his company has no real plan in place to cover a long-term disability like dementia, see if he's eligible to apply for a state-run disability program. He may also get *supplemental security income* (SSI) if his income level is low enough. Patients with early-onset AD can really suffer financially because income, retirement, and insurance benefits may be lost or reduced as the result of early termination of employment — all at a time when the cost of medications and treatment are increasing.

Sharing the diagnosis

Whether or not to tell the boss or any coworkers is a personal decision that your loved one must make. Of course, HR must know the truth about your loved one's condition in order to help him plan his departure, but by law, they can't share any of your loved one's private medical information with anyone else, not even with his boss.

REMEMBER

The most important consideration is to make sure your loved one doesn't try to hang on too long at work. Even though it's great to keep getting that paycheck, staying at work past the point where your loved one can do the job properly creates more problems than it solves.

Evaluating Insurance Coverage

Insurance coverage regulations can be complex and confusing. Trying to figure out what's covered by a particular policy and what isn't and who covers what practically requires a PhD in handling paperwork and reading hundreds of lines of tiny type. But if you're tempted to throw in the towel, don't: Buried somewhere in that type that you can barely see may be a sentence that has profound implications for your loved one's financial situation.

Insurance companies can either be one of your biggest allies in the fight to provide good care for your loved one, or they can be the biggest thorn in your side. In these sections, we review some of the most common forms of insurance coverage and tell you how to deal with your insurance providers effectively and, if necessary, fight them to get the coverage you've paid for.

Medicare

Medicare is a federally sponsored healthcare insurance intended to help provide medical services for people aged 65 and over. It's also available to some disabled people and some people with end-stage kidney disease.

Medicare is divided into three parts: Part A, Part B, and Part D. *Medigap* insurance is also available through private insurance companies, which is so named because it helps to fill in the gaps in current Medicare coverage.

Part A coverage

Part A is available for all people ages 65 or older or anyone who's receiving Social Security benefits. If you receive these benefits, you automatically receive a Medicare card. Part A covers inpatient hospital stays, hospice care, some skilled nursing facility care, and some skilled level home healthcare services. (Long-term nursing home care, assisted living, and memory units aren't considered skilled nursing units.) This part, funded by a 1.45 percent payroll tax collected from both employees and employers, is provided free of charge. It covered an estimated 52 million recipients in 2013 (43.1 million seniors and 8.8 million permanently disabled adults). Part A Medicare beneficiaries pay part of the cost of the medical services they receive through co-insurance payments and deductibles.

Part B coverage

Part B Medicare is optional coverage. Americans have seven months to sign up for this coverage, beginning three months before their 65th birthday and ending four months after their birthday. To enroll, simply call the Social Security Administration's toll-free number: 800-772-1213. If your loved one doesn't enroll during this initial period, the cost of the coverage goes up 10 percent for each 12-month period he waits.

The Part B monthly premium is taken out of his Social Security check each month before it's mailed. It covers doctors' fees, diagnostic tests, outpatient hospital care, and some other outpatient services, such as physical and occupational therapy. Low-income seniors may be able to get their states to pay part of their monthly Part B premium and may also be eligible for assistance with medications through Medicaid.

Part D coverage

Medicare Part D provides coverage for prescription drugs after a deductible is paid ($360 in 2016). The premiums for Medicare Part D are paid monthly in addition to Part B premiums and both can be deducted from a Social Security check.

Like Part B, the patient needs to sign up for Part D coverage when he is first eligible for coverage or he'll have to pay a late enrollment penalty.

Another way to get prescription drug coverage through Medicare is to be in a Medicare Advantage Plan (Part C) such as an HMO or PPO that offers prescription drug coverage. Starting in 2016, the healthcare providers (doctors, nurse practitioners, or physician assistants) prescribing medications will have to be enrolled in Medicare in order for the prescriptions to be covered by the Medicare drug plan.

The rules, paperwork, and hassle

Although Medicare was a good idea on paper, in reality, it's grown into a dense tangle of sometimes conflicting rules and regulations — as many as 132,000 pages of them at last count — that doctors and hospitals must adhere to in order to get reimbursed by the government for the services they render to patients. Many doctors and hospitals complain because they aren't reimbursed in a timely fashion or never get reimbursed at all for the services they provide because Medicare denies the claims. They then have to try to collect the entire balance owed from their patients who are often seriously ill and unable to satisfy their 20 percent co-pay, much less the entire bill.

As a result of this bureaucratic nightmare, more doctors today are refusing to accept Medicare patients, making it increasingly difficult for senior citizens to find good healthcare at an affordable price. To make matters worse, Congress keeps adding new Medicare regulations, price controls, and coverage limits, clouding an already murky picture.

So how do you thread your way through the Medicare maze? The specific dollar amounts that Medicare covers are at the mercy of congressional budgets. For the most current information, go to www.medicare.gov. The website is user-friendly and provides the detailed information you need to know.

Click on "Sign Up/Change Plans" to find out more about how and when to apply online for Part A, Part B, and more. The website can explain your costs for coverage, what Medicare covers, as well as the claim and appeal process.

If you need more assistance, contact the State Health Insurance Assistance Program for one-on-one counseling and assistance with Medicare problems. The people there can help you select the right coverage for your situation, solve billing and claim problems, and provide referrals for seniors to receive assistance from a variety of community organizations. To find the nearest local chapter, call 800-MEDICARE and ask for health insurance counseling or visit www.medicare.gov/contacts.

Medicaid

Medicaid is an insurance program that's jointly sponsored by the federal government and individual states that provides medical services for low-income individuals. Although the federal government funds the program, states administer it, and each state establishes its own eligibility standards and determines the type, amount, duration, and scope of services. They also set the rate of payment for services.

Most Medicaid services are delivered to families with children, but they're also available to certain older people who meet their state's guidelines for assistance. To qualify, a person must

>> Be 65 years of age or older, or blind, or disabled

>> Be a U.S. citizen with a Social Security number and be a legal resident of the state where the application is made

>> Have total gross assets, income, and personal property that meet certain poverty standards. To look up federal poverty level guidelines for your state, visit www.elderweb.com and click on the "Regions" tab

>> Fill out and sign an application and undergo an interview with a Medicaid specialist

REMEMBER

Because Medicaid eligibility may change from month to month because of changes in income or resources, Medicaid cards originally were supposed to be valid for one month only and had to be renewed every month. However, as a practical matter, eligibility is re-determined on an annual basis. If you have questions, call your state's Medicaid office or seek out an attorney that specializes in Medicaid qualifications.

Medigap

Medigap, also known as *Medicare plus Choice,* is private insurance intended to help people cover the cost of the gaps in Medicare coverage. Medigap covers co-insurance payments and deductibles and, in some cases, covers medical supplies and prescription drugs. Consult your insurance agent to see what coverage is available in your location.

Be aware that if you purchase a Medigap plan, it must cover at least the same benefits offered under Part A and Part B Medicare. Depending on the type of coverage you select, you may have additional benefits.

If you're having trouble locating a Medigap plan provider, head to www.medicare. gov/find-a-plan/questions/medigap-home.aspx, which can help you locate suitable insurance carriers in your state.

Private insurance

Private insurance can include health insurance as well as long- or short-term disability coverage. If your loved one is still employed or recently retired, accompany him to talk to his employer's HR benefits counselor to see what sort of coverage he already has or can obtain.

Get copies of your loved one's health insurance and disability policies and read them through from the first page to the last, paying particular attention to information about coverage of chronic illness and long-term disability.

Disability insurance is different from health insurance in that it provides a cash payment to help people cover their basic living expenses in the event that they become ill and are unable to work for an extended period of time. Short-term and long-term disability policies with different terms and benefits are available. Extended or long-term care insurance policies are also different from health insurance and are used to help pay for home care, adult daycare, assisted living, or chronic nursing home care for your loved one as his memory loss progresses and care requirements increase.

Long-term care insurance

Long-term care insurance is meant to help families cover costs of caring for a loved one who has a degenerative condition or a chronic illness like AD or dementia. According to AARP, about 70 percent of seniors older than 65 will ultimately require long-term care, either in the home or in a care facility.

Long-term care policies usually cost several thousand dollars per year, depending on age, the benefits selected, and location. Some people are under the impression that the government pays for long-term care through Medicare or Medicaid, but it doesn't. Medicare only covers skilled nursing care for a short period of time after surgery, an accident, or a period of acute illness and only if certain criteria are met. See www.medicare.gov/coverage/skilled-nursing-facility-care. html for details on whether skilled nursing care will be covered for your loved one in their specific situation. Although Medicare will cover up to 20 days of skilled nursing care in a skilled nursing facility each year, there has to be documented skilled need to qualify for this benefit. After covering 20 days at 100 percent,

Medicare will cover up to 100 days with a daily co-insurance charge ($157 in 2016). Skilled needs include intravenous fluids or medications, complex wound care, physical therapy, occupational therapy, and speech therapy. However, the beneficiary has to show continued improvement in function for Medicare to cover it.

Regular health insurance policies and Medigap insurance policies make no provision for long-term care either, so if it's something you think your loved one will need, you should get it right away. After a diagnosis of AD, dementia, or any other chronic, incurable illness is made, your loved one is no longer eligible to purchase a long-term care insurance policy.

Depending on which options are selected when the policy is purchased, services can be provided in a variety of settings, including your home, adult daycare centers, assisted living centers, or nursing homes. Long-term care policies usually take effect when the insured is unable to perform basic self-care tasks after a waiting period of 90 days or longer. Although exact coverage varies from company to company, long-term care insurance may provide a daily benefit to help cover the cost of hiring someone to provide in-home assistance with the activities of daily living such as bathing, toileting, dressing, and eating as well as residential care.

Insurance experts recommend long-term care coverage for families with extensive assets they want to protect. Because premiums are expensive, it's not something that every family will choose.

TIP

Before you purchase a policy, visit www.longtermcareinsurance.org. This site, sponsored by the National Advisory Center for Long-Term Care Information, features lots of information to help you make the best decision when purchasing a long-term care policy. Remember, a long-term care policy must be in place before your loved one is diagnosed with dementia or AD.

Help for veterans

Individuals who served in the military may be eligible for a variety of benefits, including healthcare and prescription benefits, along with some limited nursing home benefits. More than 50 percent of men older than 65 are veterans, and with today's coed military, that figure will soon include a high number of women as well.

For complete information about veterans' eligibility, visit www.va.gov/health benefits.

Running Out of Resources: What Next?

No matter how well you plan, you may one day have to face the fact that your loved one is running out of money to cover his monthly expenses. Perhaps your loved one didn't have enough resources to begin with or maybe he's outlived your best projections and has already chipped away at his capital. You can try several strategies to buy yourself a few extra months.

Using permanent assets

The most likely place to turn when looking for additional funds is your loved one's home, particularly if the mortgage is completely paid. A home equity loan can provide a line of credit based upon the value of the house. The advantage of this type of credit line is that it's flexible to you to use whenever needed without having to go back to the bank to reapply for another loan.

If the house isn't completely paid off, refinancing the mortgage may be a good idea if interest rates are low. Lower monthly house payments can put an additional hundred dollars or more back into your monthly budget. Call around to find the best rate and ask for a loan analysis to make sure that refinancing is a smart move for your loved one's situation.

Taking out a second mortgage on the home is also something to consider. A second mortgage may allow you to consolidate your loved one's debts at a lower rate of interest. Depending on how much equity has been built up in the home over the years and how much money is needed, a substantial sum of money could be collected to help cover monthly bills.

If none of these ideas is practicable and your loved one has reached the point where he can no longer live on his own, you may want to consider selling his home. Doing so may be the best way for you to access the cash you need to pay your loved one's long-term residential care and other expenses.

While you're thinking about ways to raise money, take a look at your loved one's unused household possessions. You may raise a few thousand selling furniture and appliances, or even more if cars, collectibles, artwork, or jewelry are available to be sold. But even if you have a power of attorney giving you full authority over your loved one's possessions, if your loved one is capable of participating in decision-making, include him. And to keep family peace, include his spouse and other adult children to be sure that they don't object to your selling those particular items.

Getting help from other family members

Don't wait until you've completely exhausted your financial resources to ask other family members to contribute money to your loved one's care. Just because you're the primary caregiver doesn't mean you should have to shoulder the entire cost of providing that care. If you need help paying for sitters, daycare, or uncovered medical expenses, say so. Your other family members don't know what you need unless you tell them.

TIP

Make copies of your caregiving budget and send a copy to each family member who is in a position to offer financial assistance. Be specific about what you need. Don't demand that your sister pay $200 a month and your brother $400; you may not know their true financial situation. Tell them what you need and ask how much they can comfortably contribute on a regular basis. Even if it's just $50 a month, that's $50 less that you have to come up with.

Discussions about financial matters go more smoothly when the participants feel like they have the full picture, so be open and honest; don't hold anything back or overstate the problem.

Turning to your community

If you've run out of resources to provide care for your loved one, you may be able to get help from a variety of local resources. Call your local Area Office on Aging to see what resources are available to help families in your situation. You can also call the nearest chapter of the Alzheimer's Association for a list of local volunteer groups and charitable organizations available to assist people with AD and their families.

You may be able to find an adult daycare center that offers rates that are based on a sliding scale according to income. Some churches in your community may offer free respite care or help you find low-cost or volunteer sitters, drivers, and other types of helpers as needed.

Your state or local community may offer free or reduced-cost home health aides or free placement in a state-run nursing home if your family meets local income guidelines.

Chapter 14

Choosing Ongoing Care for Your Loved One

For people with early dementia and their caregivers, the subject of residential care can be a tricky one. Older people often utter the phrase "don't you dare put me in a nursing home" to their relatives. They figure if they move to a long-term care facility that they'll be out of sight and therefore out of mind.

As a caregiver, making the decision to place your loved one into a residential care facility invariably involves feelings of guilt. You don't want your loved one to be unhappy, but know that the increasingly complex needs of this person with dementia or Alzheimer's disease (AD) make it too difficult to continue to provide care at home. This is especially true when you have to hold down a job outside the home and care for the rest of the family as well as be a caregiver for your loved one.

You must also consider the financial aspect. What care can the person with dementia afford? Will the house have to be sold to pay for her care?

These are all important considerations, but the bottom line is that the needs of the person with dementia must come first. This chapter looks at the options — from care in the person's own home, to assisted living to full-time care in a nursing home — and the advantages and disadvantages of each.

Reaching a Realistic Decision

When you sit down to start planning what sort of care would be most appropriate for your loved one, the first thing you must do is look at your goals and identify your options. Maybe you and your loved one discussed options when she was still able to make her wishes clear. If so, you can consider this info as you decide on what care setting is best for her at this time. But realize what seemed reasonable when your loved one had only mild symptoms may not be appropriate when symptoms are more advanced. If you have financial concerns, your local Area Office on Aging and Alzheimer's Association can point you to some community resources that may be able to help.

First, establish your goals. When making a plan for care, consider immediate, short-term, and long-term needs. Decisions about care may be influenced by many factors, including

>> Patient safety

>> Your health

>> Your loved one's health

>> The presence of certain behavioral symptoms

>> The level of care needed on a daily basis

>> Financial considerations

REMEMBER

An option that suits the person with dementia 100 percent is unlikely to exist, so you have to be prepared to accept an option that fits most of your criteria. Otherwise the whole process can be extremely frustrating.

These sections can help you consider all of the information to make a decision that is realistic for you and your loved one.

Being guided by how well someone is doing

How well someone is doing is by far the most important factor to think about when planning someone's future care setting. When people with dementia are still living independently at home much of the time, but just need help with personal hygiene, cooking, and shopping, moving to a nursing home is inappropriate overkill that isn't warranted. Doing so would be a poor fit because they don't warrant this level of care. Likewise, if they're severely disabled by end-stage dementia or AD, then a caregiver popping in to their home twice a day to wash their face and put a meal in front of them will be wholly inadequate (especially if the person with dementia can no longer hold a fork).

These scenarios may seem obvious, but with the panic engendered by a deteriorating situation, common sense can fly out of the window. You can avoid making the wrong care-setting decisions by asking some straightforward questions, such as:

» If the person needs help, how much does she need to make life simple for her?

» What are her main disabilities, and what can be done to work around them?

» Where do you need to draw the line to avoid stifling the independence she has left?

» Do you want to help your loved one maintain her independence for as long as possible, or would you prefer to get her into a more controlled environment right away so she can get used to a new setting?

» Do you want to keep your loved one in her own house, bring her to yours, or place her in a residential care facility?

» Will you be shouldering the bulk of the care, or will you hire someone else to come in and provide care?

» Is she going downhill fast, or is her deterioration slow and stepwise?

TIP

We're sure you can think of your own questions, but they should all be aimed at solving the following equation, where X stands for level of care:

Current level of disability + X = Best quality of life possible

REMEMBER

According to the experts, one guideline regarding whether a person with dementia/AD (or physical disabilities) is safe to live alone (or be left alone) is whether she is cognitively and physically able to exit the house in the event of a fire. This guideline may help with making your decision.

REMEMBER

As the caregiver, you want to make every effort (insofar as is practical and possible), to honor your love one's wishes. However, you may have to be the bad guy and make unpopular decisions in order to provide the living setting most appropriate for your loved ones needs. This is especially true if your loved one wants to continue living alone (and driving) despite clear evidence that it's no longer safe for her to do so.

Considering whether symptoms are rapidly progressing

If someone has rapidly progressive dementia or AD, you have to factor that into the decision-making process to avoid having to move her from one setting to another in quick succession to meet her increasing needs. Allowing your loved one to get settled somewhere and shortly afterward putting her through the upheaval and confusion of another move is the worst thing possible for her. And it's equally frustrating (and financially costly) for families to think that the process is over and their loved one is settled, only to have to go through it soon all over again.

You may be lucky and find some residential facilities locally that cater specifically to dementia patients and can alter levels of care as things progress, which is referred to as *stepped* care. Another option is to keep someone at home as long as possible by arranging in-home nursing care (although it can be prohibitively expensive). Options vary throughout the country, which may prove limiting, but the process can certainly be made easier by planning ahead and speaking to the professionals involved in the person's care to get their views on the matter.

Deciding whether existing help is sufficient

Carrying out a mental review of the support a person already receives can be helpful. Can this support be tweaked here and there if things start to go downhill? Maybe nothing more is needed at this point. Remember, you don't have to rush into anything.

However, in the midst of a seeming crisis, you may be tempted to do something. But a knee-jerk reaction can lead to premature decisions that either isn't necessary or, worse still, are more disruptive than helpful. Remain calm and don't panic. And if you're seeking advice about what to do, always speak to the person's physician. She should have a good idea of the levels of help needed and is the best person to carry out a thorough, objective assessment of your loved one's needs.

Identifying your options

Your loved one won't require as much care in the early stages of dementia or AD as he or she will in the later stages. For someone with very mild memory loss, perhaps all you'll need is someone to ensure that medications are taken as prescribed. The care plan you start out with will change and become more comprehensive as your love one's condition progresses. Tables 14-1 and 14-2 present the various care options that are available for patients.

WARNING

A common misconception exists that after someone reaches the age of 65, Medicare will pay for all that person's medical needs, including long-term care. Unfortunately, that's simply not true. See Chapter 13 for more info on what Medicare covers.

TABLE 14-1   Respite Care Choices for Patients

Respite Care Choice	Care Provider	Location	Cost
Informal unpaid care	You or another family member, friend, or neighbor.	Your home or your loved one's home.	No out-of-pocket cost other than medical bills, but you may have to adjust your work hours, take FMLA, or give up your job to provide care, depending on your loved one's level of need.
Paid caregiver or companion service	You may contract with an individual or hire a paid caregiver from an agency.	Your home or your loved one's home or elsewhere depending on need (for example, acute illness requiring hospital stay — hire a sitter to stay with patient overnight in the hospital).	Average about $20/hour, but range is $15-25 per hour. More to hire from an agency.
Home healthcare aide for patient with co-existing medical needs	Home health aide, LVN, RN licensed to provide medical services.	Same as paid caregiver.	$25 to $50 per hour, depending on certification and need. May be covered by Medicare for limited time for skilled needs.
Adult daycare	Paid staff and volunteers.	Free-standing center for adults with dementia or affiliated with a hospital, church, or care facility.	Average cost in 2015 is $69 per day with different state averages ranging from $35 to $124 per day. May include transportation; services such as bathing cost extra.
Day healthcare for patients with dementia and co-existing medical illness that requires nursing services	Paid staff.	Free-standing facility or hospital-based.	Average $85 to $90 per day; services such as bathing cost extra.

TABLE 14-2   **Residential Care Choices for Patients**

Residential Care Choice	Care Provider	Location	Cost
Assisted living	Paid staff.	Assisted-living center.	Wide variation, $2,500 to $6,000 monthly average. May have additional costs based on personal care needs.
Licensed residential care home (also called a personal care home)	On-site nonmedical staff.	Neighborhood home licensed to provide care for a certain number of people on site.	$850 to $4,000 per month, depending upon location and client need.
Dedicated Alzheimer's care center or memory support unit	On-site medical and nonmedical staff, visiting medical staff.	Alzheimer's care center; may be free-standing or be part of a continuing care retirement community that offers all levels of care from independent living to assisted living to AD care; some also have skilled nursing on site.	Assisted living setting can range from $4,000 to $7,500.
Nursing home	On-site medical and nonmedical staff, visiting medical staff.	Nursing home.	Shared room $220 daily average. Depends on level of care at nursing home. Monthly can range from $4,200 to $11,000.

Considering Options for Providing Care at Home

Early on, the vast majority of dementia and AD patients lived in their own homes with support from others. Although 20 to 30 percent of patients now live alone, many live at home with spouses or relocate to live with a relative, usually an adult child. As cognitive abilities decline and the need for supervision and assistance with day-to-day activities of living increases, more time is required of the caregiver. In addition to the financial impact of paid care (Medicare doesn't pay for someone to come to your home and provide companion care), providing care at home can be stressful to the caregiver.

Remember that you don't have to provide all the help that is needed yourself. A complete care plan for your loved one may be a combination of multiple care options. It may include a combination of adult in-home unpaid care that you provide plus enrollment of your loved one in adult daycare program three days a week and paid companion care two afternoons a week to be possible for care at home to continue.

These sections examine some of the pros and cons for providing care for your loved one at home or hiring in-home care and how about finding the right home health aide for you and your loved one.

Caring for your loved one at home

Many families feel that they don't have any other choice but to care for their loved ones at home without outside assistance. According to the Alzheimer's Association, 28 percent of caregivers have annual incomes less than $20,000. Financial constraints force them to personally shoulder the burden of providing care for their loved ones. Even families with higher incomes may find themselves caught in that proverbial sandwich between the financial needs of their elderly parents and the financial needs of their college-age children. When money's tight, providing in-home care rather than spending thousands of dollars for care outside the home may be the best choice. In fact, two-thirds of families caring for a dementia or AD patient choose in-home care as their initial care option.

The benefits

Providing in-home care in your loved one's home or in your own home does have some concrete benefits:

>> You may worry less because you believe you can better keep an eye on your loved one.

>> You have the opportunity to spend more quality time together.

>> Your loved one may feel more independent.

>> You know that your loved one is being well cared for and treated with love and compassion.

>> Other family members may be able to help provide care as needed.

>> You may feel a unique, deep sense of pride and accomplishment in your role as caregiver.

>> If your loved one is your parent, you're giving back by providing reciprocal care for the parent who cared for you as a child.

>> You may discover things about yourself that you may have overlooked had you not become a caregiver. For example, you may find that you're more caring, supportive, nurturing than you knew, or perhaps you find out that you're an effective problem-solver who possesses great organizational skills.

>> You get in touch with your ability to advocate for yourself and your loved one.

>> You may discover that you're resilient.

The drawbacks

Now for the cons:

>> You may have to invest some money in refitting the house to accommodate your loved one's needs if the disease is severely advanced or if they have a co-existing medical illness. For example, your loved one may need a grab bar in the bathtub and a toilet seat booster.

>> The strain of providing round-the-clock care by yourself and or overseeing paid caregivers can create tremendous physical and psychological stress and lead to health problems for you as the caregiver.

>> Serving as a primary caregiver can negatively impact your marriage and your family relations due to less time available for you spouse and children.

>> Serving as a primary caregiver can adversely affect your career if it takes you away from your work.

>> Creating space for your loved one in your home can lead to crowding for other family members. For example, siblings who previously had their own rooms may have to share a room to allow Grandpa to have his own room, which can lead to other problems.

>> You may have to prepare a special menu to address your loved one's nutritional needs.

>> You may have very little free time for yourself and your family.

>> The additional costs associated with caring for your loved one may impose a financial strain on your family. (See the next section for more specifics.)

>> No matter how diligent you are, your loved one may still wander away or have an accident, which can lead to feelings of guilt for you as the caregiver.

TIP

Although it may sound like a lot of negatives are associated with providing in-home care, you can do many things to make it a more positive experience for the whole family. See Chapter 10 for an overview of what's involved in in-home caregiving and how you can make it as stress-free and rewarding as possible.

Cost issues

Common directs costs to care for your loved one at home may include ongoing medical and doctor care, prescription and over-the-counter drugs, incontinence supplies, and any paid help. However, indirect costs include your own time as an unpaid caregiver including time lost from outside work.

Here are a few of the specific costs that you'll also have to consider:

>> **Mobility and medical equipment:** If your loved one's mobility is limited, a wheelchair can be a lifeline for use both inside and outside, thus ensuring that he can still get some fresh air and that friends and relatives can still take him out and about. Check with local medical supply companies because costs can vary throughout the United States.

>> **Different types of wheelchairs are available:** Some fold up so they fit in the car trunk; others are electric and can be operated by the person. Note: It takes cognitive ability to safely operate an electric wheelchair (just as it does to drive a car), so a wheelchair will no longer be appropriate as dementia progresses. Doorframes can be adjusted to accommodate a wheelchairs and a ramp can be installed to allow easy access to entrance doors, bypassing stairs.

>> **Home adaptations:** A large number of special aids and home adaptations are available to make life easier for people with increasing cognitive and physical difficulties. Of course, these adaptations come at a cost. A physical or occupational therapist from a local home health agency can assess a person's needs and suggest suitable aids, including

- A walk-in shower with a seat

- A shower chair

- Raised toilet seats (with or without arms)

- Handrails throughout the house

- A chair stair lift installed on stairs to facilitate going up and down

- Bedside commodes

- Large-faced clocks for better visibility

Some funding may be available for these alterations and adaptations through local agencies or organizations. However, more likely you'll need to purchase them privately. Call your local Area Office on Aging or Alzheimer's Association.

Hiring paid in-home care

Perhaps you want to keep your loved one in his own home for as long as you can, but you're unable to directly provide any of the care yourself. In that case, you can hire a home companion, also known as a paid caregiver, to provide the care.

Your loved one's condition and social needs determine the number of hours required for the outside help. If your loved one is in the early stages of dementia or AD and lives alone, she may be able to handle most if not all of her day-to-day responsibilities. You should let her know you're going to monitor how effectively she's handling these responsibilities and discuss the possibility of eventually hiring a paid caregiver to come a few hours in the morning to make sure she gets dressed, eats properly, and takes her medications as directed. You and your loved one can define a paid caregiver's role according to current needs. Perhaps she needs or would enjoy having someone come in to cook or do laundry and other household chores, which can also provide company for a person living alone. If your loved one has been told to stop driving, a paid companion can serve as a driver/chauffer.

Although home companions can perform a variety of tasks, they aren't licensed to provide skilled nursing care. Their primary responsibilities will be to help your loved one with his or her more complex and basic *activities of daily living* (ADLs) — shopping, food preparation, household chores, driving, errands, personal hygiene, exercise coach, medication oversight, and so on. If your loved one needs something like a daily insulin shot, a service that provides home health aides rather than home companion/homemaker/paid caregiving services is required.

The types of services provided by paid caregivers vary between agencies and also depend on what your loved one needs and how much you're able or willing to pay. You may also hire paid caregivers directly that work independently from agencies. Generally speaking, the more services an aide provides, the higher the hourly rate. Here are a few types of services:

>> **Personal care or ADLs:** Assistance with personal hygiene, such as bathing, dressing, and toileting. Some may be willing to supervise light exercise and get your loved one in and out of bed.

>> **Household chores:** Light cleaning, shopping, laundry, dishes, meeting and supervising repairmen, and so on.

>> **Nutrition:** Meal preparation and cleanup, supervision of meals and snacks, shopping or ordering of meals from outside sources like Meals on Wheels.

>> **Sitting service:** Home care agencies can provide day sitters to keep the person with dementia company while spouses and family caregivers go out.

>> **Supervisory:** Transportation to doctor's appointments, daycare, and senior centers, and so on.

>> **Social services:** Companionship and activity planning.

>> **Safety:** Ensuring that medication is taken appropriately. Inspection of premises for safety hazards, establishment of routine to ensure the safety of the patient. Making sure that the patient doesn't get injured, lost, or disoriented.

The benefits

The pros of hiring a home health aide:

>> Relieves you of the responsibility of providing care all by yourself

>> Can help maintain your loved one in a familiar and comforting environment

>> Can establish a daily routine for your loved one, which may include in-home and outside activities (that is, going to museums or the park, shopping, visiting friends, eating out for lunch, or going to the hair dresser)

>> Can help broaden your loved one's social network

>> Can help safeguard your loved one

>> Can help ensure that your loved one doesn't become exclusively dependent on you for care

>> Companion may become like a member of your family after a long period of employment

The drawbacks

The cons of hiring a home health aide:

>> An aide can't provide medical services. You'll have to hire a visiting nurse if you need this type of service.

>> The cost of service — Medicare doesn't pay for the cost of a home health aide.

>> Even with careful screening, occasionally, a home health aide turns out to be unsuited to the job, either by reason of dishonesty, neglect, roughness or abusiveness, failure to perform the job adequately, or just a bad personality match with your loved one

>> If your paid caregiver is unable to come on short notice (due to her own or their family member's illness or transportation issues), then you may be stuck without coverage. However, this issue is more likely with privately hired caregivers than agency-based home care aides because agencies often offer a back-up aide in these situations.

REMEMBER

Although aides that you hire yourself can cost much less to employ, you do run a higher risk of encountering problems than you would with an aide from an agency because all reputable agencies have rigorous screening protocols to ensure a consistent quality of service.

Finding a home health aide

You can start by checking the bulletin board in your local senior center or community center. People looking for work as aides often post their credentials there. If you can't locate any potential candidates that way, place an ad in the local paper or post a notice at the senior center. If you're a member of a church or synagogue, ask around to see if anyone is interested in the job or has used such a service. Talk to friends or coworkers, ask your doctor's office staff for suggestions, call assisted living or other care facilities to see if someone is seeking part-time work, or call the Alzheimer's Association for information on local agencies.

TIP

The Family Caregiver Alliance has an excellent webpage entitled "Hiring In-Home Help" located at www.caregiver.org/hiring-home-help. This guide can help you assess your needs, write a job description, rehearse a sample interview, and determine whether to use an agency or privately hire a home health aide. It also helps you locate resources within your own community that may be able to assist you in your search. Or look at New LifeStyles: The Source for Senior Living at www.newlifestyles.com for an area guide to senior care options in your area. Their home page can help you find senior care providers and options, just by searching with your zip code.

You and your loved one should interview several candidates. If he is able, allow your loved one to ask questions of the candidates and interact with him to assess whether they could be compatible. Also be sure to do the following:

>> Ask for a work history and references, and actually call them, even if the person is someone you know.

>> Discuss salary requirements and pay frequency.

>> Ask whether the candidate has dependable transportation.

>> Ask what services the aide will provide and what hours he or she is available to work.

>> Clearly outline what the aide's responsibilities will be and invite her to ask any questions about the job and about your expectations and requirements.

>> Describe a difficult scenario and ask her how she would handle it.

>> Ask her if she knows what AD or dementia is and what it means to her. This will give you a sense of her knowledge and experience of the disease, as well as her personal perception of those afflicted by it.

>> Ask her why she chose to go into this line of work, particularly her desire to work with patients with memory disorders.

>> Ask her if a free training program for caregivers of patients with memory disorders is available through your local Alzheimer's Association, would she be willing to attend.

>> Ask if she would be willing to read literature about ways to care for patients with dementia or AD.

TIP

For a different approach to finding a home health aide or companion, eldercare. com maintains a database of aides seeking employment caring for seniors in their homes as well as other senior care options.

Tell the aide about your loved one's condition, but don't make the mistake of talking about your loved one as if he wasn't right there in the room with you — this dehumanizes the person with the memory disorder and can make him angry or unhappy! If you need to share things with the aide that may upset your loved one, do so privately. Also tell the potential employee about any special needs your loved one has, such as requiring assistance with toileting, bathing, or dressing, and your routine for doing these tasks.

Check with your insurance agent to see whether you need to adjust your home insurance policy to cover an in-home employee. When you do hire someone, make the job offer in writing, specifying hours, duties, and salary. Tell the aide how often you'll pay her and on what days. Make a copy of the aide's Social Security card and driver's license. You'll need the card for tax purposes and the driver's license copy as a security measure. These steps can avoid a lot of confusion later on.

If, for whatever reason, the aide you hired doesn't prove to be a satisfactory choice and you find it necessary to replace the aide, give her written notice and a couple of weeks' severance pay to tide the aide over until she can find another job. Although you're not strictly required by law to offer notice and severance pay, doing so is a generous gesture that can go a long way toward smoothing out any difficulties that the firing may bring up.

REMEMBER

If you pay the aide $1,900 or more during a year, you must deduct Social Security and Medicare taxes from her wages. Once a year, you're required to report the income to the IRS and pay the taxes you've deducted. By law, you must provide your employee with copies B and C of IRS form W-2, outlining her wages and the taxes withheld by January 31 of the year following the year the wages were paid. You have until the last day of February to send Copy A to the Social Security Administration.

WARNING

After you hire someone, make sure you pay the Social Security and Medicare taxes that are due on the wages you pay her, or else Uncle Sam may pay you a visit. Consult your financial adviser or visit the Social Security website at www.ssa.gov/pubs/10021.html for information about the financial responsibilities of people who employ household workers. If you don't pay the taxes on time, you'll have to pay the overdue taxes plus a penalty.

Considering a live-in

You may prefer to have someone live in the house with your loved one, especially if your loved one is living alone. Providing room and board should allow you to negotiate a better hourly rate for services.

WHAT TO LOOK FOR IN A CAREGIVER

Everyone's personality is different, but you should look for a few key personality characteristics when seeking a caregiver for your loved one. The candidate should be

- Cheerful, upbeat, positive
- Patient and understanding
- Even-tempered
- Mature, sensible, cool-headed
- Caring, compassionate, empathetic

Follow the same procedures to find a live-in aide as you would for one who comes into your home to work. After you've made your selection, you need to figure out where you're going to house the person you've chosen.

REMEMBER

Hiring someone to live in your or your loved one's home and then trying to cram that person into a broom closet is unfair. The aide should have her own private, clean, furnished room with adequate space to store personal belongings. Get your junk out of there before she moves in. The aide should either have her own bathroom or access to a nearby bath. You should discuss your expectations for use of the kitchen and other common areas of the house.

Just because someone is living in your home doesn't mean that she is available to work around the clock seven days a week. The aide is an employee, not a slave. Agree on her duties and draw up a written schedule before the aide starts work, and then stick to it. If you require the aide to work more than 40 hours in one week, you should be prepared to pay her overtime, which is generally one and a half times her regular hourly rate.

Keep in mind that your live-in will need a certain amount of time off per week and may have an emergency that requires immediate attention. When you rely on others to provide care, you have to be ready to fill in or have a contingency plan in place to cover their responsibilities. See the following for options.

FINDING A HOME HEALTH AGENCY

If you don't want the hassle of screening candidates and have neither the time nor the inclination to deal with tax forms and Social Security, you should hire your aide through an agency. Home health agencies take most of the work out of finding an aide because they've prescreened all their candidates and send out only the people who meet their standards to interview for jobs. Best of all, you pay the agency, and they pay their aides, so you don't ever have to worry about collecting Social Security taxes and dealing with the IRS at least not on your aide's account. Realize that using an agency may be more expensive then hiring a caregiver yourself, but it can be a lot less hassle so it may be worth it.

WARNING

But using an agency does have a downside: Agencies frequently use a rotation of personnel to provide care, so the person sent to look after your loved one on Monday may be different from the person sent on Tuesday. This lack of consistency can be upsetting and confusing for AD and dementia patients.

On the other hand, if one aide is sick, a qualified substitute is automatically sent, which means you don't have to scramble trying to arrange last-minute care the way you would if you'd hired an aide privately. Make sure the agency agrees to provide this backup service ahead of time so you don't get stuck.

You need to give the agency a complete overview of your loved one's physical and mental status so the agency can assign someone who's qualified to handle your needs. Review the information we provide under "Finding a home health aide" earlier in this chapter and use it to discuss terms of employment with your agency aide. Let the aide know your loved one's schedule and preferences, preferably in writing, and the duties you expect her to perform. Writing down these expectations and leaving them available for reference on the kitchen counter or under a magnet on the refrigerator can be helpful, especially if a backup aide comes.

You can find a listing of home health agencies by doing an online search for "home health agencies" with your city or zip code, but that doesn't give you much information about an agency's track record. Ask your loved one's doctor for a referral to an agency that he trusts and ask friends who've used an agency and if they were satisfied with the care provided. You can also check with the Better Business Bureau, Angie's List, or your local Chamber of Commerce to check out the agencies reputation.

If, for whatever reason, the first aide the agency sends over doesn't work out, you can simply call the agency, explain the problem, and ask for new candidates for the position. Of course, you want to make it clear from the beginning that you'll be expecting the same aide to come each time for consistency, if at all possible.

Knowing when you need a visiting nurse

Sometimes your loved one needs more care than a home health aide can provide. If your loved one has multiple health issues, such as dementia and diabetes or AD and heart disease, he may also require a visiting nurse. A visiting nurse can provide medical services that a home health aide can't, such as changing dressings, reinserting catheters, giving injections, monitoring vital signs, and so on. Visiting nurse agencies provide services ranging from highly skilled nursing care to physical and occupational therapy, as well as hospice care for terminally ill patients.

TIP

Members of the Visiting Nurse Associations of America have a mission to provide compassionate, high-quality, cost-effective home health and hospice care in their respective communities through skilled nursing and therapy services and home health aides. To find a Visiting Nurse Association near you, enter your zip code in the search box at www.vnaa.org/find-a-provider.

Medicare may cover nurse visits for short term, especially if your loved one has just been discharged from a hospital and has a specific skilled nursing need. But generally speaking, hiring a visiting nurse is an expense that you'll have to cover out of pocket.

Contemplating adult daycare

If your loved one isn't yet ready for an assisted living facility or a nursing home but you don't feel that your situation is conducive to providing 24/7 in-home care, adult daycare is for you. Adult daycare for people with dementia and its newer cousin, adult day healthcare, can be a real godsend for a two-career family that simply can't provide in-home care during work hours and doesn't like the idea of leaving their loved one alone at home all day alone or with an aide. Adult daycare provides some real benefits for dementia patients as well, giving them the chance to socialize and participate in enjoyable activities with their peers in a safe and controlled professional environment.

Adult daycare evolved from the child daycare model, but it should never be confused with childcare. These programs are geared toward adults, with adult activities tailored to meet the capabilities of the participants and an atmosphere designed for adults. Adult daycare programs are usually open five days a week during traditional business hours. These programs are designed to meet the needs of both functionally and cognitively impaired older adults, though programs can vary depending on the population that they target. In other words, some daycare programs are designed for patients with mild to moderate dementia, whereas others cater to the needs of those with more advanced dementia. Some adult daycare facilities provide transportation. Most programs provide at least lunch meals on the premises as well as some support services such as medication reminders and blood pressure monitoring. In addition to providing respite for the caregiver, these programs provide enjoyable and appropriate social activities and engagement for those with memory disorders. Having AD or dementia doesn't mean you no longer have a need to feel meaningful or socially connected to others. Attendance at an adult day program can provide a sense of purpose and a reason to get up in the morning for your loved one.

REMEMBER

Dementia and AD patients are often leery of change, so you may encounter some resistance when you first pose the idea to your loved one. Acknowledge that they have some healthy skepticism, and reassure them that you'll preview the program together. If you ask whether they want to go, you're almost certain to get a no. You would be wiser to ask if they would prefer to preview the "wellness center, senior center, or activity center" on Monday or Wednesday, thereby giving them a choice and sense of control but not the final decision about whether to go. Keep in mind that it may not be necessary for your loved one to know that he isn't formally enrolled in the program. You can tell him that he is attending on a volunteer basis. The staff of the day center is probably familiar with this approach and will be willing to acknowledge him as a helper or volunteer rather than a paid subscriber. As a transition, you may want to start off with attendance just twice a week and over time increase the number of day your loved one attends. After you initiate enrollment, try to stick with it for a few weeks before quitting. After your loved one settles in, makes a few friends, and starts participating in the activities, he may begin bugging you to go to daycare even on the weekends.

TIP

Adult day healthcare programs offer more comprehensive care than regular adult day programs for patients who require specific medical or psychiatric supervision. They provide services, such as on-site nurses, social workers, physical therapists, and other medical and caregiving professionals, in addition to the social activities, meals, and transportation services offered by regular adult daycare.

The nice thing about these programs is that they don't use a one-size-fits-all approach. Activities are tailored to your loved one's interests, needs, and abilities. One patient who has mobility problems may do crafts whereas other patients who are more mobile participate in a light exercise class. Another patient may visit with a nurse for a blood pressure check and then join his fellow patients for a snack or musical entertainment. But the most important function adult daycare serves is that it eliminates the problem of social isolation that can overwhelm a person with a memory disorder who stays at home all the time. These places offer so many enjoyable planned activities, from crafts to music to exercise games, that your loved one is sure to find something to enjoy.

Finding a daycare center

Adult daycare programs are licensed and regulated by the states where they're located, so you can be assured of a fairly consistent quality of care. But you should still visit several centers in advance and interview the personnel. This way, you'll be able to select a center that best fits your loved one's interests and personality, which gives you a better chance of a successful experience.

TIP

The following sources can help you find a good adult daycare center:

>> The National Adult Day Services Association (NADSA) maintains a searchable directory at http://nadsa.org. For more information on choosing an adult daycare center, see "Choosing a Center" at http://nadsa.org/consumers/choosing-a-center/. The NADSA also offers an excellent site visit checklist at http://nadsa.org/wp-content/uploads/2015/08/Site-Visit-Checklist-for-the-web.pdf.

>> You can visit the federally sponsored Eldercare Locator at www.eldercare. gov and enter your state and zip code to obtain a list of organizations in your area that can help you locate appropriate care for your loved one.

Knowing what to look for in a center

Look for a pleasant, secure, comfortable atmosphere that has plenty of space and good lighting. The facility shouldn't be cluttered or crowded because that can lead to falls or other accidents. Patients should be attended to and well supervised to make sure they're engaged and safe. The staff should be courteous, compassionate and caring, and experienced in dealing with the needs of older adults with dementia.

If the center provides transportation, inspect the center's vehicle to make sure it has an adequate number of seat belts and that the driver takes the time to assist passengers getting on and off the bus or van and to belt in each passenger. If your loved one uses a walker, wheelchair, or scooter, does the center have a way to transport the mobility equipment back and forth? Watch the driver for a few minutes to satisfy yourself that safety considerations are being observed.

Here are some other questions you should ask:

>> What's the ratio of paid staff to attendees?

>> Are the activities provided stimulating, enjoyable, age, and cognitively appropriate?

>> Are activities available for both large and small groups?

>> Is the dining area clean? Are the meals nutritious and appealing?

>> If your loved one has special nutritional concerns, such as a diabetic diet, can the center accommodate that?

>> Can the center provide emergency medical care if your loved one needs it?

Don't forget to ask your loved one for input if she can still express a choice. Then, if you're considering two or more centers, ask your loved one for her preference, which may enable a more successful transition to adult daycare. However, if you anticipate difficulty in getting your loved one to go to an adult daycare program, don't discuss it much ahead of time or agitate her with a visit before she's actually enrolled. In these situations, the key is to get her to go the first time and ask staff to make her feel welcome and at ease so she will want to return. This method often enables a more smooth transition.

Making the Transition to Residential Care

No matter what sort of care approach you ultimately decide on, the first few weeks after you start the new care arrangements may be difficult because it represents a change for both you and your loved one. Some older people are happy to get out from under the burden of caring for their home and into a more protected and supportive environment, but others will fight you tooth and nail if you so much as bring up the topic for discussion. You may encounter anger, bitterness, tears, grief, and accusations that you don't really care for your loved one and are just trying to shuffle her off into a corner somewhere to get her out of the way. Just knowing that these problems may crop up and having a plan in place to deal with them is half the battle.

REMEMBER

Don't beat yourself up if the biggest feeling you experience after placing your loved one in a residential care facility is a huge blast of relief. Caregiving places profound burdens on the caregiver. If you've provided care for a number of months or even years, feeling relief at such a time is perfectly natural. Now your relationship with your loved one will evolve into something new. You aren't finished caring for your loved one, but the nature of your work changes as you go from being a direct, hands-on caregiver to a care manager overseeing those providing the direct care.

REMEMBER

Don't be surprised if you find yourself battling some difficult feelings of your own. Even if the thinking part of your brain knows that changing care settings is the best thing for your loved one, the emotional part of your brain may be weighing you down with guilt and an overwhelming sense of loss. You may feel like you've abandoned your loved one. Nothing could be further from the truth. Keep in mind that what's changing the caregiving situation is dementia, not you.

Making sure that your loved one feels included in the decision-making and preparation process can help the transition. Generally speaking, this is much more likely to be possible if you select an assisted living facility rather than a nursing home (because when your loved one needs a nursing home, their dementia is already quite advanced). Here are some tips to help:

>> Take a tour of the facility with your loved one and encourage her to ask any questions she may have.

>> Give your loved one the opportunity to meet other residents and staff members and socialize.

>> Visit at lunchtime so you can enjoy a meal together.

After you decide on a residential home, you can make the transition easier for your loved one. Consider these suggestions:

» Help your loved one choose a few truly meaningful things to bring to her new home, like family photographs or a favorite afghan blanket. Understand how giving up most of what she owns in order to move into a care facility can be difficult for someone who's lived in the same house for years, surrounded by family keepsakes and treasured possessions. But don't bring valuable family heirlooms or expensive collections that are irreplaceable and could be lost or even stolen in this setting.

» Reassure her that you'll make sure that other belongings will be kept safe and allow her to grieve the loss of a way of life she may have cherished. Offer support and hope for a new chapter in her life and reassure her that you'll be a constant part of that chapter.

» Make a scrapbook with favorite family photographs and include pictures of the family home, inside and out, to remind your loved one of the happy memories associated with the house. However, don't be disappointed if the person with memory disorder shows little interest in this, or if reviewing it together sparks a negative reaction or no reaction at all.

KNOWING WHEN IT'S TIME FOR FULL-TIME RESIDENTIAL CARE

The goal of effective management of dementia or AD is to keep the patient independent and living in a familiar environment for as long as possible. But you can watch for some signs that signal the time to place your loved one in a residential facility:

- You can no longer control your loved one's wandering.

- His nighttime restlessness is keeping the rest of the family from getting a good night's sleep.

- Your loved one's behavior is becoming increasingly unmanageable.

- He is frequently incontinent.

- When you assist your loved one with personal care such as bathing or toileting, he becomes agitated or combative with you.

- Your loved one's had a fall or some other sort of accident.

- The strain of providing round-the-clock in-home care is threatening your health or your family's stability.

If you do use it, use it to reminisce, not to quiz your loved one on her recall of their previous residence.

>> Move the furniture and other belongings in before your loved one moves in. This way, when she arrives at her new living quarters, the room will be well organized and inviting. Arranging two or three pieces of furniture in a familiar setting with some of the same decorative objects that she had at home is a good way to bring a little piece of her former surroundings with her into her new life. Maybe there is room for her favorite recliner or bedside table. Familiar objects can be comforting and help cut down on the feeling of strangeness your loved one may experience when he first moves into his new place.

Patience and understanding can go a long way toward helping your loved one make a smooth transition to her new home. But if either one of you still has difficulty coping with your emotions after a few weeks, seek the advice of a professional counselor to help you over the rough patch. And if absolutely necessary, you can always transition to another residential facility if you and/or your loved one are totally dissatisfied with the first selection.

Eyeing Residential Care Options

No matter how wonderful the care you give and your willingness to use respite services, the day may come when you simply can no longer provide the kind of care your loved one requires in your home. Full-time residential care is a necessary consideration for many families caring for someone with a memory disorder. For many, it becomes a necessary step to keep their loved one safe and healthy. It's also a step that caregivers take when the level of care required becomes overwhelming. In these sections we discuss the various kinds of residential care available for dementia and AD patients. Even if you never intend to use this, it's wise to know about residential care and explore the options for placement in your community. This way you know what options are available if you need them on short notice down the road. Knowing what facilities to turn to can be a great relief. It's better to be prepared to make a decision and do so before a crisis precipitates one.

Don't let anyone fool you: Making the decision to place your loved one in a full-time residential care facility is probably one of the most difficult a caregiver can experience. You may realize that your loved one is nearing the end of his fight with dementia or AD, and you may be disappointed that you can't provide all the care he needs right up to the end. It becomes even more difficult if you promised your loved one to never put him in a home. You may encounter some stiff resistance from him when you first broach the subject of residential care, but don't let that sway you. You must make the decision based on what's best for your loved one, you, and your family.

In all residential care situations, you'll have some basic questions. For example:

>> Will your loved one have a private bath or have to share a bath?

>> Will you be able to install a private phone line in his or her room, or will your loved one have to use a community phone?

>> Is a cellphone acceptable (if your loved one knows how to use one and can keep it charged)?

>> Are the doors of individual rooms or suites equipped with locks?

>> How often are housekeeping and laundry services provided?

>> What social and entertainment activities are provided?

These questions are just the beginning. You can locate good checklists online at the following locations:

>> **AARP:** "Comparing Nursing Homes" contains an excellent checklist. You can find it at www.aarp.org.

>> **American Health Care Association:** You can find its well-written consumer guide, "Choosing an Assisted Living Residence 2013" at www.ahcancal.org by inserting the title of this document into the homepage search bar.

>> **Assisted Living Checklist:** Download the PDF at www.alfa.org/alfa/Checklist_for_Evaluating_Communities.asp.

>> **Medicare:** Medicare also offers a 17-page detailed checklist with great practical tips at www.medicare.gov/nursinghomecompare/checklist.pdf.

>> **The Natural Center for Assisted Living:** This organization offers two free guides about choosing and making a successful transition upon moving to a facility at www.ahcancal.org/ncal.

After you've made the decision to place your loved one in a residential care facility, you need to decide what kind of facility is right for his needs and your financial situation. The following sections describe the various types of facilities that are available for patients with a memory disorder.

Assisted living facilities

Some people are confused by the idea of assisted living, thinking it means that someone comes into your home to assist your loved one. Actually, assisted living facilities are full-time residential care centers where the residents have their own room/suite/apartments and are assisted with the activities of daily living. Your loved one's privacy and some sense of independence are maintained, but he has an added level of security and access to services needed to stay healthy and independent, yet supervised and safe.

REMEMBER

The *Assisted Living Federation of America* (ALFA) defines *assisted living* as the following: "A special combination of housing, personalized supportive services, and healthcare designed to meet the needs — both scheduled and unscheduled — of those who need help with activities of daily living."

What they offer

Placing your loved one in an assisted living center has many advantages. Perhaps the best, at least from your loved one's point of view, is that your loved one will still be living in his own space in a home-like setting surrounded by familiar and comforting furniture and many of his belongings, such as family photographs and keepsakes.

You may find that moving to an assisted living facility is even cheaper than keeping your loved one in his own home with a home health aide. If your loved one's home is sold after the move to assisted living, then all the expenses associated with maintaining his residence — mortgage payments, taxes, upkeep, and repairs go away. Prices for assisted living facilities vary greatly. The cost is often based on the level of services provided. The more services (medication oversight/administration, laundry, bathing assistance, toileting assistance, incontinence care, supervised trips to see the doctor, housekeeping, blood pressure or blood sugar monitoring, and so on), the more the cost. In addition, if you've been paying a home health aide to watch your loved one, that expense disappears as well.

Assisted living centers are able to offer a high level of comprehensive services through economy of scale. Whereas it might be prohibitively expensive for 25 families to each hire a visiting nurse, when a 25-unit assisted living facility hires a full-time nurse to monitor the health needs of its residents, it makes good economic sense. Not every resident needs to see the nurse every day, but the nurse is there and quickly available when residents need medical attention. According to the National Center for Assisted Living, more than one million residents are currently living in approximately 36,000 assisted living residences throughout the United States with an estimated annual income of $15 billion!

What should you look for in an assisted living residence? The Assisted Living Federation of America says that the following services are required for a balanced and effective assisted living program:

>> Three meals a day, served in a common dining area

>> Housekeeping services

>> Transportation

- » Assistance with eating, bathing, dressing, toileting, and walking

- » Access to health and medical services

- » 24-hour security and staff availability

- » Emergency call systems in each resident's unit

- » Health promotion and exercise programs

- » Medication management

- » Personal laundry services

- » Social and recreational activities

WARNING

Assisted Living isn't a good choice for patients who require around-the-clock nursing care or extensive medical care and monitoring.

What they cost

Depending on your location, assisted living facilities cost between $2,500 and $6,000 per month. Except for medical services and the cost of prescriptions, all your loved one's basic needs, including food, social activities, household services, and basic medical monitoring, can be covered by the monthly stipend depending on the level of care selected. Assisted living isn't covered by Medicare, but in some states, Medicaid patients may qualify for help in covering assisted living expenses. Consult your local Area Office on Aging for information regarding your state's regulations.

You can search online for "Assisted living facilities" and add your zip code for a list of the facilities nearest you. Some states have what's called *licensed residential care homes* or *board and care homes,* where patients are cared for in a small, private home setting. We discuss this form of care in the next section.

Board and care homes

Licensed residential care homes are known by many names — board and care homes, personal care homes, adult family homes, adult foster homes, or adult group homes — but they all provide similar services, such as room and board, assistance with daily activities, and, in some cases, minimal nursing services. Unlike nursing homes and assisted living facilities, board and care homes don't have to be licensed in all states.

In smaller communities, board and care homes may well be the only nearby choice available to families looking to place a loved one in a full-time residential setting. Care is frequently provided in single-family residences that have been modified to accommodate the needs of elderly residents. Generally, such homes care for no more than six patients at a time.

Although many such homes provide excellent care for their residents, instances of abuse have been reported, particularly in unlicensed homes. Before you decide to place your loved one in a board and care home, visit the facility several times at different times of day. Note whether the other residents seem clean, content, and well cared for. Ask to see the room your loved one will be occupying and if you'll be allowed to bring some of her furnishings into the room. Ask for a written list of the services provided for a list of references and call them. Talk to other families that have had loved ones in the facility to see if they were satisfied with the care their family member received.

Finally, if you do decide to place your loved one in a board and care home, make sure the fees and all the services your loved one will receive are laid out in writing in a formal contract so there's no confusion about what you expect. Most of these homes offer different levels of services for varying fees; make sure you don't sign up thinking you're getting one level of service only to find out that the facility charges additional fees to provide the services, such as laundry, that you thought your loved one would be getting.

Dedicated Alzheimer/dementia/ memory care centers

If your loved one's memory loss is advanced or she has developed additional behavioral or physical health problems, you can put her in a dedicated Alzheimer's, dementia, or memory care center where she can get the care she needs. These facilities are designed specifically to meet the needs of AD and other dementia patients, with special services aimed at creating personal satisfaction, preserving self-esteem and dignity, and creating a sense of independence — all in a secure and nurturing environment.

Although some centers provide adult daycare only, most are residential facilities that also provide some level of medical services. Frequently, dedicated Alzheimer's, dementia, or memory care units are part of a larger facility, such as a nursing home. Often these units are housed in a separate wing of the facility and are *locked units* to prevent unsafe wandering issues or elopement.

Nursing homes

Just like hospitals, nursing homes are staffed 24 hours a day by healthcare professionals and support personnel who provide medical and personal care services for residents. Generally speaking, at least three different levels of care are available: basic care (also called *custodial* or *intermediate care*), skilled nursing care, and sub-acute care, as well as dedicated Alzheimer's units in some locations. According to a National Nursing Home Survey, the average length of stay in a nursing home is about two and a half years.

Residents in nursing homes or *nursing facilities* as they're sometimes called, get a furnished room, meals and snacks, housekeeping and laundry services, and basic medical services such as monitoring and the administration of medications. They also receive supervision and help with their daily activities, usually from nursing assistants who are supervised by *licensed practical nurses* (LPNs). Additional services, such as transportation, physical and occupational therapy, and doctor visits incur additional charges over the basic monthly rate.

Patients who require high-level medical care, such as after a knee replacement, hip fracture, or severe pneumonia are placed in nursing units where registered nurses (RNs), therapists, and rehabilitation specialists can provide for their special medical needs like intravenous therapy, wound care, or aggressive rehabilitation with physical and occupational therapists. Skilled nursing services are more expensive than basic custodial care services.

AARP'S SIGNS OF A BAD NURSING HOME

Not every nursing home is a great place. AARP published the following list of warning signs of a bad nursing home. If you encounter one or more of these negative indications, run, don't walk, out of there and definitely *do not* place your loved one in that facility.

- **Odors:** A strong smell of urine and feces indicates a shortage of staff to help residents to the bathroom or to keep residents and the facility clean.

- **Lack of privacy:** Residents should not be undressed or partly dressed in rooms or hallways in view of guests and other residents. Staff should knock before entering rooms.

- **Lack of dignity:** No resident should be spoken to disrespectfully.

- **Unanswered calls for help:** Every call bell or cry for help should be attended to promptly.

- **Loneliness and inactivity:** People-watching is fun, but residents shouldn't spend hours on end sitting at the nurses' station, front door, or in front of a TV.

- **Lack of help with eating:** Residents who can't feed themselves shouldn't spend mealtime with full trays in front of them.

- **Restraints:** Restraints are no longer allowed in nursing homes so you shouldn't see them in use. Vests and other devices that tie or otherwise hold people down in their beds and wheelchairs are dangerous and humiliating. Good nursing homes seek safe and respectful ways to protect residents from falls and wandering.

Patients who are recovering from major surgery, a serious illness, or severe traumatic injuries may require placement in a *sub-acute unit,* which means that they're not as sick as they were while they were in the hospital, but they're still much frailer and require much more care than residents receiving custodial care in the nursing home.

WARNING

Medicare may pay for some portion of nursing home care, but only if the home is Medicare certified and only under certain qualifying circumstances. Medicare only covers care in a skilled nursing facility that follows a qualifying hospital stay, not custodial care, which is how most nursing home care is classified. If your loved one is financially eligible for state-based Medicaid services and meets the care requirements necessary to justify custodial care, then Medicaid may foot the bill. Otherwise, families that don't have long-term care insurance coverage must pay for their loved ones' nursing home care out of their own pockets.

Nursing homes are the most expensive type of care, costing anywhere from $4,200 to $11,000 a month, depending upon the level of services your loved one requires, your location, and how upscale the nursing home is. If you're considering a nursing home for your loved one, refer to the next section for more information.

TIP

Information on more than 15,000 Medicare- and Medicaid-certified nursing homes is available for comparison on Medicare's website at www.medicare.gov/nursinghomecompare/search.html.

Identifying a Quality Nursing Home

Choosing a nursing home for a parent or relative is as important as choosing a good school for a child. For a school, you probably consider small class sizes, excellence in exam results, and top sporting facilities. You would choose one that checks off most or all of those boxes. Looking for schools is something many people are used to doing, but looking for nursing homes is often virgin territory.

TIP

In order to achieve a successful nursing home placement, you should visit several facilities to see which one you like best and to determine which one would be the best fit for your loved one. Try to schedule at least one visit at night and one on the weekend so you can see how the nursing home performs outside the 9-to-5 timeframe.

The Foundation for Health in Aging website (www.healthinaging.org/resources/resource:eldercare-at-home-choosing-a-nursing-home/) lists the following of what to look for in a nursing home:

>> Is the nursing home clean? Are there any unpleasant smells?

>> Is it well maintained?

>> Do the residents look well cared for? Check to see if the residents are clean and properly dressed. Do they seem content or agitated?

>> Are the rooms adequate?

>> What recreational and private space is available?

>> Are there safety features, such as railings and grab bars and elevated toilet seats?

>> Is the home licensed by the state and certified by Medicaid/ Medicaid?

>> How many nurses and nursing assistants are there compared with the number of residents? This staff ratio is provided for each individual nursing home at www.medicare.gov/nursinghomecompare.

>> Are the administrators accessible to family members actively involved in day-to-day facility operations?

>> Do the medical professionals have special training in geriatrics or long-term care?

>> Are key professionals full time or part time?

>> What type of medical care is provided, including after-hours and on weekends and holidays?

>> How close is the nursing home to family members? How close is it to the nearest hospital?

>> What is the food like? Eat a meal or two to test the quality of the food.

>> How much do basic services cost? What services are covered?

>> What additional services are available? How much do they cost?

>> What happens if a person runs out of money and needs to apply for Medicaid? Does the facility maintain the resident or require discharge?

>> How long have the managers and medical professionals been with the nursing home?

In addition, consider the following when choosing a nursing home:

>> What type of activities does the staff offer residents? Are sufficient activities available, or do most residents just seem to be parked in wheelchairs and staring off into space?

>> Are residents offered appropriate assistance with activities like eating and toileting?

>> Does the staff treat residents with courtesy and compassion, or are they short-tempered? When working with residents, do staff members seem patient or impatient?

REMEMBER

Not all good homes observe all these things, but you need to be satisfied that those items most important to your loved one's care are addressed and provided by the facility your select. The final step before making a decision is checking out the home's reputation (refer to the next section for help).

Assess your loved one's needs and select a nursing home that seems best suited to fulfill those needs. Give the placement at least a month to see whether it's working out, but if you're unhappy with the care or your loved one doesn't like the facility and isn't making a good transition, don't be afraid to change facilities.

Checking the Home's Reputation

In the United States, state government inspectors regularly assess nursing homes to ensure that they meet appropriate standards. Each state has its own set of surveyors, but they all use federal guidelines for evaluating facilities. Thus, they all provide similar reports that you can refer to when checking a potential nursing home's suitability for a relative.

The state surveyors go about their task by

>> Carrying out unannounced inspections

>> Using inspectors typically from health and social services backgrounds

>> Assessing whether the homes are safe, caring, responsive to people's needs, and well managed

>> Speaking with people who live in the homes, as well as their caregivers and staff members

>> Observing what goes on in the homes and interviewing the management teams

If problems are found, the state surveyors issue deficiency citations that the facility is required to correct within a certain period of time. Medicare's Nursing Home Compare website (www.medicare.gov/nursinghomecompare/search.html) allows families to check out facilities. The five-star rating system gives each facility a rating that is determined by a combination of the state survey results, staffing ratios, and quality measures. As with any rating system, not every participant can get 100 percent or five stars, so take the rating system for what it is and include that info in your decision-making process, but don't make it your only criteria. Most important is the facility's reputation among the residents that live there and their families. Understand that just because a facility had a deficiency on a survey or doesn't have a five-star rating doesn't mean that it isn't a good nursing home. Do your homework and investigate what deficiencies were cited and how they were addressed. Was the citation for a critical patient care problem a minor maintenance issue?

WHAT STANDARDS DO REGULATORS LOOK FOR?

To be part of the Medicare and Medicaid programs, nursing homes must meet certain requirements set by Congress. The Centers for Medicare and Medicaid Services (CMS) has entered into an agreement with state governments to do health and fire safety inspections of these nursing homes and investigate complaints about nursing home care. The inspections assess whether the nursing home meets certain minimum standards. Inspections don't identify nursing homes that give outstanding care. Here are some of the standards that are looked at:

- **Proper management of medications:** Whether medications are given on time and in the correct manner.

- **Resident protection from physical and mental abuse:** Assuring that staff and caregivers treat residents with respect.

- **Storage and preparation of food:** Assuring that food is cooked to the proper temperature and prepared in a safe environment.

- **The care of residents and the processes used to give that care:** Facility staff engages in performance improvement projects and develop care processes based on known best practices.

- **The nursing home environment:** Residents live in a clean and uncluttered environment that allows them to live with dignity and safety.

- **Fire safety inspections:** Fire safety specialists evaluate whether a nursing home meets Life Safety Code (LSC) standards set by the National Fire Protection Agency (NFPA). The fire safety inspection covers a wide range of fire protection concerns, including construction, protection, and operational features designed to provide safety from fire, smoke, and panic.

Chapter 15

Easing the Transition to New Surroundings

eciding to place a loved one in a residential facility is one of the most difficult decisions that family members and caregivers have to make. Residential facilities run the gamut of personal care homes, assisted living facilities, and nursing homes. Although it's normal to have concerns about moving your loved one into any of these types of residential facilities, the additional structure that they provide for a person with dementia or Alzheimer's disease (AD) is generally is quite valuable.

After you've decided on the best care setting for your loved one, it's time to help her move and settle in. The more information you can give the new caregivers, the better able they will be able to make the person with dementia or AD feel at home. Your loved one will likely feel unsettled by having to move out of a familiar home into an unfamiliar setting. She may be leaving her own home, which she may have shared with a spouse for many years. Or maybe she's leaving your home if she's been living with you due to care needs. Either way, her surroundings are now different as are the faces of those caring for her. Now she's in an unfamiliar place and will have a lot to get used to that is different from home.

One meaningful change is that other people are sharing this new residence with her. These are new people including other residents and the facility staff that she must get to know. She may be sharing a TV, dining table, and toilet facilities with others for the first time. Even if she has her own room, she'll still have to get used to communal living. This chapter helps you smooth out some of the common bumps in the road that may occur when moving your loved one to a new home.

Helping the Home Care Staff Get to Know Your Loved One

The first thing to do after moving your loved one to a residential facility is to help the manager and staff to get as clear a picture of your loved one as soon as possible. Take time to inform staff members about the person's history and family background, diagnosis, treatment needs, likes and dislikes, personal quirks, and anything else you think they should know to ease the transition for everyone involved.

TIP

The facility staff members will keep a file on each resident containing this sort of information. And no doubt there will be a standard set of questions to be answered during the admission process. But there's no harm in you anticipating the admission process by making a list of things you want to tell them and that they may not think to ask.

Providing important biographical details

The amount of information provided to the staff needs to be somewhere between the sort of things the person may have told a stranger at a dinner party about herself and a printout of her resume. You don't want to leave the staff with any lingering questions about the person, but you don't want to bore them to death with details of how she loved annual trips to San Diego to keep up her shell collection. The following sections examine more closely what types of information to share.

Background and family

"No man is an island, entire of itself," wrote John Donne. Everyone has connections with other people. Everyone has a life story that explains how they got to where they are today. To be able to understand your loved one, staff members need to know where she came from. Caregiving staff will find it useful to have at least the following pieces of information about their new resident:

>> **What she likes to be called:** This detail may seem obvious, but not all Margarets like to be known as Peggy. Maybe her given name is Irene, but she has always been called Marge. She may get really upset when someone calls Irene even though that is what is printed on her Medicare card. So, make sure the staff members know what names or nicknames are preferred to help your loved one feel at ease.

>> **Her age, date of birth, and where she was born:** Remembering someone's birthday is a vital way to show you care, and the staff in the home will want to celebrate her birthday each year. Doing so makes her feel special. It helps her to know that her new caregivers have a genuine interest in her.

>> **Where she's moved from and why:** Numerous reasons may account for the person moving into the residential facility. Maybe she is unable to live safely at home any longer. Maybe her needs are becoming too much for a family caregiver to manage. Maybe she needs short-term rehabilitation after a hospital stay for a sudden illness. Maybe her family caregivers just need a temporary respite so they can have a vacation. Knowing the reason for the move helps the staff ease her transition. And remember, if your loved one has moved to residential care because you were struggling to look after her at home, the staff can support you in your decision as well.

>> **Whether she's been married, and if so, whether her spouse is still alive:** If her spouse is living, will her spouse be visiting? Or has her spouse recently died? Knowing when her partner died helps the home anticipate when she may be sad, withdrawn, or perhaps a bit touchy. Maybe she has a same-sex partner or spouse who is involved. Help the staff members to know the personal relationships important to your loved one so they can better understand and support your loved one.

>> **Who's who in the family:** Identify who may visit. Highlight the person who has power of attorney and any tricky relationships that exist within the family. Be sure the staff members know whom to call in the event of an emergency. In most homes, they may ask for the family to select a "responsible party" meaning the one person will be notified in the event that any issues arise with your loved one during her stay.

>> **Previous occupation and military service, if applicable:** Some dates or situations may trigger specific emotions and memories. Seeing TV footage of battles or soldiers may bring back difficult memories for veterans who saw military action. Tell staff members what your loved one did for a living. Knowing a person's prior work can help new caregivers make her feel comfortable. A former homemaker may like to fold towels. A former journalist may still like to read the newspaper even if she doesn't remember what she read.

>> **The names and species of past and present pets:** Possibly she's had to leave beloved dog or cat behind and would greatly appreciate having them visit. Or she may talk about deceased pets as though they're still alive.

>> **Drinking and smoking habits:** Just because someone's older and has dementia doesn't mean that she doesn't drink alcoholic beverages. Maybe she's used to having a glass of wine with dinner each night. Certain assisted living facilities and most nursing homes don't allow alcoholic beverages, so check this out ahead of time. If the staff members know about her alcohol consumption, they can anticipate and deal with this issue.

Likewise, if the person smokes and smoking isn't allowed indoors, she may need regular supervised trips outside for a puff to avoid withdrawal symptoms and associated irritability. Some facilities don't allow smoking at all (including on the grounds), so this may be the time she has to give up cigarettes. Sharing this information is essential to share with staff members because they may be able to arrange medication to assist her to avoid the issues of quitting cold turkey.

Likes and dislikes

Although residential facilities or nursing homes can't cater to absolutely every one of their residents' dietary likes and dislikes, it certainly helps them to know if a certain food makes a person feel sick and what she particularly enjoys for a special occasion. Likewise, if they know about a person's interests, they can plan trips and activities that may at least tickle most people's fancies.

Do tell the home's staff about the person's

>> **Favorite food and drink:** Supplement this information with details of things she absolutely can't bear and any allergies or special dietary requirements she has. Many facilities can cater to special diets, such as those for people with celiac disease or diabetes. Some facilities prepare meals suitable for people of different religious faiths especially if a large number of people of that faith reside there.

>> **Her hobbies:** Maybe your loved one has always liked painting or knitting. Maybe she'd enjoy gardening or doing crafts. Many homes have gardens that residents are free to putter around in and craft time.

>> **Musical tastes and dislikes:** If someone fails to show up to see a jazz band playing in the activity room, the staff members will find it helpful to know that the person isn't ill or being moody, but simply doesn't like that type of music.

>> **TV programs and films she enjoys watching and those she doesn't:** Such information may help explain why she starts shouting when football comes on or she flips the channel to watch the latest hit crime series instead.

>> **Sleeping habits:** Is she an early bird or a night owl? Does she require a special pillow or bed position?

>> **Wandering habits:** Does she have a tendency to wander? If she tends to wander or has been known to leave home and get lost, telling the staff is essential. If so, staff members need to be extra vigilant to avoid *elopement* (meaning your loved one leaves the facility without staff knowledge). Many facilities have special bracelets that alarm if the wanderer tries to leave the building so staff members can make sure that residents don't get outside unattended.

>> **Things that always make her upset or happy:** Let staff members know if certain circumstance upset her, like if she throws a tantrum at shower time. Tell the staff the best way to cheer her up if she's grumpy.

>> **Her religious beliefs, if any:** Inform the staff if someone is a member of a local church, mosque, or synagogue, along with the name of the clergy person. A member of the congregation may be able to pick up and take the person to services each week. If that's the case, the staff members need advance notice to get the person ready in time. Some facilities offer religious services in-house with visiting clergy. Tell the staff if you think your loved one would enjoy attending these services.

Covering medical details

Although medical notes usually accompany new residents to the facility, if they're transferring from a hospital, the staff members need additional medical information that often isn't covered in the hospital notes. The facility staff members rely on relatives to bring them up to speed with the most relevant parts of the new resident's medical history.

REMEMBER

Your loved one is suffering from memory loss and won't be able to remember enough to tell her medical history accurately to the staff, which is why it's so important for you to make sure her medical records come to the facility and you fill in the gaps from your own knowledge of her health history. If she is coming from home rather than the hospital, ask her primary care physician and any specialists to send copies of their records to the facility for continuity of medical care. Doing so is necessary even if she'll have the same doctor in the facility as she did in the community because it helps the facility staff learn her background.

REMEMBER

Getting medical records requires a written release to be signed by the resident or her power of attorney. In general, there is no cost for this service if the hospital or doctor's office is sending or faxing the medical records directly to the facility for continuity of care. However, realize that many hospitals and physician offices now charge by the page to provide medical records directly to patients or families. So, you may want to avoid this expense by having the records transferred directly to the facility.

Ongoing medical conditions

Even with medical records from the hospital or physician's office, the facility staff will want to know details of your loved one's medical history and what health issues she currently has, including

>> Allergies to any food or medications

>> Arthritic joints, which may be painful and affect mobility

>> Bowel troubles from simple indigestion and constipation to stomach ulcers or inflammatory bowel diseases such as ulcerative colitis or Crohn's disease

>> Breathing problems such as asthma, bronchitis, or chronic obstructive pulmonary disease (COPD)

>> Cancer history, including surgical and chemotherapy treatments

>> Diabetes

>> Hearing problems (if she wears hearing aids, make sure she has them there to use to maximize communication)

>> Heart disease, including angina, high blood pressure, heart failure, or a history of heart attacks

>> Mental health conditions (on top of their dementia) such as anxiety, depression, or bipolar disorder

>> Neurological conditions such as Parkinson's disease, epilepsy, headaches or migraines, strokes, or ministrokes

>> Skin conditions like eczema, dermatitis, psoriasis, skin cancer, or leg ulcers

>> Visual difficulties (if she wears glasses to help her see, make sure she has them there to wear)

>> Rare or unusual conditions that aren't covered by the preceding items in this list

>> A complete list of all past surgeries

>> A complete list of past medical problems including prior hospital admissions

Providing this information to the facility staff members helps them to monitor your loved one's health and to address any issues that arise. Such information is especially important for the in-house attending physician who will care for her in the assisted living or nursing home setting.

Pills and prescriptions

If they're going to be dishing out pills and applying creams from the person's regular prescription list, the caregivers obviously need to know exactly what's on that list. They also need to understand which medicines are to be given daily regardless of symptoms and which are prescribed for use as needed when a problem exists.

The primary care physician's office can provide a printout detailing all current medications to give to the facility staff. Be sure to tell the staff members if your loved one is taking other over-the-counter medications, herbal supplements, or vitamins that may not be on the doctor's medication list.

In personal care homes or assisted living facilities, you may be able to (or be required to) provide your loved one's prescriptions and over-the-counter medications for the staff to administer. In other facilities including all nursing homes, the in-house pharmacy will assume responsibility for providing the medications for the staff to administer to your loved one. Be sure you ask what process the facility follows.

Identifying who's already involved in care

If the person with the memory disorder has moved to a residential facility in a new area, knowing what professionals have been involved in the person's care isn't so important for the facility staff because her supporting medical team will probably change due to distance. (But in this instance, be sure that you arrange to have medical records from these providers sent to the facility for use by the new care team). However, if the residential facility is nearby where the person has been living and she's not changing doctors, give the staff the following information:

>> The primary care physician's name, to ensure continuity of care, along with the name of another doctor at the practice whom the person may request to see if the first physician is unavailable

>> The name and location of the person's dentist, podiatrist, optometrist, dietician, physical therapist, or speech and language therapist, if applicable

>> The name and contact details of the social worker or care manager who has coordinated the person's care

All nursing homes and some assisted living facilities have specific attending doctors on staff members who provide care for residents of that facility. Usually the resident or family is asked to select one of these attending physicians from a list at the time of admission. That physician (or sometimes their nurse practitioner or physician assistant) will provide the medical care for your loved one at the facility. Shortly after admission, this doctor will see your loved one for an admission history and physical. Then the doctor will make periodic medical visits for regular follow-up or to address acute issues. If your loved one is admitted to the nursing home at night or on a weekend or holiday, realize that it may be a covering doctor that provides the initial medical evaluation because the selected attending physician may not be on-call.

Most of the time, care from specialist physicians (such as cardiologists or neurologists) will require you to arrange to bring your loved one to their offices for appointments. Sometimes, the assisted living facility or nursing home arranges to have a podiatrist, audiologist, or dentist come to the facility once every few months to tend to residents there as a convenience, but this isn't always the case. If there isn't an in-house physician at all, such as in some assisted living facilities, then you'll need to arrange to bring your loved one to the primary care physician's office to be seen for regular appointments.

REMEMBER

Let the staff members know there are any pending follow-up appointments scheduled with these medical professionals so they can make sure your loved one is ready in time to go to the appointment. Be sure that you tell them if you'll be taking your loved one to these appointments. If the facility needs to set up transportation and arrange a staff member to accompany her to the appointment, then arrangements must be made in advance. Note that such services may involve added expense, so be sure you discover the details ahead of time.

Visiting Regularly

Many people fear that when they're "put in a home," their family and friends will neglect them and they'll be forgotten about. Sometimes relatives defend their lack of visits to elderly relatives by saying, "Well, they don't know whether I've been in or not, so it doesn't matter how often I go."

Even though your loved one has memory loss, she may well remember whether you've put in an appearance and be upset if you don't turn up for months. And even if she doesn't remember whether or not you have visited, the staff members do. Possibly, you're worn out from serving as the main caregiver and see the person's admission to a residential facility as the green light for some well-earned rest. That's understandable. However, don't leave extended periods between visits, especially when the person is getting used to a new environment. Your visits may be just what she needs to help her settle in. These visits also can give you peace of mind, knowing that she's well looked after and happy. Plus, even a person with memory loss may retain emotional memory, so enjoying a visit may leave her feel happy, even if she doesn't remember why. Remember, a person may not recall an event, but she may remember how it made her feel.

Your visits can be ad hoc to fit your own schedule, but given the benefit of routine for people with dementia, visiting on set days is probably a good idea if you can manage it. Involving other members of the family is also beneficial, especially grandchildren, who are likely to bring a lot of pleasure to the person with dementia or AD.

TIP

Tell the person's friends where she's living and encourage them to visit too. Receiving old friends in this new environment will make it feel more like home for your loved one. The friends may also be able to take the person out for a walk or to lunch if she's still able to get in a car.

Residential facilities aren't scary places to visit and aren't intended to feel like prisons to their residents. Bring in familiar things from the person's previous home, such as favorite books, family photos, and other objects that may help her reminisce and feel at home.

Try to visit regularly and to make the person's life more interesting by taking her out on trips if she's up to it. Or bring in a special homemade dish that she really likes to share with you during a visit. Such efforts can help your loved one get used to her new surroundings.

Taking Part in Care and Activities in the Home

Research suggests that good relationships play a vital role in improving the quality of life of people with dementia living in residential facilities. Good relationships cover those with other residents, facility staff, family, and friends are all important. Even people with severe dementia have been shown to benefit from building and maintaining these relationships.

When you visit the facility, don't just make a quick visit every time — try to hang around and participate in activities with her. Such involved visits improve mood and reduce anxiety of the person you're visiting. Residents who have been surveyed say that an engaged visit improves their feeling of hope. This level of involvement also helps you get to know the staff better.

In order not to get under the feet of the staff members when they're most busy, avoid visiting at bathing and dressing times. As you get to know your loved one's schedule, you can get involved in the following kinds of activities:

>> Social hours

>> Visits from entertainers

>> Trips out for the day

>> Knitting or sewing groups

>> Music therapy

>> Exercise classes

>> Mealtimes

>> Palliative care at the end of life

TIP

As you spend time with your loved one in the care facility, you'll meet and interact with many staff members. The more often you're at the facility, the better you'll get to know them, and you'll also see how they interact with and treat your loved one. For those staff members who go above and beyond the call of duty or those who treat their patients with special care, consider doing something to show your appreciation. Bring in cookies or donuts for the staff. Buy flowers for their desk, write a thank-you note, or look them in the eye, say thank you for all that they do, and give them a hug. Little kindnesses on your part toward the staff will likely be returned to you, which can go a long way to making your loved one's transition easier for you.

Acting as an Advocate If Problems Occur

By visiting regularly and taking an active part in some of the facilities activities (see the preceding section), you send a clear message to the person with dementia or AD that even though she has moved into a residential facility, she's never far from your mind.

You may also notice things that you're not happy with regarding the way your loved one is treated or the way the facility is run. By visiting, you'll be more available for your loved one to tell you about issues that perhaps annoy or upset her too. Some people don't want to make a fuss; they stiffen their upper lip and put up with the upsetting situation. But given some recent high-profile news reports of treatment of residents in U.S. residential facilities and nursing homes, you know that mistreatment of residents can occur. Hence, you need to be vigilant.

Thankfully, cases of resident mistreatment and neglect are rare. Regular inspections by state surveyors in facilities throughout the United States mean they're likely to become even less frequent. People who choose to work in residential and nursing homes are generally extremely patient, kind, and caring individuals who do a physically and emotionally demanding job to the best of their ability.

REMEMBER

People with dementia are vulnerable and need others to speak up for them. Little difficulties can become significant problems if such people can't speak for themselves and nobody is looking out for them. That is why it's so important for you to serve as an advocate for your loved one.

Considering typical problems

Problems affecting your loved one at a residential facility can be of a physical, emotional, psychological, or even environmental nature. Some particular areas for concern are

>> **Level of personal care:** Are people in clean clothes? Are they changed quickly if they have incontinence accidents or food or beverage spills? Do they have regular baths and showers?

>> **Quality and quantity of food:** Does everyone get their fair share at mealtimes? Are decent portions offered? Do the meals vary? Are residents helped to the dining table if needed? Is food cut up if necessary? Is food taken to residents' rooms if they're feeling ill? Are they assisted at meals or spoon-fed if they're unable to feed themselves?

>> **Cleanliness:** Are bathrooms thoroughly cleaned? Does the home smell of urine? Does the housekeeping staff keep the floors clean?

>> **Staff professionalism:** Do staff members behave appropriately and professionally at all times or are they rude to residents or even neglectful? Do they talk over or about residents without acknowledging them? Do they address residents respectfully?

>> **Resident behavior:** Do people seem happy and relaxed, or are they stressed, anxious, and uncomfortable in their surroundings?

If you find yourself providing a few negative responses to these questions, you need to share your concerns with someone in authority to make sure they're addressed swiftly and appropriately.

SOURCES OF SUPPORT WHEN MAKING A COMPLAINT

Complaining isn't something (most) people do lightly, and the process can be difficult and stressful. The following organizations provide advice and support on navigating complaints processes:

- You can file a complaint with your state survey agency. For more information, go to www.medicare.gov/NursingHomeCompare/Resources/State-Websites.html.

- Locate an ombudsman at http://theconsumervoice.org/get_help or http://ltcombudsman.org. An *ombudsman* is an individual who serves as a liaison between you and the residential facility. An ombudsman investigates your complaint and brings it to the attention of higher authorities (such as state regulatory and licensing agencies) as necessary to get a resolution. The ombudsman serves as the advocate for facility residents and their families protecting resident rights and working to assure residents get good care.

Making a complaint

If you have concerns about your loved one's care in the facility or the condition of the home itself, speak to an administrator, head nurse, or other staff member informally at first. An honest conversation is often the simplest (and least stressful) way to deal with things. But if your concerns aren't dealt with to your satisfaction, a formal complaint is necessary.

TIP

You can express your complaint in writing (in a letter or email) or verbally (over the phone or in person). If you lodge your complaint verbally, make a written note of what's said, who took part in the conversation, and the date the conversation took place.

Escalating the complaint

If you make a complaint and it's brushed aside, or not dealt with to your satisfaction by the residential facility staff and management, then you have to move your complaint to a higher level. The best approach is to contact your state ombudsman's office. You should consider doing this if you have complaints about any of the following issues:

>> Poor-quality care

>> Financial concerns

>> Poor complaint handling

>> Unsatisfactory care needs assessment

>> Resident safety

You can also contact your state health department and file a complaint through the state survey agency. Depending on the severity of the complaint, this may initiate a *complaint survey* in which state surveyors come to the facility to investigate directly the issue to see if it's warranted and if so, to require the facility to make necessary changes to address the problem.

Of course, if you're really unhappy about the care someone has received, you can seek advice from an attorney. However, dealing with the residential facility management directly and/or involving an ombudsman are both more likely to resolve the situation to the benefit of your loved one and other residents who may have similar concerns. The services of the ombudsman are free, so you can therefore avoid the cost of pursuing legal action.

4

Respite Care for the Caregiver

IN THIS CHAPTER

Understanding that caregiving is hard work

Looking at the emotional and physical costs of caregiving

Making time for yourself

Asking for help

Chapter 16

Coping While Caregiving

t's difficult to comprehend the mind and body-numbing exhaustion a person can experience when confronted with the multiple responsibilities of caring for someone with dementia or Alzheimer's disease (AD). Caring for a dementia or AD patient can literally be a 24-hour-a-day job. If you don't develop a good support system early on, serving as a family caregiver can damage both your mental and physical health, divide your family, and even hurt your career. Caregiving has also been associated with lowered immune system functioning and increased mortality.

While serving as a family caregiver, you easily can overlook your own needs and the needs of others who depend on you (but who aren't as dependent on you as your patient). You can get caught up in the cycle of endless demands and crises and lose sight of the other important things in your life, which may lead to burnout. You'll have days when you wish you could clone yourself because you don't know how you're ever going to get everything done. All this responsibility weighs heavily and can eventually exact a high toll. Caregiver burnout leaves everyone in the lurch and only adds to the feelings of overload, failure, and isolation you may be experiencing. Your burnout is also a source of distress for your loved one and can trigger behavioral problems and frustrations for him.

In this chapter, you discover the ways that caregiving can impact you and some smart ideas to help you cope. You discover the importance of taking time for yourself and some good ways to lift your spirits when you're having a tough time. We also cover the special considerations involved in caring for a parent or a spouse. You also see how isolating yourself from your normal support system can lead to trouble.

Caregiving Is Hard Work

When you first take on the role of caregiver, you may have misgivings or you may feel confident that you can handle the job no matter what. After a few weeks of on-the-job experience, you'll probably see things more realistically. Even if you feel up to the job, you can't get around the fact that taking care of a cognitively impaired adult is one of the hardest things you'll ever do.

The United States has an escalating trend toward community-based care rather than institutional-based care for aging seniors. As a result, family members and friends increasingly are providing informal caregiving for the growing number of American elderly. According to the Family Caregiver Alliance (www.caregiver.org), as of February, 2015, 43.5 million Americans were providing informal caregiving for someone age 50 years or older. Of these caregivers, 14.9 million were caring for someone with AD or other dementia.

TIP

Numerous studies point to caregiver attitude as a predictor of stress level and burnout. If you have a positive outlook and remain calm, you're less likely to suffer from depression and other health problems than caregivers with negative attitudes who see themselves as overburdened by responsibilities. Respite care isn't a luxury or an option; it's a critical part of good caregiving.

You can avoid caregiver stress, burnout, and other potential problems if you take good care of yourself. Try the following strategies:

>> Confront your feelings head-on and deal with them before they boil over.

>> Be kind to yourself, get help, and schedule time off.

>> Acknowledge that what you're doing is very hard work; don't try to pretend it's nothing.

>> Realize that it's not all sheer drudgery.

If you can manage the balancing act, caregiving can pay off in a big way psychologically, giving you the satisfaction of performing a compassionate service for someone you love. Some caregivers report learning more about their own strengths as a result of caregiving. They may find that they are better problem solvers; have stronger organization and management skills; and are more flexible, tolerant, resilient, nurturing, and affectionate than they thought possible. Perhaps these attributes were always there but went unrecognized or unappreciated until the person became a caregiver.

Considering the Challenges of Caregiving

The challenges involved in being a caregiver for someone with dementia are many, varied, and ever changing as time goes on. And millions of people are facing these challenges around the clock, every single day.

Look at this anecdote: When Sadie first developed dementia at age 80, her 55 year-old daughter helped care for her. It wasn't an easy task. As Sadie became less independent, her daughter needed to do more for her. She cleaned Sadie's house to keep it clean and tidy the way she knew her mother would like it. As Sadie became more forgetful and anxious, the frequency of her phone calls to her daughter increased. Sadie would ask her daughter the same questions again and again, day after day and night after night.

Sadie became more frightened about what was happening. Her personality simultaneously changed: She became increasingly aggressive. Her daughter bore the brunt of it, often being shouted at in shops when Sadie became muddled and confused, and once even being shoved into a wall as they walked down the street. Fortunately, Sadie's daughter loved her mother dearly and was only too happy to reciprocate for the care she'd received while she was growing up.

But the job was a difficult one and it kept getting harder, because the goalposts constantly moved. Just as Sadie's daughter felt that she'd got the hang of dealing with her mother's behavior, either Sadie's behavior would change or she would respond differently to her daughter's attempts to help. As her role became increasingly challenging, Sadie's daughter began to find her mother annoying. She resented having to get a bus across town to see her a couple of times a week only to be shouted at when she arrived — and then felt extremely guilty as a result.

Ultimately, Sadie had to go into a nursing home, and her daughter felt guilty and stressed about that decision too.

The following sections examine the stress and guilt often associated with caregiving and what you can do to help alleviate them.

Caregiving and stress

Most people become stressed in any situation where they feel they have little control over what's going on. And although some stress is thought to be good, prolonged and persistently high levels of stress can be bad for your health. Adrenaline, the *fight-or-flight hormone*, is responsible for creating this sensation. When you're stressed and feel under threat, the adrenal glands release more adrenaline into the blood stream to prepare your body to either fight it out or flee.

Even though a regular shot of adrenaline was useful for early humans thousands of years ago who regularly needed to run from marauding saber-toothed cats, it's not so helpful when you're helping a person with dementia. As a caregiver helping your loved one get dressed, changing her soiled sheets for the tenth time in a day, or finding her when she's gone wandering, you don't need the increased levels of adrenaline that results from this stress.

Examining the effects of stress

In the short term, excessive adrenaline produces the symptoms you're probably familiar with as the time for an important exam or a job interview approaches: a sick feeling, a frequent urge to go to the bathroom, butterflies in the stomach, a racing pulse, a tight throat, and an inability to catch your breath.

In highly stressful situations such as caregiving, high levels of adrenaline and its close compatriot, the hormone noradrenaline, can produce a range of unwanted physical and emotional symptoms:

>> **Physical symptoms:** These include tension headaches that radiate up from the back of the neck and make the skull feel as though it's in a vise; heart palpitations; nausea; daily bowel upset, ranging from chronic constipation to abdominal pains and diarrhea; and widespread bodily aches and pains that aren't the result of injury or overexertion. Over the long term, blood pressure may rise, leading to an increased risk of heart attack and stroke. It's not uncommon for people experiencing unrelenting stress-related physical symptoms to start to believe they're actually seriously ill, possibly with cancer. Doctors frequently encounter such patients seeking reassurance.

>> **Emotional symptoms:** Long-term stress can play havoc with someone's mental health. Depression and anxiety are common and can lead to a whole range of other emotional responses, such as anger, irritability, sleep problems (insomnia or excessive tiredness), changes in appetite (going off food altogether and losing weight, or comfort eating and piling on the pounds), loss of interest in life (hobbies, socializing, reading, television), poor concentration for even the simplest tasks, reduced sex drive, and even suicidal thoughts.

Depression and anxiety can also lead to alcohol or drug abuse and increased cigarette consumption. And stress and anxiety are the most common reasons for work absenteeism in the United States.

Recognizing the types of stress that caregivers experience

Research has shown that the stress experienced by caregivers differs according to the type of dementia the person they're caring for is suffering from and the particular symptoms she's exhibiting. According to a 2012 study, caregivers report the following:

» Looking after people with Lewy body disease and frontotemporal dementia is more stressful than caring for people with AD or vascular dementia.

» Psychiatric symptoms such as hallucinations, depression, anxiety, and apathy in the person with dementia are a particular cause of stress.

» Fluctuations in the cared-for person's cognitive symptoms (unpredictability) are more stressful than a steady deterioration in memory and ability to plan.

» The person with dementia's age and gender and the degree of impairment in relation to carrying out activities of daily living and mobility are less likely predictors of caregiver stress than these factors.

Dealing with guilt

Many caregivers feel a sense of guilt when they're looking after loved ones with dementia. This feeling can arise for a variety of reasons, but can be dealt with when it's acknowledged.

Everyone is different, and depending on your personality, you may feel guilty about some thoughts, feelings, and failures and not about others. Perfectionists probably feel guilty about anything that falls below the tough high standards they set for themselves, whereas those with a more relaxed attitude probably cope better when things don't go as well. Caregiving is a tough role whatever your personality, but particularly so if you're looking after the person with dementia 24 hours a day.

Caregivers feel guilty for a whole range of reasons, including

» **Comparison with other caregivers:** Evolution has made humanity a competitive species. From school days onwards, you're encouraged to compare yourself with others. Doing so as caregivers isn't helpful, though. Other people may appear to be doing a better job, but that doesn't mean they actually are. They're likely to be experiencing their own struggles, doubts, and guilty feelings.

>> **Negative feelings toward the person being cared for:** People with dementia can be aggressive, demanding — and dirty. Caring for someone who smells, is wearing dirty clothing, looks grubby, and — worst of all — is incontinent, sometimes doubly so, is very difficult. Caregivers may feel a sense of disgust, swiftly followed by guilt. Couple that with challenging or embarrassing behavior, and the caregiver may find it difficult to like, let alone love, the person they're caring for.

>> **Emotional baggage from the past:** Not all caregivers share a rosy history with the person they're caring for. Possibly, they feel guilty because they didn't pick up on the person's early symptoms quickly enough and were impatient and cross with her as a result. Maybe the caregiver treated the person with dementia as if she was crazy, muddled, and intentionally annoying rather than unwell.

Even further back, maybe the caregiver has always had a troubled relationship with the person with dementia or AD. Maybe the person was a poor, neglectful, or abusive parent. Seeing that person become helpless and vulnerable can stir up all sorts of emotions, particularly about the caregiver's feelings toward her.

>> **Feelings of failure when the caregiver can't manage alone:** Accepting help from others can be difficult, and people often feel guilty when they can no longer cope alone and have to call in the professionals. This guilt is invariably magnified if the person with dementia ends up in an assisted living facility or nursing home. Sometimes the guilt arises from caregivers' personal beliefs that they should do more and therefore shouldn't need such help. Other times, the guilt can bubble up because of pride and the notion that others will think badly of them if they relinquish daily care to paid caregivers in a care facility.

>> **Feeling trapped:** Trying to fit caring on top of a job, family responsibilities, socializing, and a sex life can be extremely stressful. Caring can understandably engender feelings of resentment and entrapment, followed by guilt.

>> **Needing time out:** You probably know of caregivers who desperately need a break but feel so guilty about leaving the person with dementia on her own or with someone else even for an evening that they don't take any time to recharge their own batteries. For these individuals, taking time for themselves can make them feel so guilt ridden that they push themselves to the point of exhaustion. They plod on without a break — benefiting no one and ultimately hurting themselves and the person they're caring for.

TIP

If you recognize any of these guilty feelings, you first need to acknowledge that they're normal, and not just in relation to caring but in pretty much all aspects of life and in many relationships. Second, rather than bottling them up, you need to offload those feelings by sharing them with others. Consider talking to a good friend, a sibling, other caregivers (who'll inevitably feel just like you!), your physician, a specialist nurse, your religious leader, or a counselor. Finally, work out ways to create some time for yourself. Doing so isn't selfish, and you're not letting down the person you're looking after. In fact, recharging your batteries means you'll be better able to care for the person afterward than if you'd soldiered on in a state of exhaustion, your guilty feelings intact.

Fearing the loss of your loved one

One of the most natural and immediate fears you face when you hear that a loved one has dementia is your worry over his or her impending death. No one, not even the doctor, can predict how long your loved one will live or how the dementia will progress. The best thing you can do is not to dwell on the idea of loss, but rather make the most of the life you now share with your loved one. Try to find some special moment in each and every day, particularly in the months and years before memory worsens.

REMEMBER

The sad truth about dementia or AD is that you actually lose your loved one long before he or she dies. Many of the ways you recognize someone you love — the funny stories, crooked smile, or infectious laugh — slip away long before death comes. The most difficult thing to deal with is the day you realize that your loved one no longer knows or recognizes you on a consistent basis.

If you're having trouble dealing with this aspect of a memory disorder, seek out a caregiver's support group or some individual counseling to help you cope.

Watching memory slip away

Problems with learning new information, new routines, and new tasks precede memory problems, which make up the hallmark symptom and often most recognizable sign of dementia and AD. Dealing with memory loss can be one of the most trying aspects of caring for a patient with a memory disorder, because he or she will ask the same questions over and over and over again and tell the same stories, word for word, without even knowing it.

TIP

Try to keep your humor and patience about you and take everything in stride. Keep in mind that dementia patients can't help their behavior; they're not misplacing their dentures and asking you the same question repeatedly to annoy you; they're doing it because they can't remember, and their minds are stuck in a sort of endless loop.

Although medication may slow the progress of cognitive loss, don't lose sight of the fact that dementia is still an incurable disease. Inevitably, your loved one's memory loss will worsen, and that will make taking care of him or her more challenging.

Fearing that he will forget who you are

Dementia patients progress in different ways. A rare few may have trouble recognizing their family and friends relatively soon after their diagnosis; others may recognize them for far longer. It depends upon how far along they are in the course of the condition when they're diagnosed.

Although some patients completely fail to recognize their relatives and friends at some point late in the course of the disease, others continue to recognize them as relatives or at least friendly faces, even if they're not exactly sure of names and relationships. Don't be surprised if your loved one (who may be your parent) thinks that you're her mother (despite her mother having died 30 years prior). Don't take offense at this confusion, which is unintentional and due to the dementia.

REMEMBER

Don't be discouraged if your loved one seems afraid of you or treats you like a stranger. She's afraid because she doesn't know who you are and is thus unsure of your intentions toward her. Be calm, approach her slowly, and speak softly and reassuringly. Remember that she's acting out of fear and uncertainty and that it's nothing personal directed at you. It's just part of the process of dementia or Alzheimer's disease.

Building a new relationship

Even if your loved one no longer recognizes you, you can still build a new relationship. If he's living in a long-term care facility, frequent short and pleasant visits may help him to associate your presence with periods of relaxation and fun. If your loved one is still in your home, don't just leave him or her isolated in a room; bring the loved one out to the family room where he or she can be part of the ebb and flow of family life.

TIP

Try appealing to the five senses to associate your presence with good feelings. Bring a flower for the loved one to smell, provide some homemade cookies to snack on, or bring a small stuffed animal that he or she can hold. Hold your loved one's hands and give lots of hugs and kisses. Let your loved one know that you think he or she is special and loved.

This sort of sensory stimulation can go a long way toward helping you build a new sort of relationship with your loved one. He or she may not remember exactly who you are, but your loved one will happily accept the visit of that nice woman who always has a hug or a smile, or a rose in her pocket.

Worrying about your loved one

Alzheimer's disease and dementia bring with them a specific list of cognitive symptoms and variable behavioral symptoms, and all the worrying in the world isn't going to change that. Although it's natural to worry about your loved one and want the best for him or her, spending too much time worrying can actually have a negative effect on your ability to provide care — not to mention that the stress of too much worry can have a damaging effect on your own health.

TIP

You can't do anything to change a diagnosis of a memory disorder, but you can make sure that your loved one feels supported and is living life as fully as possible. You can make sure he or she has good care and good food and the correct dosage of medication at the right time. You can help your loved one fulfill his or her needs for socialization and stimulation. You can see to it that your loved one stays pleasantly occupied and that his or her living quarters are free from any obvious hazards, such as throw rugs or matches. You can take steps to make sure your loved one doesn't have access to household poisons or sharp objects, such as knives or scissors.

Worrying about yourself and your family

Don't feel selfish if you're worried about yourself and your family. Taking care of a chronically ill person, particularly someone with a condition like AD or dementia, can be a frustrating experience for a family. You and your family will have to work extra hard to maintain your relationships and to make sure you don't let your loved one's condition take over your entire lives.

You may go through times when you feel isolated, particularly if you're the sole caregiver. At other times, financial worries will crowd into your tired head, or in a state of exhaustion, you may worry that your life will never be the same.

REMEMBER

Hundreds of thousands of families have lived through this ordeal, and you and your family can do it as well — and perhaps even come out stronger on the other side. Remember to keep the lines of communication open and share whatever is bothering you. If you do start to feel completely overwhelmed, reach out for help from your church, friends, or the community. You don't have to go it alone.

BEING A "GOOD ENOUGH" CAREGIVER

No one's super-human; you can only ever do your best. Although this revelation shouldn't be seen as an excuse to drop your standards, it's nonetheless reassuring to know that being "good enough" still means you're doing a good job.

British pediatrician and psychoanalyst Donald Winnicott (1896–1971) developed the concept of "good enough" during his work with mothers and their babies in the 1950s. He wanted to reassure these women that falling short sometimes is fine and striving for perfection is merely frustrating. According to Winnicott, a "good enough" mother does her best to give her baby appropriate attention, physical care, and emotional support and creates a safe environment in which her child can develop independence. She's not a quitter, and when she fails at something, which she inevitably does, she gets right back in the saddle and gives it another go. In short, she demonstrates a sacrificial love that makes allowances for getting things wrong. This concept allows mothers to acknowledge feeling resentful about the stress of their role and having to put their own needs to one side in order to look after their baby, all for very little thanks. It also allows them to be annoyed with their baby at times without subsequently feeling that they're bad mothers.

This concept can clearly be applied to everyone who has a hands-on role as a caregiver. Caregivers can never perform the role perfectly, and at times they'll feel angry, frustrated, and resentful. They'll do some things badly and forget to do others. But most of the time, their desire to do their best means that things will be fine and the person they're looking after will be safe and well cared for and know that she's loved.

If you're a caregiver for someone with dementia, take Dr Winnicott's wisdom to heart and recognize that being a "good enough" caregiver is good enough.

Looking At the Emotional Effects of Caregiving

People react to behavior caused by severe memory loss in many different ways. It can bring out your best or your worst. You may become angry and take your feelings out on your loved one. You may feel helpless and depressed. Or you may be broken-hearted, grieving for what you have lost, for what AD or dementia has taken from you and your loved one. Or you may feel strong and composed, burdened but not overburdened. In fact, you may feel all these emotions to varying degrees.

REMEMBER

In a 1999 study, researchers found that the more hours of care a person provides and the more problem behaviors her loved one demonstrates, the higher the caregiver's risk for depression and burnout. However, caregivers who had a good relationship with the person they were caring for, good emotional support, and a high level of confidence in their own abilities were less likely to experience burnout, even if their patients exhibited difficult behaviors.

The following studies explain how you can handle these negative emotions and how you can cope with your changing relationship with your loved one so you can reach some serenity in your life.

Dealing with negative emotions

Your attitude toward your caregiving responsibilities depends on many factors, including the following:

» Your personality

» Your relationship with the person you're caring for, both in the past and in the present

» Whether you volunteered for the job or were recruited by circumstances beyond your control

» Who else is depending on you for support and care (including other family members including children)

» The amount of support you seek and receive

» Your competing occupational responsibilities

REMEMBER

If you find yourself dwelling on negative thoughts or feelings, deal with them as soon as possible to keep them from spiraling out of control. If you do experience a crisis of negative emotions, it could seriously impact your own health and lead you to abuse your loved one in some way. The following sections give you tips for dealing with some specific negative feelings.

Anger and frustration

Anger and frustration are usually a result of feeling put-upon, as if the whole situation were just plopped in your lap without anyone asking your opinion. A common source of anger for adult children of dementia and AD patients is the sense that the caregiving responsibilities aren't equally divided, they don't feel that their other siblings do enough. If you're angry, get those feelings under control because angry caretakers can trigger aggressive behavior from dementia patients.

You're more likely to experience anger if

>> The caretaking role was thrust upon you.

>> You have or have had a difficult relationship with the person you're caring for.

>> You're isolated and don't have the support of other family members or friends to help you shoulder the burden of caregiving.

>> Your loved one exhibits difficult behaviors, such as irritability or repetitive questioning, or if he resists your efforts to help care for him.

Here are some steps to take if your negative emotions start to overwhelm you:

>> **Get help for your anger.** Talk to a therapist, enroll in an anger management course, or talk to your spiritual advisor. Don't let your anger fester and build until it explodes in a crisis situation.

>> **Join a support group.** Joining a support group for dementia caregivers gives you a healthy outlet for your anger and the opportunity to be heard and feel validated. As an added bonus, other members of the group are likely to have good suggestions for handling angry feelings based on firsthand experience. (See more about support groups in Chapter 17.)

>> **Don't isolate yourself.** Caregivers with the angriest feelings are often those who feel cut off from the rest of the world because of their responsibilities. If you feel this way, ask a family member or friend to relieve you for a few hours on a regular basis. Use that time to connect with friends old and new — attend a club meeting, a church social — anything that puts you in the company of other people you enjoy. Staying connected in this way keeps feelings of isolation to a minimum.

>> **Take care of yourself.** Anger can also build when you're neglecting your own needs and not taking care of yourself. No matter how tough your situation, if you make it a priority from the beginning, you can and should find time every day to care for yourself. Exercise, read a magazine, dig in the garden, pursue your hobbies — just make sure whatever you do is something that will relax and de-stress you, make you feel good, and take your mind off your caregiving chores for a while.

Depression

Depression is a serious problem among caregivers. Depending on which study you read, 30 to 50 percent of dementia caregivers are depressed. Depression is more common among caregivers who have lower incomes, care for patients who exhibit more problem behaviors, feel overburdened, are female, and have had a bad relationship with the patient in the past.

TIP

You may be suffering from depression if you

» Feel tense or irritable

» Have frequent headaches or stomachaches

» Sleep or eat more or less than usual

» Lose interest in activities you once found pleasurable

» Have feelings of hopelessness

According to the National Mental Health Association, approximately 12 million women a year are clinically depressed in the United States — about double the rate of men. But 41 percent of the women surveyed didn't seek treatment because they were embarrassed, ashamed, or thought that it was normal for menopausal women to feel depressed. If you have any of the symptoms mentioned previously, you may be clinically depressed. Get help! You don't have to keep feeling bad.

WARNING

Many studies have shown that unresolved long-term depression can have a devastating effect on physical health, with higher incidences of heart disease, hypertension, and stroke in depressed caregiver populations than in control groups who are not caregivers.

To overcome depression, try some or all of the following strategies:

» Seek personal or group counseling.

» Ask your doctor whether an antidepressant medication is appropriate for you.

» Find regular relief from your caregiving duties to take care of yourself and your own needs.

» Avoid isolation; seek the company of your friends and peers.

» Enroll your loved one in a respite or daycare program, which is not only good for the patient's social wellbeing but is a key way for you to get a break and therefore manage stress over time.

In other words, give yourself a break. Wallowing in the blues only makes them worse — seek help, and you can overcome depression.

Grief

The odd thing about the grieving process regarding a person with dementia or AD is that you're grieving the loss of someone who isn't dead. But instead you're grieving for the person you knew before the cognitive and functional impairments of dementia began taking their toll. Because caregiving responsibilities can last for many years, the grief you feel can also persist. You're not likely to be able to work your way through grieving unless you make a conscious effort to do so.

REMEMBER

As with other negative feelings, the best relief for your grief is to seek appropriate counseling. Unresolved grief can not only negatively affect your ability to provide appropriate care for your loved one, but it can also damage your mental and physical health.

Accepting altered relationships

Everyone has unique relationships with each of the special people in their lives. One of the toughest aspects of dealing with a patient with a memory disorder is watching that relationship change before your very eyes; all the things that made it so wonderful — the shared memories, the secret jokes, the facial expressions — can fade as dementia continues its inevitable march.

It can be incredibly difficult for a caregiver when the person she cherishes begins to regard her differently due to progressing memory loss. Even if your loved one still recognizes you as a friendly face, he may not know exactly who you are or remember your familial relationship on a consistent basis. But no matter how much you accept this situation, having your mother think you're her mother or her sister and not her child isn't easy.

Losing your life partner

When the patient you're caring for is your spouse, you have an additional emotional burden because you're losing your life partner. As dementia progresses, your loved one may lose most of your shared history, perhaps even forgetting that you had children together, and that loss can be very difficult to handle.

TIP

You can help recall old family memories by sitting together and sharing old photo albums and memory boxes containing mementos of special times you shared. Although these aides can help with reminiscing, they don't "boost" memory, so don't use them to quiz your loved one — quizzing may upset him.

Your relationship with your spouse during her illness will be shaped by the relationship you've both shared throughout your life together. The kinds of behavior that your spouse displays over the course of the illness will also impact it. Obviously, caring for a person who has angry outbursts is more difficult than it is caring for someone who sits quietly and smiles sweetly all the time and has retained the capacity to express appreciation.

REMEMBER

If you have adult children, be sure to enlist their help. If you don't have grown kids to ask, then ask good friends to help you. Don't try to handle all the caregiving chores by yourself. And take a few minutes each day to talk quietly with your spouse, recounting some favorite shared memory from long ago to reinforce your bond.

Becoming a parent to your parent

Taking care of a parent can be a real challenge, even if the child is 50 and the parent is 72. Role reversal is never easy, and assuming the caregiving role is especially difficult if you're used to depending on your parent.

If you've had a difficult relationship with your parent all your life, you may not want to or be able to provide care. Don't feel guilty. Hiring someone to provide care is better than forcing yourself to do it in this situation because your negative feelings may build to neglect or explode in an abusive incident.

TIP

If you don't live in the same town as your parent and aren't able to be part of the caregiving team, you still have many ways to help your other parent or your siblings provide care. See Chapter 20 for ways you can help even if you live halfway across the country.

Finding serenity

Although you can't control or change AD or dementia, you have control over how you handle your caregiving responsibilities, how you interact with your loved one, and how you let the situation affect you. As difficult as caregiving is, you do have choices. With a positive attitude that empowers you and make you feel good, you not only survive the caregiving experience but you also thrive and grow as you rise to meet the challenges of caring for your loved one in new and creative ways. If you have a bad attitude, you end up feeling overwhelmed, over-burdened, burned-out, resentful, depressed, physically ill, and miserably unhappy.

TIP

Serenity isn't going to find you; you have to actively pursue it. Make time for yourself, even if it's just 15 minutes. In 15 minutes you can

>> Take a bubble bath

>> Read a chapter in a book

>> Read and answer email

>> Call a supportive friend

>> Massage your feet with peppermint lotion

>> Pick some flowers and arrange them in a vase

>> Listen to your favorite song — several times!

>> Make a fruit smoothie

>> Pet or brush your dog or cat

Alaskan dog sledders have a popular saying: "The pace of the pack follows the pace of the leader." As a caregiver, you are your loved one's leader. If you're always crabby, impatient, snappish, angry, short-fused, and martyred, how do you think your loved one (and the rest of your family members) is going to react? But if you're patient, kind, loving, and compassionate, you'll find that you get an entirely different response from your family and your dementia patient. The choice of how you act is up to you.

Taking care of your spiritual health

Although the number of people attending a place of worship is apparently dwindling, surveys invariably show that far more people say they believe in God (74 percent, according to a 2013 poll). If you're in either of those groups or drift into them as life becomes a struggle, make sure you find a way to maintain your spiritual health too.

TIP

If you normally go to a church, mosque, or temple, do your best to maintain that attendance. Also consider going on a religious or spiritual retreat to regain your equanimity or mental strength. If you can't leave the person with dementia for long enough to get to your place of worship, make every effort to stay in touch with other people who share your faith so they can support you.

Remembering Your Physical Health as a Caregiver

You may find it hard to believe, but taking care of a dementia or AD patient can have a significant impact on your physical health. Whether your health is affected depends on how well you care for yourself while you're taking care of your loved one. If you let yourself go, overlook your own needs, eat a poor diet on an irregular schedule, and are constantly sleep deprived, the combination of physical neglect and increased stress can make you sick.

Caring for another adult is hard work. Depending on the severity of your loved one's condition, you may be doing the work of an entire staff of an assisted living or memory care center, from director, business manager, nurse, aide, housekeeper, cook, and maintenance man to lawn attendant. You may be constantly bending, lifting, twisting, and straining, which can lead to muscular injuries such as strains, sprains, or even skeletal problems resulting in back, neck, or knee pain.

Unrelenting stress constantly bathes your system in the stress hormone cortisol. Although cortisol is quite valuable in normal concentrations, researchers at Stanford University found that caregivers had irregular levels of cortisol, which may raise their risks for heart disease and some types of cancer.

WARNING

A study conducted at the University of California at San Diego concluded that mortality from all causes is 63 percent higher in spousal caregivers than in non-caregivers. A Stanford University study concluded that 40 percent of all AD caregivers die from stress-related disorders before their patient dies. The University of Pittsburgh estimated that 25 percent of nursing home placements are a direct result of caregiver illness or death.

Caregivers are also subject to higher rates of weight gain or loss, adult-onset diabetes, anemia, ulcers, high blood pressure, insomnia, and alcohol or drug abuse than non-caregivers.

REMEMBER

All these undesirable effects can be negated by taking care of yourself. If you eat a balanced diet, exercise regularly, get support for your stress, sleep six to eight hours every night, take a few minutes every day to pamper yourself, and strive to maintain a positive outlook, then you should be able to bring your physical health risks back to normal. See the following sections for tips on how to take of yourself while taking care of your loved one.

Focusing on you first

Although it may seem selfish, you absolutely must put your own health and sanity first. Why? Well, if you run yourself into the ground and end up in the hospital with a heart attack or stroke, or you're so tired you fall asleep at the wheel and have a bad car accident, who's going to care for your loved one then? When you have another human totally dependent upon you for everything, not putting yourself first can put them last.

REMEMBER

By putting yourself first and making sure all your needs are met — physical, emotional, and spiritual — you're making yourself a better caregiver, not to mention a better spouse and parent. You're not only preserving your own wellbeing, but you're also sending a powerful message to the people around you: you're doing an important job, but that doesn't mean you will neglect yourself, so nobody else better neglect or marginalize you either.

Enlightened self-interest can have a whole host of unexpected benefits, so start practicing it today. Being your own advocate doesn't mean you always get the biggest steak or the piece of cake with the most icing; it means you care for yourself as much as you care for your loved one, and you won't sacrifice your health or the quality of your life in order to take care for her. It means you understand that with some planning, you can assemble a support team that will help you to do it all — a spouse, kids, a career, and still serve as a caregiver. It's not easy, but you can do it.

Seeking professional support

Prevention is always better than cure. Healthcare professionals would rather advise patients about how to stay fit and healthy before they head off on their travels than have to treat them on their return because they didn't take malaria pills or get vaccinated and now have a potentially life-threatening mosquito-borne illness, rampant diarrhea, and the after-effects of altitude sickness. These things are preventable with the correct physical preparation, vaccines, and pills.

Likewise, healthcare professionals are always happy to chat with someone who's about to become a full-time caregiver to offer advice about what to expect and the physical and mental challenges ahead. Being a caregiver is like competing in an endurance sport: people wouldn't head off to run a marathon or climb a mountain without knowing they were physically up to the job and had prepared in advance.

Don't think that asking for a check-up is wasting the doctor's time. They're happy to have the opportunity to dish out the following advice:

>> **Eat a healthful, balanced diet.** Ensure you get adequate portions of fruit and vegetables and plenty of water every day, and stop what you're doing and actually sit down to eat. Stay away from cigarettes and excessive alcohol.

>> **Exercise.** Just a short walk around the block every day will help keep you in shape and raise the endorphin level in your brain to boost your feeling of wellbeing.

>> **Have a good night's sleep.** You need your rest if you're to keep going day after day, so try not to wait until the person you're caring for goes to bed before you start doing chores. Do jobs like washing and folding clothes together as long as your loved one is able to do so. This gives the person with dementia a sense of purpose. It also allows you to finish necessary tasks

before too late an hour. That way you'll have some down time in the evening and get to bed at a reasonable hour.

>> **Take care of your back.** If you have to help the person with transfers into and out of bed, on and off the toilet, and out of chairs, you need to be very careful with your back. Although primary care physicians can offer advice about back care, seeing a physical therapist or massage therapist might also be worthwhile. Not only can physical therapists check out your spine in more detail and treat existing problems, but they can also show you the best way to lift and maneuver someone to avoid throwing your back out and then being no good to anyone for weeks.

>> **Get your flu shot every winter.** Because you're caring for someone, you really should consider getting this vaccination at your doctor's office or local pharmacy. It protects both you and your loved one.

>> **Don't neglect your own medical condition.** Have the relevant health check-ups and blood tests when needed. See your dentist and optometrist for regular checkups. If you're on any medications, make sure you take them regularly.

TIP

A Caregiver Self-Assessment Questionnaire is available on the Health in Aging website (`www.healthinaging.org/resources/resource:caregiver-self-assessment`) that allows you to give yourself a self-evaluation. This obviously isn't a substitute for seeing a clinical professional, but it can act as a useful guide to whether you're as managing as well as you think you are or actually need to see a doctor, unload some of your caregiving responsibilities to get respite, or join a support group. Be honest in your responses.

Fighting fatigue and illness

Unless you're careful, the stress of long-term caregiving can lead to fatigue, and ongoing fatigue makes you more susceptible to illness. You can help yourself stay healthy if you pay attention to your body's need for rest. If you feel yourself getting over-tired, do whatever is necessary to get a few nights of good sleep to relieve your fatigue. Here are a couple of ideas:

>> Ask a family member to take over your loved one's care for a few nights so you can catch up on your sleep.

>> If you don't have a relative nearby, hire a home health aide for a couple of days or check your loved one into an overnight respite care center.

Taking Time Out

When you work a paid job, be it 9-to-5 or shift work, you expect to have breaks and holidays. Without them, both you and your bosses are well aware that your efficiency and productivity will suffer.

You always know when a vacation is overdue because you become more easily stressed and irritated by small things and are perpetually tired. After some time off, you invariably return refreshed, invigorated, and ready for whatever the boss throws at you.

Being a caregiver may be an unpaid job, but the stresses and pressures it presents are no less exhausting than those experienced by people in a paid occupation — if anything, they're more exhausting. You thus need to ensure that you take some time out, and doing so is doubly important if you're still working as well as acting as a caregiver.

REMEMBER

You don't have to do the same thing every week. One week you may want to see a movie, and the following week you may want to have lunch with your spouse or a close friend. What's important is that you schedule regular breaks for yourself and then actually take them.

TIP

Before you get started on ways to treat yourself well, try a little exercise to get rid of any lingering feelings of guilt you may have about taking some time for yourself. The AARP developed a Caregiver's Bill of Rights for its members who are caring for a family member (see the nearby sidebar). Read through it, then print it out and tape a copy in several places around the house — the bathroom mirror, the refrigerator, and the laundry room — to remind yourself that as valuable as your services are, you're much more than just a caregiver. You're an individual with unique needs and desires, and you have every right to take care of your needs.

Treating yourself to a little pampering

Pampering yourself doesn't have to be expensive or time-consuming (although nothing is wrong with splurging now and then). Here are some ideas to get you started. Most of them can be completed in 15 minutes or less, and some cost absolutely nothing.

>> **Watch the birds.** Buy a small bird feeder with a suction cup and attach it to a window where both you and your loved one can see it. The comings and goings of birds and all their little dramas as they fight for spots at the feeder, chase each other, and sing and chirp will bring a smile to your face. Birdwatching is a great activity for your loved one.

TIP

» **Try something fishy.** A study at Purdue University found that tanks of brightly colored fish curtailed disruptive behaviors and improved eating habits of AD patients. Another study from the University of Pennsylvania reported that watching fish in an aquarium reduced stress and lowered blood pressure of AD patients.

» **Get private.** Take 15 minutes of absolute solitude to get yourself re-centered. Go outside, turn your face to the sun, and soak up its warmth, or lock yourself away in your study with your journal or a good book. Set a timer for 15 minutes and let the tension flow out of your body.

» **Burn an aromatherapy candle.** All sorts of wonderful fragrances are available. Select a fragrance you especially like, and light the candle in a protected place so your loved one can't get to it. In about 15 minutes, its soft fragrance suffuses an entire room.

SCENTS AND SENSIBILITIES

If you're afraid to light a candle around your loved one, set out a dish of potpourri or buy a fragrance diffuser that plugs into an outlet. Add a few drops of your favorite fragrant oil to a ceramic diffuser or buy diffusers with fragrance gels already packed inside. Can't make up your mind about which fragrance to choose? Lavender is very soothing and calming.

- **Try chocolate therapy.** When you're feeling stressed, indulge in some really tasty dark chocolate and eat one piece very slowly. Take the time to notice the chocolate's fragrance, color, and texture. Savor the delicious taste as it melts in your mouth. Why does chocolate make you feel so good? It's just science: chocolate contains a mood-enhancing chemical called *theobromine,* the same chemical our brains manufacture when we think we're falling in love. Don't eat dark chocolate more than once or twice a day, or you may have to buy *Dieting For Dummies*!

- **Dig in.** Plant some flowers in a spot where you can easily see them from the window. If you don't have a yard, buy a bouquet of inexpensive flowers from the grocery store or buy a flowering potted plant in full bloom, such as a geranium, miniature rose, chrysanthemum, or an African violet.

- **Act like a baby and have a good cry.** No fooling. Many caregivers bottle up their feelings in order to stay focused on their tasks. But repressing emotions can have detrimental health effects or lead to depression, a lapse in care for your loved one, or even an explosion of anger or inappropriate behavior. Even if you're the sort who never cries, rent a tearjerker to get the old waterworks going. Lock yourself in your room and scream, cry, and beat your pillow to a pulp — do anything you have to do to get the emotions flowing. You'll feel better afterward.

Making time for coffee or tea

When you're busy looking after someone else, your own basic needs can fall by the wayside. You can easily get to the end of the day hungry and thirsty because you've had nothing to eat or drink. As a caregiver, you need to ensure that you're fed and watered in order to be any good to the person you're looking after. Having a cup of tea or coffee both provides an opportunity for rehydration and acts as a trigger to sit down for five minutes and take a breather. Making a cup of tea is also a task you can share with the person with dementia.

Going out for coffee or tea with friends is an even better way of getting some respite, whether you go alone or take the person with dementia with you. On your own or with friends, it's a chance to get troubles off your chest or to have a laugh and forget about everything. Going out together with your loved one is a source of stimulation and a change of scenery for you both.

Meeting friends

Friends can be your greatest source of moral and physical support, so staying in touch with them is very important. Unfortunately, if you're caring for someone 24 hours a day, you may end up cutting friends out of your life. Denise's story illustrates how important the lifeline of friends is to a caregiver.

Denise is in her 50s, but still lives at home because she looks after her dad who has vascular dementia. She does everything for him, from cooking meals to rinsing soiled underpants. Her life is tough. When she tries to go out, he becomes upset and tearful, and she responds by staying at home as he wants her to, becoming ever more isolated in the process.

Recently, however, an old school friend has begun dropping in to see Denise every Tuesday evening for a couple of hours. Her dad's happy because she's at home, and she's happy because she gets a chance to share a couple of glasses of wine, reminisce about the old days, have a laugh and a cry, and get things off her chest. That one evening per week with a good friend has made a huge difference to her life.

Enjoying a hobby

Finding a hobby that you enjoy shouldn't be too difficult. Consider knitting, bowling, birdwatching, cake baking, bridge or poker nights, tennis, swimming, dog walking, oil painting, creative writing — the list goes on.

You can take up a solitary hobby that allows you to simply enjoy time on your own, or you can engage in group hobbies that also provide an opportunity to meet new people and make friends. Choosing a hobby that you have to sign up and pay for is even better because you then feel duty-bound to attend. In effect, you're forced to take a break and have the psychological permission you need to leave your caring duties for a short while to go out and have fun.

Alongside the general benefits you experience from taking up a hobby and belonging to a group, a significant amount of research suggests that hobbies also increase a person's social capital. In simple terms, social capital refers to the collective and economic benefits that result when people cooperate in groups. Such groups can be closely interacting neighbors, members of clubs and societies, or people who belong to faith groups. Those with high social capital are demonstrably healthier, happier, and less stressed.

So what have you got to lose? Whether you decide to take up a new hobby or re-engage in an old one, that activity can help keep you sane and fit enough to continue with your caring duties.

Getting away from it all

Although short weekly breaks from the psychological and physical rigors of caring have obvious benefits, nothing quite beats taking a week or two off work. Packing a suitcase or backpack and getting away from it all can give you a new perspective. And whether that involves putting your feet up poolside in Miami, basking in the sun in Bermuda, or skiing in Colorado doesn't matter, the prolonged period of time out is what's important.

Taking short breaks alone

Stepping away on your own may well be a great way to recharge your batteries so you can return to your caring role with more energy than you left it. You can choose from a whole range of short breaks, and some organizations actually provide breaks with caregivers in mind. If you're a full-time caregiver for someone with dementia, you may need to arrange for additional assistance while you are away.

Going on vacations together

You can also consider going away with the person you're looking after. This can work well particularly in the early stages of dementia if the person isn't too disabled by her symptoms. You have to do a lot of planning, however, to anticipate difficulties and find a way around them (borrowing a commode from the Red Cross, for example) to ensure the vacation is as relaxing and stress-free as possible. You don't want to spend the time desperate to get home for a rest.

TIP

Here are some useful tips from the Alzheimer's Society, an organization in the United Kingdom, website (`www.alzheimers.org.uk`):

>> Go on vacation with your extended family so the caregiving tasks are shared among the group and you, as the main caregiver, still get some time off.

>> Check out hotels in advance to ensure they're welcoming to someone with dementia. Picking smaller hotels or B&Bs is a good idea because fewer guests will be staying there and the building is less likely to have identical, and therefore confusing, corridors. Also check on disabled access and facilities, such as larger bathrooms and toilets, which make life easier too if your loved one has mobility issues.

>> Choose a vacation specifically designed for people with disabling conditions and their families.

Pampering yourself macho style

About now, male readers are probably saying, "Enough with this girly stuff! How about some pampering for guys, too?" There's no reason why men can't light a candle or indulge in chocolate, too. But here are some ideas for ways men can pamper themselves:

>> **Splurge on take-out.** Order your favorite take-out food — Chinese, pizza, ribs, or whatever you like.

>> **Putter around.** If you enjoy golf but rarely have time to get out to the links anymore, buy an indoor putting green and practice your putts in the den for 15 minutes.

>> **Rock out.** Put on your favorite playlist, plug in your headphones, and listen to music. Or tune the radio to your favorite station. If you're really feeling ambitious, dance to the music. Dancing is a great way to relieve stress.

>> **Take a virtual trip.** Set your timer for 15 minutes, sit in your favorite, most comfortable chair (preferably a recliner or a rocker), and lean back and put your feet up. Look at a travel brochure or read through a magazine article about your preferred destination. Pay particular attention to the photographs. Now close your eyes and envision yourself at that place you've always wanted to visit — on the white beaches of Hawaii, climbing the Mayan ruins in Mexico or the Eiffel Tower in Paris, photographing the Grand Canyon, or going to the sporting event of your dreams to watch your favorite team. After your 15 minutes are up, you feel more relaxed and refreshed.

>> **Put up your dukes (or watch someone else put up his).** Order a favorite pay-per-view sporting event on television or watch a ballgame.

>> **Whack some weeds.** Grab a weed whacker and mow down as many weeds as you can find in 15 minutes or trim the edges of your driveway, sidewalk, or patio.

>> **Clean up your act.** Remember to take a bath or shower every day. No, this tip isn't a joke. One of the first things caregivers do when they get overloaded is let go of their personal hygiene. Even if you have only five minutes for a quick shower, make that time special and associate it with renewal and re-energizing yourself. Get a nylon body scrubber, fill it with your favorite shower gel, and as you scrub yourself down, pretend you're washing away all your worries. Do this, and your bath cleans more than the outside of your body — it washes away the cobwebs from your spirit as well.

REMEMBER

You can pamper yourself in many other ways, too. You're the best judge of what it takes to bring a smile to your face and help you feel more calm and more in control. Pampering empowers you to be a better, more dedicated (and less distracted) caregiver.

Using Humor to Cope

When you're at your wit's end and don't think you can fit one more thing piled on your plate, take a few minutes to laugh. No, really. Why do you think someone made up that cliché: "Laughter is the best medicine"? When you're laughing, you can't be frowning at the same time.

Laughter takes your mind off your problems, if only for a few minutes. It increases respiration, relaxes tense muscles, and makes you feel good. Seeing you and other family members laughing also makes your loved one happy. It reminds him of good times from the past and helps distract him from his own worries and fears.

TECHNICAL STUFF

One of the best remedies for a bad mood is a good dose of laughter. According to a 1996 study, laughter lowers blood pressure, reduces levels of stress hormones, boosts immune function (by raising production of infection- and disease-fighting cells), and triggers the release of endorphins (Mother Nature's natural painkillers and mood enhancers). So pull up a funny video online and watch it with your loved one. You'll soon feel better after a good laugh.

Even if you couldn't make a living as a stand-up comic, you can find plenty of ways to inject a little humor into your day.

>> **Find humor in some of the situations that arise because of dementia or AD.** Your loved one can say and do some pretty funny things. Just remember

to laugh with them and not at them. If you have cable or satellite television, check out Comedy Central.

>> **Think of your all-time favorite comedies and buy a few on DVD or check them out of your local library.** Stay away from the heavy dramas — caring for a patient with a memory disorder probably provides enough drama on a daily basis.

>> **Laugh at funny jokes or videos on the Internet.** Visit a few humor sites until you find one that matches your sense of humor. Some are risqué, some are corny, but only you know what makes you laugh. Or spend a few minutes watching funny clips on YouTube — but remember, funny is subjective.

>> **Watch a late-night talk show.** The best jokes are in the opening monologues, so you can grab a few laughs without staying up too late.

Lots of things can make you laugh. Find something that works for you and use it whenever you feel down or overwhelmed. A hearty laugh may be just what you need to get going again.

Avoiding Isolation

Given the multiple responsibilities a caregiver must juggle, shutting yourself away in your house with your loved one and all your problems might seem like the simplest thing to do. In fact, self-imposed isolation is a common reaction among caregivers exposed to long-term stress. But isolation is bad for several reasons:

>> Humans are social creatures, designed to interact with one another. Depriving yourself of the company of others and trying to go forward without maintaining any meaningful relationships has the same effect on your body as stress.

>> If you keep to yourself to avoid stress, you're still stressing your mind, body, and spirit through the act of isolation.

>> Interacting with others gives you a sounding board. Problems can seem worse than they really are if you don't have anyone to discuss them with. Talking through a particular situation with a sympathetic friend helps in many ways — you come up with different solutions, compare the advantages and disadvantages of each, and ultimately realize you do have options.

>> Self-imposed isolation keeps you from asking for other's help, which adds to your caregiving burden.

As your loved one's cognitive function declines and he requires more care and attention, shutting yourself away becomes particularly easy to do. Even when caring for someone in the most advanced stage of dementia, taking time out for yourself on a regular basis is important; otherwise your mental and physical health suffers. Staying connected to other family members and friends is one of the best ways to keep you primed for the caregiving role.

Understanding why you really do need people

As a caregiver, you may find that keeping up friendships with people who can go anywhere they want any time they want is difficult, but you can do it. Some friends are going to drift away after you tell them you're caring for your loved one. But many friends step forward and volunteer to help you in any way they can. Joining a support group may be most gratifying of all. After you get plugged into such a caregiving circle, you find many new friends who are also caring for a loved one with AD or dementia.

After you make friends with other caregivers, a world of new possibilities opens up. Perhaps you can share the cost of a paid caregiver for your loved one or enroll your loved ones in a daycare center together after they get to know one another. You can also alternate providing transportation to daycare programs.

No matter what your situation, you've no good reason to shut your friends out of your life just because you've become a caregiver. If you tell yourself that none of your other family members or friends can possibly understand your situation or how stressed and overwhelmed you feel, you're giving yourself an excuse for cutting others off and making your own fears about isolation come true. To avoid isolation, you must help your friends and family understand your feelings; they can't read your mind.

TIP

TALKING TO OTHERS WHO'VE BEEN THERE

Looking for someone who really understands your situation and can lend a sympathetic ear? Join the online message boards available at www.alzconnected.org. You can meet other caregivers there. Some are looking for answers to specific questions. Others are just searching for a good listener or a few minutes of understanding and sympathy. But it helps to realize that you aren't alone in your caregiving challenges. Remember you also need real face-to-face human contact. Despite being helpful and accessible from your home computer, online message boards are no substitute for direct human contact. Relying strictly on this sort of impersonal communication can be almost as isolating as never going out of the house at all.

How others see you is determined mostly by how you present yourself and your situation. If you play the martyr and reject help or are angry and blaming, then of course you're going to drive other people away. Friends will offer support and assistance if you just ask them for help. As your loved one's condition progresses and he requires more care and attention, it's particularly easy to lose contact with other family members and friends. Even when caring for someone in the most advanced stage of a memory disorder, it's important to keep taking time out for yourself on a regular basis or your mental and physical health will suffer. Staying connected to other people you care about is one of the best ways to keep yourself primed for the caregiving role. Call, write, send them an email — make sure they know you care about them and think about them regularly. Regular communication keeps your support network active.

Numbing your feelings to avoid the pain and frustration of dealing with an AD or dementia patient is another negative coping mechanism. By cutting yourself off emotionally, you also miss out on many joyful moments, like when your loved one smiles sweetly at you or remembers a funny story from the past. The other people in your life don't want you to be cold and remote either; they want the same warm, wonderful person they've come to rely on over the years. Don't lose yourself — caregiving is a demanding job, but by its very nature it's a temporary one.

Keeping good friends around

Let your friends know that you need their love and support now more than ever. After news gets around that you're serving as your loved one's caregiver, a few of your friends will voluntarily step forward to offer assistance and a few others will fall away. Losing touch doesn't mean they're bad people; maybe they just don't know how to handle your situation.

If someone offers to help, don't be shy about accepting his offer. And don't be shy about asking for help when your responsibilities threaten to overwhelm you, either.

If you're not getting the responses you expect, check your own attitude. If you're ashamed or self-conscious about your loved one's condition, that sends a negative message to the patient and to others, and they respond accordingly.

WARNING

Relying on one friend or family member for all your assistance can overwhelm her and maybe overtax your friendship as well. If you have weekly errands to do, try getting two or three people to assist you at different times. Then, rotate your requests for help among your friends so one person isn't being asked to help you out all the time.

TIP

Writing down the list of chores you need assistance with is helpful. Then, show the list to other family members and close friends and ask them which items they can be responsible for. When you're well organized, you make a more effective team leader. Your friends and family members may be only too willing to help you, but are waiting for you to ask them. You must mold your team in the ways that best serve your needs.

Sorting Out Your Own Finances

As a caregiver, particularly if you have durable power of attorney, you're involved in making sure your loved one's finances are in order. Making sure you don't neglect your own finances is equally important. You may still need to work because you'll certainly have bills to pay.

With the possibility of your caregiving role expanding over time, you may well have to change your working pattern or even consider early retirement, and both situations have a potential negative effect on your income.

The following sections explore your options where your own employment is concerned and look at allowances you may be entitled to and whom to turn to for the best advice.

Changing to flexible working

You may need to alter your working arrangements if you're also acting as a caregiver for a person with dementia. Alternative working patterns might include approaches such as:

>> Flex-time

>> Staggered hours

>> Compressed hours

>> Working from home

>> Job sharing

A 2014 report published by The Council of Economic Advisers (www.whitehouse.gov/sites/default/files/docs/updated_workplace_flex_report_final_0.pdf) lays out a variety of approaches that businesses in the United States have developed for employees seeking flexible work hours. Flexible work schedules have been shown to reduce absenteeism and to improve health and productivity. Explore these options in your workplace. Discuss alternatives with your boss or human resources. You won't know what approaches are realistic options until you ask.

Applying for tax deductions

Relatives are eligible to become a dependent on a caregiver's tax return if their total income was less than $3,950 a year in 2014, excluding nontaxable Social Security and disability payments, and if the caregiver provided more than 50 percent of the relative's support. If you meet the criteria, you can take a $3,900 tax exemption for each dependent. If you claim a relative as your dependent, you can also claim medical deductions if you're providing more than 50 percent of support and if your total medical costs represented more than 10 percent of your adjusted gross income in 2014.

Getting financial advice

Whenever your life circumstances change — for example, when you get a job, get married, or become a caregiver — asking an independent financial advisor to review your finances is a good idea. A financial advisor can make sure your savings and insurance policies are in order for your maximum benefit. Use the advice offered to make sure you can cope financially in your new circumstances.

TIP

Go to the National Association of Personal Financial Advisors (NAPFA) website at www.napfa.org to find a fee-only financial advisor in your area.

Chapter 17

Finding Support

M anaging the care of your loved one without any support from others is like being Sisyphus, who was condemned by the Greek gods of Mount Olympus to roll a heavy boulder up a mountain, only to see it roll back down to the bottom again and again. Sisyphus is the symbol of endless labor. Unless you want to vie for his job, you need to find some support early on while taking care of your loved one.

Support can and should come in many forms — it can be a friend's voice on the phone, a strong neighborhood teen who comes to lift your loved one into bed every night, a church friend who cooks dinner one night a week, a sister who flies in from across the country every three to four months so you can have two weeks off, or even a group of strangers who are struggling with the same problems as you. The kind of support you seek depends on the kind of help you need. What form the support takes isn't important; what's important is that you have support. Taking care of a dementia or Alzheimer's disease (AD) patient by yourself is an overwhelming job. Keeping yourself up to the task requires regular breaks, and that's where support comes in.

In this chapter, we discuss the kinds of support that are available for caregivers and help you tune in to local resources. You find out how to identify possible sources of support and figure out whether a formal caregivers support group is right for you. Finally, you discover the importance of seeking a counselor or a confidante to help you shoulder the burden of taking care of your loved one. This chapter focuses on emotional support and physical respite for the caregiver; if you need information about possible sources of financial support, see Chapter 13.

Figuring Out What's Available

AD and dementia are becoming so prevalent that even smaller towns are likely to have some support services available for caregivers within the area. Obviously, if you live in a metropolitan area, your choices are more extensive. Even suburbs sometimes have a surprising array of support services available.

REMEMBER

Support falls into two categories — formal and informal:

>> *Formal support* is provided by governmental agencies, nonprofit organizations, healthcare providers, and church and volunteer groups.

>> *Informal support* is provided by relatives, friends, and neighbors.

These sections take a closer look at these two categories of support.

Formal support — enlisting the experts

Organizations that provide formal support for caregivers are the first places to turn to for help when taking care of your loved one. Because these groups specialize in offering support, the assistance they provide is usually on target and helpful. On the other hand, working with bureaucracies can be frustrating, and you may have to deal with delays. But if you are persistent, patient, and calm, you can usually get the help you need.

Government agencies

A number of federal and state agencies deal with caregivers' and senior citizens' issues. The type of help you're seeking determines which agency you contact.

The U.S. Department of Health and Human Services created the Administration for Community Living (ACL) in conjunction with the Administration on Aging (AOA) in 1965 with the passage of the Older Americans Act (OAA).

In turn, each state then provides services to caregivers including information, assistance in accessing services, support groups, caregiver training, and respite care. Some of the caregiving training helps caregivers understand their roles, make good caregiving decisions, and solve their caregiving problems.

On the websites you can find detailed lists of resources and useful links to services:

» `www.aoa.gov/aoa_programs/hcltc/caregiver/index.aspx#resources`

» `www.acl.gov/Get_Help/Help_Caregivers/Index.aspx`

TIP

To find services and resources for caregivers in your community, call the AOA's Eldercare locator toll-free at 800-677-1116. The AOA coordinates caregiving information for a number of other agencies and organizations, both publicly and privately funded. All that information is available through this one number.

Nonprofit organizations

The local chapters of the Alzheimer's Association and the Family Caregiver Alliance provide excellent resources for caregiving questions and crisis resolution. In addition to the best and most current information on AD and dementia, the national Alzheimer's Association (`www.alz.org`) offers the *Safe Return* program, which enrolls people with memory disorders who may wander away from home. For a nominal fee, you receive a bracelet or pendant for the patient and a 24-hour emergency response system to assist you in the event your loved one becomes lost. In some communities, local sheriff or police departments offer similar programs with GPS tracking bracelets.

The Alzheimer's Disease Education and Referral Center (ADEAR; `www.nia.nih.gov/alzheimers`), sponsored by the National Institute on Aging (NIA), offers education for families caring for an AD patient and sponsors support groups for both caregivers and dementia and AD patients.

TIP

If you need a quick answer to a question about your loved one's memory disorder, your role as a caregiver, or locating community resources, you can talk to an ADEAR Alzheimer's Disease specialist at 800-438-4380 toll-free Monday through Friday from 8:30 a.m. to 5 p.m. Eastern time. Or email your questions to `adear@nia.nih.gov`.

The Family Caregiver Alliance has fact sheets on dozens of topics related to dementia and AD at `https://caregiver.org/fact-sheets`. The alliance publishes an informative monthly newsletter that is packed with the latest information about AD research, caregiving, funding, family issues for caregivers, and a host of other topics.

The Caregivers Action Network (`http://caregiveraction.org`) is an advocacy group that supports and trains caregivers. Caring.com (`www.caring.com`) provides a wealth of online resources including a comprehensive directory of caregiving services.

Many nonprofit organizations sponsor Alzheimer's Caregiver Support groups online, which have message boards where caregivers can communicate. These sites usually have resource centers and some, like the University of Florida (http://alzonline.phhp.ufl.edu), offer excellent learning centers that provide professional quality online training for Alzheimer's caregivers.

The American Association of Retired Persons (AARP) has excellent resources for caregivers including connect with an expert, care for the caregiver and locating services. See its website www.aarp.org/home-family/caregiving/ for details.

In addition, the Alzheimer's Disease Centers (ADCs) offer valuable websites with information on treatment, research, and practical information on caregiving. Go to the ADEAR website (www.nia.nih.gov/alzheimers) for links to various ADCs and other important websites.

Many smaller organizations provide online support and fellowship for caregivers across the United States, and family caregivers themselves host some sites.

Healthcare providers

If your loved one has an overnight hospital stay for any reason — even a bad cough — take advantage of a little-known service provided by hospitals called discharge planning. *Discharge planning*, overseen by social workers and case managers, will assist in coordinating appropriate post-hospital care including rehab stays in a skilled nursing facility, outpatient testing, and follow-up physician visits. They can also arrange home care if needed including visiting nurses or physical therapists to follow the patient at home. In the case of elderly patients, particularly those with dementia, discharge planners want to make sure the patient's basic needs are met after she returns home.

Discharge planners can connect you with community services — everything from counseling to meal delivery to support groups to caregiver training. Some hospitals as well as local community agencies provide free or low-cost round-trip transportation for seniors and disabled people who are visiting a doctor or having outpatient tests. This service can be a tremendous help for caregivers who work because it keeps them from leaving work to provide transportation. However, most dementia and AD patients require supervision when using these services to avoid confusion and disorientation in unfamiliar settings, so if you have to work, be sure someone is accompanying your loved one. Keep in mind though, that you (or another responsible family member or friend) should be present at your loved one's doctor visits to ensure compliance with the doctor's medical recommendations.

Religious and volunteer groups

Although churches, synagogues, and volunteer groups may not have the vast resources provided by the federal government, many of them do offer valuable services for people struggling with caregiving issues. Ask your pastor or rabbi if your church or synagogue has volunteer sitters or respite care, and take full advantage of these programs if available. Many of these faith-based programs are very affordable and may even be free for families with limited finances.

TIP

Many churches, synagogues, and volunteer groups also offer hot meal delivery for seniors and transportation services for doctor's appointments, shopping, and errands. Call your local senior center to see what volunteer groups are active in your area.

Informal support — getting by with a little help from your friends

Informal support can come from a variety of people. Informal support doesn't even have to involve the care of your loved one; it can be someone doing something for you, such as running an errand so you can stay with your loved one and not hire a sitter. For example, perhaps a coworker is willing to cover your desk for two hours once a month when your loved one has a doctor's appointment so you can go with her. Perhaps you have an understanding boss who allows you to take an hour off here and there or rearrange your lunch breaks to accommodate your loved one's needs.

Whether help comes from family, friends, neighbors, or people online you've never met, informal support helps you do a better job of caring for yourself and your loved one.

Family

You may not think you have to ask family members for help; you assume they're just going to step right up to the plate and volunteer. But that may not always be the case, especially if they perceive that you've taken over and have things in hand. If you want help from a family member, be specific about what you want him to do and ask nicely; don't demand assistance and don't try sending him on a guilt trip. A lot of stress, resentment, and anger among adult children providing care for a parent is caused by the perception that other siblings aren't doing their part. It's true that responsibilities are rarely shared equally; so many factors like work, family demands, distance, the quality of the relationship and how it affects the people involved, and personal strengths and weaknesses play a role that equal division is almost impossible.

TIP

The best way to get help from someone is to communicate clearly what you want him to do. Look him in the eye, and in a pleasant tone, tell him what chores have to be done. Instead of assigning chores, give your family member a choice of chores. Ask whether he wants to pick up the prescription or sit with your loved one for half an hour while you do it. Let him choose what he's most comfortable doing, and you're more likely to get his help. Every person responds differently to the news that someone he loves has dementia. Don't push someone who is uncomfortable with the situation beyond what he's comfortable doing. (See more about family dynamics in Chapter 19.) If your brother is squeamish about bathing your mother, ask him to shop for groceries instead. Accomplishing any task is valuable and helps relieve you in some way. By being flexible and willing to accept help in whatever form it's offered (as long as it's a reasonable offer), you encourage people to help you even more. But if you're bossy, picky, and constantly nagging people to help and then criticizing the way they do things when they do help, don't be surprised if they're nowhere to be found the next time you ask for help.

Friends and neighbors

Friends and neighbors can sometimes be even more helpful than family members because they don't have to contend with the history and baggage of your family dynamics. They can just step right in and do whatever needs to be done. But like family, friends have to know that you need help before they can offer assistance. Let your friends know what your needs are, and you may have a veritable army of people running errands, cooking meals, and offering to sit with your loved one for a few hours so you can have a break.

Online support

Oddly enough, the people who offer you the most emotional support may be people you never even meet. Members of online message boards who serve as caregivers for a loved one with dementia or AD know just how you feel because they feel the same way. They're facing the same day-to-day problems, the same worries about money, and the same feeling of overload that you are. This shared experience can make for some very nurturing friendships. Refer to earlier sections in this chapter for specific URLs.

Knowing When to Ask for Help

Even with the best routines in place and good stress management techniques, you're still only one person with one set of hands and 24 hours in your day. If after establishing routines, you find that you still can't get everything done, don't stress out — ask for help.

Early on, schedule regular time off from your caregiving chores. Having a few hours a day to yourself, at least two to three days a week, is critical if you plan to provide care for your loved one for the duration of his illness. If money to hire help is tight, ask local day care centers if they have scholarships available or have sliding scale fees based on financial need.

REMEMBER

Nothing's wrong with asking for help. Most caregivers are unpaid family members, not trained professionals. You're not supposed to know everything or cope by yourself in what can be very difficult circumstances. If you're in that position, bear in mind that if you become ill yourself because you don't get the help you need, your loved one may then have no one to care for him.

The following sections examine some specific ways that you can ask for help as a caregiver of a loved one with dementia or AD.

Making a volunteer list

Make a list of everyone in your family and close friends and neighbors. Beside each name, write an honest assessment of his ability to contribute to the care of your loved one. Hopefully, two or three people will stand out as those you can trust to help with your loved one's care.

Call each person and ask for help, or invite everyone to your home for a meeting. Lay out your schedule, explain where you need help, and ask for volunteers. Perhaps you can't get to the dry cleaner to pick up your clothes, but your neighbor who uses the same dry cleaner may be happy to get them for you. Maybe you don't have time to shop for groceries, but your sister is happy to get what you need when she goes shopping.

WARNING

If your loved one has special care needs such as incontinence, it's not fair to expect an untrained volunteer to manage that problem. When you need some time off, try an adult day care center or hire a home companion/caregiver.

Getting help for abusive tendencies

The National Center on Elder Abuse (NCEA) estimates that 1 out of 10 seniors is abused in some way every year. With the number of seniors in America increasing exponentially, this problem is growing, and 90 percent of those abusing elders are family members. See the NCEA website at www.ncea.aoa.gov/ for more details.

Many situations can cause a caregiver to lose control and strike out physically or verbally at the person they're caring for. People who haven't spent much time around a dementia patient in the later stages of the disease have very little understanding of just how maddening it can be to have to answer the same question 20 or 30 times a day, or be constantly accused of stealing, or clean up an incontinent person time after time. Add an isolated, overwhelmed, rundown caregiver and a few financial, job, or marital problems to this mix, and you have a recipe for abusive behavior just waiting to come to the boil.

WARNING

If you don't deal with your anger, it can grow to the point where you may abuse your loved one. If you exhibit any of the following warning signs, get help immediately! Schedule emergency respite care for your loved one until you can get your angry feelings under control.

>> You feel indifferent or angry toward your loved one all the time, not just occasionally.

>> You blame your loved one for all your problems and negative feelings and don't accept responsibility for your own behavior.

>> You isolate your loved one from other family members to retain control of the situation.

>> You habitually exhibit aggressive behavior; for example, you shout, name-call, threaten, or insult your loved one.

>> You feel a desire to hit or hurt your loved one.

>> You have a history of alcohol or drug abuse that is getting worse.

REMEMBER

If you do lose control, call your local senior center for information about anger management and stress relief classes. Join a support group, seek counseling — do whatever it takes to make sure it doesn't happen again. If despite your best efforts, you find yourself abusing your loved one, make other care arrangements to ensure her safety.

Looking into Support Groups

Many different organizations sponsor support groups for AD and dementia caregivers, including the Alzheimer's Association, assisted living residential care facilities, churches, and senior centers. Support groups provide a comfortable and accepting atmosphere where caregivers can talk openly about their concerns and problems and gather new information about memory disorders and caregiving.

If you're looking for a group in your area, call your local chapter of the Alzheimer's Association or ask your loved one's doctor or counselor for a recommendation. Your local Area on Aging and senior center may also have some good suggestions.

Visit several groups before deciding on which to join. Some groups may appeal to you more than others. If one group has a bunch of whiners who dominate the discussions, that won't be much help, so keep looking. If you join a group and come away from the sessions feeling worse and not better, try another group. The ideal group is comprised of a nice cross-section of caregivers who exchange information and tips, listen compassionately to other member's problems, and offer reasonable suggestions.

The two main types of support groups are

>> Groups led by a professional, such as a doctor, nurse, or social worker who has direct experience dealing with memory disorders.

>> Self-help groups led by someone who is currently caring for an AD or dementia patient or has cared for one in the past and has become a volunteer advocate for caregivers.

Depending on the type of group you join, meetings may be educational or emotional in focus or both. Educational meetings offer a variety of speakers on different topics related to care for those with memory loss. One night a speaker who is a political activist and AD advocate may fill you in on the latest legislation affecting seniors or caregivers. Another night a nurse may tell you tips for basic self care and medication management strategies or a website with good resources and information for caregivers. A registered dietitian may give you nutritional tips and hints to get your loved one to eat well. Or you may hear a doctor involved in a clinical trial for a new drug telling you the latest news from the research front.

Groups that offer emotional support for caregivers usually have a less formal structure to the meetings. Members may sit in a circle and share stories, shed a few tears, hug each other, offer advice and solutions to specific problems, and allow each other to vent in a safe atmosphere.

TIP

If you have trouble getting out of your house to attend a meeting, dozens of online support groups are available — formal, moderated, and informal. Just enter "Alzheimer's caregiver online support" in any search engine and you get a huge list of sites. Check out several until you find one with people who are on your wavelength.

Support groups may be available for both caregivers and patients. Many centers schedule meetings for both groups at the same time so caregivers can relax and enjoy the meeting, knowing their loved one is in an enjoyable and secure situation at the same time. In some larger centers, the group for your loved one may be a true support group for people with mild AD, or a respite service offered to those with varying levels of AD so the caregiver can attend his or her own support group meeting without worry.

Finding a Counselor

Seeking the help of a professional counselor, such as a psychologist, psychiatrist, social worker, pastor, or doctor, may help you and your loved one make the most of your situation and stay on a more even keel. People in the early stages of dementia or AD can benefit tremendously from counseling. Just having a sympathetic ear really helps sometimes. If you don't want to see a counselor regularly, consider visiting one to help you through a crisis situation.

Ask your doctor to recommend a counselor who has experience working with dementia patients and their families. Scrolling through a list of names on an Internet search engine and ending up in an office with someone who specializes in truant teens isn't going to help you much. Call the counselor and ask about their experience in counseling patients and families dealing with memory disorders.

Counseling provides many benefits, including the following:

>> You can talk through your feelings about your caregiving role and express any doubts or fears you have in a safe, controlled situation to a person who is qualified and experienced enough to offer you real solutions.

>> A good counselor teaches you better ways to cope with the stress of caregiving and teaches you proven stress reduction techniques.

>> Counselors can help patients look at their situation in a more positive light and can also encourage patients to actively to maintain their health.

REMEMBER

The best approach to managing your love one's care is to take advantage of ongoing education and support. Don't wait until a crisis arises.

Chapter 18

Knowing What to Do If the Person with Dementia Goes into the Hospital

H ospitals are unnerving, strange, and scary places for most people, particularly if you've associated them with trauma or the loss of a loved one. So imagine how much scarier they can be for people with dementia who may not recognize the people around them. Understanding what's happening to them and why can be difficult.

This chapter has suggestions for ways in which you as a family member or caregiver can help someone with dementia during a hospital admission.

Understanding the Emergency Room and Hospital Admission Process

If the admission is planned, the person with dementia will probably go straight to the hospital floor where he's staying. If it's an unplanned emergency admission — for example, for an acute issue like injury from a fall, shortness of breath, or chest pain — the admission may not be so smooth.

These sections explain what happens when you and your loved one arrive at the hospital and what you can expect to occur while you're there.

Undergoing the initial exam

The first stop will be the Emergency Room (ER). After a nurse conducts an initial evaluation, the healthcare provider (doctor, physician assistant, or nurse practitioner) on duty at that time will question and examine your loved one. However, the process isn't always in order of time of arrival. Your loved one will be *triaged*, which means he'll be seen in descending order of severity of the problem. The sickest patients will be seen first, and those less ill will wait in line. If a severely injured car accident victim arrives after your loved one, he'll be pushed to the head of the line for care. As a result, sometimes you and your loved one may be waiting in the ER for a period of time before a provider sees you. Other times, if your loved is the most ill (such as having chest pain), he'll be seen before others who were there before him.

After the healthcare provider initially evaluates your loved one, he'll order appropriate diagnostic tests and blood work to evaluate the problem. Such tests may include X-ray studies like CT scans or chest X-rays that require the patient to go to the radiology department. Other tests like EKGs (electrocardiograms) and blood draws are conducted at the bedside.

Then you have to wait for results from all the tests. The nurse assigned to your loved one's care will follow his blood pressure and pulse and stop in to check on him during this time. Sometimes results are ready quickly; other times they take a while before they're available. After the test results are available, the healthcare provider will discuss the diagnosis and treatment plans for your loved one. It's important for you to be present with your loved one at this time so you can understand what the tests showed and get your questions answered about the diagnosis and treatment plans. You then make decisions about admission to the hospital at this time.

REMEMBER

This time is one of the most important when you serve as patient advocate for your loved one. If he can't speak up for himself due to dementia, then you need to ask the questions he would have asked about the diagnosis and treatment plan. Make sure you understand what is going on and the prognosis or expected outcome of the situation.

Imagine how unsettling this process is for a patient with dementia. Regardless of how a hospital admission takes place, your loved one will be seeing multiple unfamiliar staff members, which can be upsetting especially when he isn't feeling well. Hence, be with your loved one, hold his hand, and provide a familiar face. Tell the staff how to address your loved one if he uses a nickname rather than the name written on the insurance cards. You need to make sure that the staff knows and understands the person they're caring for.

Giving the staff some background history

Doctors, nurses, and other hospital staff members who come into contact with patients try to treat them as individuals and not according to their problems such as "the heart attack in room 300." Unfortunately, hospital staff members are all human, as well as busy dealing with many patients over the course of a day, so the ideal situation doesn't always match reality. To facilitate the best care for your loved one, speak up for his needs. Be polite but persistent when you talk with hospital staff. Ranting and raving in anger isn't effective. Remember the old adage, "You get more flies with honey than with vinegar."

TIP

A danger also exists that when staff members hear the word *dementia*, they'll jump to conclusions about the condition. To avoid misunderstandings, give the staff as much information as you can about your loved one as early on in the admissions process as possible. Let the staff members know what type of dementia your loved one has been diagnosed as having. Tell them if it's mild, moderate, or severe dementia and review your loved one's mental capabilities so they know what he can normally do. Keep the following points in mind:

>> **Inform staff members who has power of attorney.** You need to provide copies of any advance directives including a *do not resuscitate (DNR) order* if one exists, which is a legal document that states the patient doesn't want any life-saving measures taken should his heart stop beating or he stop breathing. A patient resuscitated against his wishes can be distressing for everyone concerned, so you need to let staff know what those wishes are. (See Chapter 12 for more details on power of attorney specifically for healthcare decision-making.)

>> **Make sure you provide your current phone numbers so that staff members can contact you in an emergency.** Give staff members the name of an alternate family member or friend to call if they aren't able to contact you.

Providing details about the person's care

In order to minimize the possible distress of new surroundings, the staff members will also appreciate knowing your loved one's established routines so they can be observed as much as possible. They'll also appreciate knowing how to reduce agitation if things go wrong. Give staff information on

>> The best way to communicate; for example, slowly and precisely and covering one important issue at a time

>> Whether the patient needs help with eating and drinking or can manage alone if the food is cut up or always served with ketchup

>> What sort of behaviors to watch out for that may suggest pain or a need to go to the toilet, particularly if the person isn't good at directly expressing these things

>> Whether the person needs help with washing or dressing, and whether he prefers to be assisted by a man or a woman to avoid distress and embarrassment

>> Ways you generally settle agitation, such as soft music or calm talk

Getting to Know the Hospital Staff and Doctors

Communication always works best when it's a two-way process, so as well as providing staff members with information about the person in their care and introducing yourself, take time to get to know them too. The hospital helps with this process, because each patient should have

>> A named doctor who's in charge of overseeing his care.

>> A named nurse who's available to talk to relatives about what's happening during the patient's hospital stay. (However, realize that the nurse will change at each shift of either 8 or 12 hours depending on the particular hospital.) Usually the name of the nurse on duty is displayed on a board in the room to help you know which nurse to talk to.

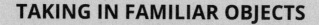

TAKING IN FAMILIAR OBJECTS

A few home comforts and familiar objects always make strange, and especially clinical, places seem less frightening. But most importantly, surrounding people with dementia who are prone to more confusion in strange and scary environments with familiar items can be helpful. Such objects can include anything from family pictures to a favorite afghan blanket. However, don't bring in any significantly valuable items because they could be lost or stolen.

The names of both these professionals will be written in each patient's chart. Ask the receptionist whom to turn to for information if you don't know.

Introduce yourself to those individuals caring for your loved one. Let them know your relationship to him. Explain that you're there to be a resource because of your familiarity with his care and you want to be helpful in any way you can.

Visiting Regularly

Your family member, spouse, or friend is just in the hospital, not in a prison. Traditionally visiting hours were quite restrictive in order to allow the staff to provide care and the patients to undergo tests and receive treatment without a crowd of people hanging around. But nowadays hospitals are much more flexible with visiting hours, especially for those patients with dementia who benefit greatly from having a familiar person present.

You may be an exhausted spouse or child for whom this time away from caregiving allows a recharging of your batteries. It may be a relief to know that someone other than you is caring for your loved one. But you need to balance your caregiving break with your loved one's needs. Remember that for your loved one, seeing familiar faces can be extremely reassuring. While you're visiting, you can provide distraction from the confusion of noise and activity that's going on around the person while he sits in his hospital bed. Of course, you don't have to stay at his bedside 24/7, but staying for an hour or so isn't so much to ask.

TIP

To avoid the awkward silences so common during hospital visits, consider the following activities to keep you both occupied:

>> Take in family photo albums to go through together.

>> Look through favorite picture books, especially those that help trigger fond reminiscences that you can chat about.

>> Do word or jigsaw puzzles together.

>> If the person is fit enough to do so, go for a walk down the hall, outside to get some fresh air or to the hospital cafeteria.

If you see the hospital admission as a chance for some well-deserved time out from the tough world of 24-hour caring, then try to share visiting duties with friends and family members. Seeing different but also familiar faces still provides reassurance and also much-needed stimulation for your loved one. But remember to be available by telephone in case of an emergency. A cell phone can be invaluable by allowing you to be accessible no matter where you are.

Don't feel guilty if you can't go in to visit every day. If you're already exhausted, trekking back and forth to the hospital won't help. To continue in your role as caregiver when the person comes home, you may need to give yourself some time off.

Helping at Mealtimes

Another important way in which you can help the person in the hospital is to visit him at mealtimes. Although breakfast is served early, you can certainly be there for lunch and dinner. And the nurses will be only too glad.

Assisting your relative or friend may only involve opening a milk carton or moving food items within reach. However, cutting up food and even spoon-feeding may be necessary. Providing help with the meal also allows the hospital staff to concentrate on other needy patients. Helping at mealtime also enables you to provide further familiar reassurance to your loved one.

REMEMBER

Everyone deserves to be treated with dignity and respect, and although this is just as likely to be provided by professional nursing staff, there's no substitute for care provided by a family member or familiar friend.

Chapter 19

Keeping Up with Work and Family as a Caregiver

People who hold down a job, take care of their families, and also care for a loved one with dementia or Alzheimer's disease (AD) may argue in favor of human cloning. Sometimes you don't have enough hours in the day or enough hands to get everything done, and having two or three of you to pick up the slack would be nice. Cloning yourself may seem like a brilliant idea — especially on those nights when you're standing over a sink full of dishes while a load of clothes spins in the washer and another waits to be folded in the dryer, and you still have to pack lunches and finish a report for an early meeting at work.

Despite reports to the contrary, human cloning is still the stuff of science fiction, and household robots aren't economically feasible for the average homeowner. So how can you juggle work and family while caregiving?

In this chapter, you find out how to enlist the help of your boss, coworkers, and family members — not just to help you care for your loved one, but also to help keep the parts of your life that don't revolve around caregiving on track. You may not mind putting your career on hold for a while, but you don't want to lose your job entirely.

The same goes for family. You may put off the trip to Disney World, but you don't want to put off weekend picnics in the backyard or trade time with your children (or spouse!) because you all need the closeness that makes you a family, now more than ever. But family dynamics can cause problems. Read on to discover the best ways to keep it all together.

REMEMBER

As you read this chapter, consider what type of care your loved one needs, such as supervision and household tasks like laundry or food preparation. Does your loved one have personal needs like bathing assistance or incontinence care? After assessing the needs, then look at whether any of the needed care can be shared with other family members or friends. If not, look at paid caregiver options and evaluate the costs of such care (refer to Chapter 13 for more information).

Recognizing the Importance of Routines

With so many tasks to accomplish every day, caregivers can get overwhelmed easily. The best defense against drowning in a sea of to-do lists is to determine what you need to accomplish each week at home and at work. Then make a schedule and stick to it. Although putting a schedule together takes time, knowing what you have to accomplish in any given time period more than makes up for the time you invested developing the schedule.

TIP

In order to prevent caregiver burnout, make sure you share the work with your family members. Make a chore schedule, divided into daily, weekly, and monthly chores. Hold a family meeting and ask your spouse and children to assume responsibility for a few of each. Let them choose what they prefer to do; if you assign tasks, they may feel some resentment. Be careful about overloading children with too many chores. Put family members' names next to the tasks they choose. For example, put your teenage son's name next to taking out the garbage or mowing the lawn — whatever he volunteers to do. Perhaps your spouse can cook dinner a couple of nights a week. By breaking tasks into manageable chunks and sharing the workload, you get a lot more done. Stay on top of your day-to-day schedule and days flow more easily. Problems develop only when you ignore day-to-day chores and let them pile up.

TIP

For easy-to-follow daily household routines, check out http://wellnessmama.com/3812/organization-checklist/ for a printable organization chart or www.homeroutines.com for an app to help you set up routines.

Routines help you stay on top of your job as well. Evaluate your workload and look at any recurring deadlines (such as end-of-month-close or sales quota periods) and factor them into your schedule. Compare your work and home schedules to avoid conflicts. For example, don't schedule a doctor's appointment for your loved one during a busy time at work. After you get in the habit of following routines, they become second nature. In the long run, routines save a lot of time and energy and let you squeeze the maximum productivity out of your days with minimal stress.

Juggling a Job and Caregiving Responsibilities

How do you see your job? Do you work just to bring in a few extra dollars, or are you passionately committed to a particular career? A person who has slowly climbed the career ladder toward a long-cherished and just-in-sight goal may feel unhappier about reducing his or her workload to provide care for a loved one than a person who temps 20 hours a week just to earn extra money. Some people see their jobs as a respite from caregiving. If you're juggling multiple responsibilities, you must schedule regular, true respite breaks to keep from burning out.

It may be that you have no choice but to work; your family absolutely needs every penny you earn, so you can't quit your job or reduce your hours. How do you cope in that situation? Here are some suggestions.

FMLA to the rescue

Until 1993, overloaded employees juggling work responsibilities with caring for an impaired loved one were pretty much on their own. Employers didn't see the need to cut caregivers any slack: either you did your job and carried out your assigned tasks in a timely fashion, or you didn't. And if you didn't, you more than likely lost your job.

This standard changed with the passage of the Family and Medical Leave Act (FMLA) in 1993. The FMLA allows any employee who has worked for at least a year for a company with 50 or more employees to take up to 12 weeks of unpaid annual leave to address family emergencies without losing medical benefits or his job. Companies that disregard this policy and fire employees who take family leaves face stiff civil penalties and open themselves up to lawsuits. Many companies allow you to use accumulated sick time toward this leave of absence.

Although the FMLA marked a milestone and caregivers across the nation applauded it, this act didn't cover the other 40 weeks a year — weeks when caregiving requirements continue, in spite of work deadlines and important meetings. More needed to be done.

In December 2000, Congress approved the National Family Caregivers Support Program, which provides free services for millions of families through local Area Agencies on Aging. (To find the AOA nearest you, call 800-677-1116 or visit www. aoa.gov/AoA_programs/OAA/How_To_Find/Agencies/Find_Agencies.aspx.)

But as more and more employees entered the ranks of caregivers, employers began getting on the bandwagon, realizing it's more expensive to recruit and train new employees than to invest money and time in retaining experienced long-term employees going through difficult times in their personal lives.

TIP

For more ways to be protected from employment discrimination, check out www. aarp.org/content/dam/aarp/research/public_policy_institute/health/ protecting-caregivers-employment-discrimination-insight-AARP-ppi- ltc.pdf for a detailed discussion by the AARP Public Policy Institute entitled "Protecting Family Caregivers from Employment Discrimination."

Throwing a rope: How employers help working caregivers

Businesses incur real costs when employees' work days are impacted by caregiving responsibilities — costs related to hiring temps to sub for absent employees, lost productivity due to workday interruptions and emergencies involving caregiving, and finding and training new employees to replace workers who quit to provide care, to name a few. Working with employees experiencing a caregiving crisis takes supervisors away from normal duties, slowing down the workflow. Employees who are caregivers and don't have good support systems in place also suffer more physical and mental health problems, meaning higher insurance claims for employers.

Most major companies have figured out their interests are best served if they have a reasonable and consistent policy to help employees who are caregivers. After all, the number of caregivers is growing. According to a 2011 Gallup Healthways Well-being Survey, more than one in six employed Americans older than 18 care for an elderly or disabled family member or friend and said it significantly affected their work life. Although there are no consistent standards from company to company for dealing with caregiving issues for employees, most employers do recognize certain caregiver needs:

>> The desire for a flexible schedule

>> Job sharing

>> The opportunity to telecommute, if the job permits

>> Access to long-term care insurance

>> On-site adult daycare (still rare, but more companies offer it every year)

>> Office-based support groups for caregivers

>> Workshops and educational programs

>> Leave of absence to meet caregiving needs

>> Stress management classes

>> Employee Assistance Programs

>> Flexibility when using benefits—for example, the ability to use accumulated sick leave as paid days off to provide caregiving services

Employers who offer understanding and flexibility to their employees who are caregivers reap benefits that they can see on their bottom lines. Bosses who are the most flexible about allowing employees to find creative ways to get their work done and provide caregiving services are rewarded with fewer work interruptions, better job performances, higher job satisfaction, and significantly lower turnover.

Larger companies with more resources usually offer more extensive support programs, but even smaller firms are willing to help valued employees however they can. Ask your benefits manager what help is available. Then explain the situation to your immediate supervisor and explore solutions to help you keep up your job performance while serving as a caregiver.

When you find coworkers willing to help, be sure to thank them and offer to return the favor whenever possible. Everyone has days when they must leave work early or take an extended lunch to run an important errand. On those occasions, offer to help your coworkers meet their deadlines. If you can't do that, write a note of gratitude, or buy them small gifts, such as a gift card to their favorite coffee shop, or treat them to lunch. How you do it doesn't matter; just let them know you appreciate their help.

Grabbing the rope: Taking advantage of employee benefits for caregivers

Employers aren't mind readers. You have to let them know your situation and what sort of relief may be beneficial. You may not get every consideration you ask for, but even a good compromise is better than juggling too many responsibilities without support.

REMEMBER

After you determine how your caregiving responsibilities may impact your job, figure out what accommodations you need to make your schedule work. Do you have to take time off to take your loved one to the doctor once or twice a month? Will you be 15 minutes late to work every day because the adult daycare center opens too late for your current work schedule? Write down your desired schedule and ask your boss for a few minutes to discuss solutions. By putting your needs in writing, requesting help, and asking your boss to be part of your team, you're giving yourself the best chance of getting the flexibility you need to make it work.

If your company is small and your employer isn't required to offer family leave, discuss other options. Perhaps your boss is open to a job-sharing arrangement that allows you to work half days. If your boss agrees to this arrangement, offer to train the person who shares your job. Even if your boss considers you to be irreplaceable, remind him that he can either help you moderate your responsibilities and work schedule or face the prospect of replacing you. If you have an hourly or part-time position, explain your situation to your supervisor and tell her you may not always be able to work your normal schedule if your loved one has a crisis. Line up other employees who are willing to cover for you as needed.

WARNING

Don't mix work and caregiving. If you're at your desk but spend most of the day on the phone with caregiving business, you aren't getting much work accomplished, and sooner or later, your boss will notice. Make personal phone calls during lunch or on your breaks and ask hired caregivers to call during lunch, except for emergencies.

Occasionally, you may come across a boss who doesn't budge an inch and refuses to even grant family leave. If you're eligible for family leave, gently remind him of the law's requirements. If you're still not getting anywhere, you may have to consider finding another job or quitting work. Keeping two full-time occupations at once — caregiving and your job — is simply too stressful without any scheduling and workload flexibility.

REMEMBER

For more detailed information on working caregiver issues, see the Family Caregiver Alliance website: www.caregiving.org.

WHAT WILL CAREGIVING COST YOU?

Businesses aren't alone in suffering economic losses from caregiving. According to a 2011 MetLife study that looked at the costs of caregiving on working baby boomers, employees who are 50 or older and provide caregiving services for their parents suffer lost wages, Social Security and pension contributions, and personal expenses.

These challenges for employed caregivers occur because there is a significant time commitment with caregiving especially for a loved one with dementia. Often caregiving is a long-term commitment, especially for people with dementia. According to the Alzheimer's Association, caregivers for people with Alzheimer's and other dementias provide on average a duration of one to four more years of care than caregivers caring for someone with other health problems. In addition, many studies have shown that caregivers of those with dementia have higher levels of caregiving responsibilities than other caregivers, which is often due to people with dementia developing increased care needs over time due to the progression of cognitive loss and consequently functional loss. Clearly, this escalating commitment can greatly affect any employed caregiver.

Making a contingency plan

Life is full of little and not-so-little surprises. A *contingency plan* helps you cover your bases when something unexpected comes up at work or at home. Write your plan on a sheet of paper and make copies for other family members, hired caregivers, your supervisor, and your coworkers. Include the names and phone numbers of people who can provide alternate transportation or be substitute sitters or temp workers who can sub for you on the job. Having this plan in place saves time and energy because then everyone knows what to do in a crisis. Try to cover all the bases and create a fallback plan for every potential crisis situation you might encounter: for your work, your home, the daycare center, and so on, and give copies of your plan to a responsible person at each location.

>> **For work:** Ask coworkers in your department who have similar job responsibilities if they can help cover your job if you have a crisis. Be sure to clear any arrangements you make with your supervisor.

>> **For home — one-time emergencies:** Write out your loved one's schedule and share it with a trusted friend, family member, or hired caregiver. Ask if she can serve as your emergency backup in case something prevents you from picking up your loved one from the adult daycare center on time or if another short-term emergency arises.

>> **Ongoing crisis situations:** For situations that may be ongoing, make more permanent arrangements. The same neighbor you rely on to occasionally pick up your loved one from the daycare center can't be expected to step into a full-time caregiving role if you become incapacitated. If you're hospitalized, you need time to regain your strength before returning to caregiving. If you have surgery, you may not be able to safely lift again for months. To prepare for such an event:

- Line up someone who can take over for an extended period of time; perhaps a sibling, your spouse, a member of your church, or a hired caregiver can take your place.

- Give that person a copy of your loved one's schedule and the duties you want him or her to perform.

- Identify suitable paid respite options. Gather information from local agencies to determine which facility you'd like to use. Most can admit your loved one within 24 hours especially if you have discussed your caregiving needs with them previously. If you've been using respite services proactively to ensure you get regular breaks, your loved one is already familiar with the paid caregiver or facility. If you do this, your crisis is managed and your loved one's routine is intact.

>> **If you die:** The last contingency plan you must make is arranging permanent care for your loved one in the case of your own death. Although it's not easy to think about, and preceding your loved one in death is unlikely, making a plan and putting it in writing is vital so everyone involved knows what to do if the unlikely event happens.

Balancing Family and Caregiving

One of your delicate balancing acts will be figuring out how to care for your loved one without shortchanging your family. According to a study by the National Alliance for Caregiving and AARP, 41 percent of caregivers have children at home. Tensions can spiral if your spouse or children think you aren't paying them enough attention, while you may think the last thing you need is more people leaning on you when you're already so pressed for time.

Your road is harder if you have young children, because they don't understand why their grandmother or uncle is acting differently and needs increasing help. They have even less understanding about why it takes time away from them and your family life, and they may not understand how to express their needs. Your children may throw tantrums, misbehave, and act out — anything to take your attention away from caring for your loved one and set it back on them.

The *sandwich generation* refers to people who are sandwiched between the needs of their parents and their children, shouldering the responsibilities of caring for both at the same time. These sections provide some guidance to help you manage your life at home with your family and caregiving for your loved one.

Smoothing things over with the kids

Try a bit of creativity to overcome problems with demanding younger kids. Explain to them that your older family member has an illness that requires a lot of care. Draw an analogy they can relate to, such as reminding them how you cared for them when they had chickenpox or a bad cold. Then tell them that's the sort of care you must provide for your older loved one. The hard thing to communicate to children is the on-going nature of your caregiving responsibilities.

Even very young children can help with light chores. Including them makes them feel important, helps them overcome feelings of isolation, and keeps them feeling connected to you. Also, pay attention to how your children interact with the person with Alzheimer's disease (AD). You may find that they relate well to your loved one, but in some cases, children aggravate AD patients.

Be realistic when estimating the time required for caregiving activities. Most caregivers underestimate the time their loved one requires by 10 to 20 percent. Underestimating your time can get worse as AD progresses and the amount and complexity of care required increases.

Making a schedule

Schedule individual time with your children and spouse every day. Even if you meet for 15 or 20 minutes, you may be surprised how much information you can exchange. You can read your child a book (at a leisurely pace) or ask your spouse about her workday. Put all thoughts of your loved one out of your mind during this special time. Really listen to your children and spouse, and express your appreciation for the support they're showing you. Ask if they have any issues they want to discuss or problems that need solutions. Make them feel special, and you'll feel better as well.

Even with the best planning, caregiving often disrupts the rhythm in a family. Everyone misses the special family activities you shared in the past and the day-to-day comforts you previously provided. In the first few weeks of caregiving, you can easily overlook your family's needs, putting them on automatic pilot and hoping for the best. However, this approach creates problems, especially when your caregiving responsibilities persist and require more of your time. When making your weekly schedule, include special family time and make getaways as a priority. Doing so avoids hurt feelings and the difficulties that may arise when other family members feels neglected or overlooked.

Being creative

If camping in the woods every weekend is no longer feasible, find new activities for your family. Think of other ways to do the same activity. For instance, put a tent in the backyard and let your kids sleep there on weekend nights. You may even join them if you have a good ghost story to share.

Perhaps you all like the zoo but haven't gone for a while because of your caregiving responsibilities. Can you take your loved one along on a zoo outing? Call ahead to see what accommodations are available. If your loved one tires after a little walking or has a tendency to wander, rent a wheelchair and push him around the exhibit areas. You can do the same for the aquarium or children's museum. If you think creatively, you can find ways for the entire family to participate in an enjoyable outing.

If your loved one is too impaired to come along or you want to spend special time with your spouse and children, ask your sibling to stand in or hire a sitter. Spending regular quality time with other family members is vitally important. If your kids are young when your loved one comes to live with you and your loved one stays for ten years, putting off family fun until your caregiving responsibilities are over means you have put off your childrens' entire childhoods. You don't want your children to graduate high school and go off to college thinking of you as an overworked shadow that flickered in and out of their lives.

Communicating

Even if you've always maintained positive relationships with your siblings and your marriage is successful, the strain of caregiving can create conflicts. Deal with problems head-on. Don't let difficult family dynamics derail you emotionally. Honest, open communication and flexibility help resolve conflicts fairly — negotiate, compromise, and ask everyone to lay their concerns on the table. Are your family members worried about your loved one's care? Do they disagree with the diagnosis or how you're handling the situation? Do they feel left out? Are they worried about being asked to pay a share of the costs of caregiving, or do they think that because you have the dementia or AD patient in your home, you get to scoop up the entire family fortune? Whatever the problem is, get it out in the open so you can address the issue together. Counseling can be helpful in resolving uncomfortable situations.

Perhaps you're the one with the problem. Maybe you feel like you're doing all the work and your siblings or spouse aren't doing enough to help. Don't play the martyr; express your feelings calmly and ask for help. Instead of whining or crying about being overworked, hand out printed copies of your schedule and ask for help with specific chores. For example, if your daughter's dance class makes it impossible for you to pick up your loved one from adult daycare one day a week, ask your sister if she can take over the driving on those days. Ask your husband if he can pick up prescriptions on his way home from work. And remember, you can't force anyone to help; some people in your family may refuse to offer any assistance. If that's the case, move on. No amount of nagging will change their minds, and your bad temper serves only to reinforce stereotypes about your family dynamic. Otherwise persistent negative interactions with other family members will only increase your own stress.

It's normal for siblings and other family members to have differences of opinion on caregiving issues such as how and when to use respite care or when to consider assisted living or a nursing home, and so on. As the primary caregiver, you may have to override their opinions. Counseling can help you make sure your approach is realistic and not a knee jerk response to old family conflicts and resentments. For more information on enlisting support, see Chapter 17.

WARNING

Don't ask the same person for help over and over. Try to build a team of helpers and rotate your requests for assistance among them. This approach circumvents burnout and saves family relationships and friendships.

REMEMBER

Keep your family members informed, ask for their help in planning and problem solving, and share responsibility equally, and you may be able to avoid most problems arising from underlying family dynamics.

Making Family Time a Priority

Finding special time for your family is a matter of priority. Make family time important, and your family stays happy and strong. Ignore family time, and you add to the heavy load of problems you're already shouldering.

REMEMBER

Don't expect your spouse to understand your situation indefinitely. Make a date night once a week to just enjoy each other's company and to get away from the house and all your responsibilities. Don't let anything interfere with this time. Be sure to involve your spouse in caregiving plans. He may have valuable ideas to contribute — ideas you won't hear if you shut him out. Ask for help and accept what help is offered. Discuss finances and worries you have concerning your ability to pay for your loved one's care. Make plans for family outings. In other words, go on with your family's normal life.

Involving your adult children in the caregiving process can reap multiple benefits: you get additional help, an increased understanding of the situation, and the opportunity for each child to develop and strengthen his or her relationship with the person with AD or dementia.

Tell your younger children the kind of behavior you expect from them. Make a list of house rules and explain why the rules are important. For example, your teen likes to listen to loud music, but has a bedroom next to your loved one's room. Instead of trying to get the volume down, buy a set of headphones so your teen can listen as much as she wants without disturbing your loved one. Look for creative solutions that preserve individual rights without upsetting other family members. Don't overreact to slip-ups or mistakes. Remind your children of the house rules and ask them to follow the rules for everyone's benefit.

You can give every member of your family the attention he or she craves, and you can do it without cloning yourself. Plan ahead, involve everyone in the planning stage, and adjust your plan as your caregiving responsibilities evolve.

TIP

You can find an excellent resource with many specific practical suggestions for all caregivers of loved ones with dementia (and especially those employed outside the home) on the Family Caregiver Alliance website at www.caregiver.org/health-issues/alzheimers.

IN THIS CHAPTER

Caregiving with family dynamics

Finding ways to help the primary caregiver

Coping with long-distance guilt

Chapter 20

Helping When You're Not the Primary Caregiver

You experience many different emotions when you hear that your loved one has dementia or Alzheimer's disease (AD) — especially if you're living far away from your loved one. Part of you may want to give up everything and rush to your parent's or grandparent's side; another part may feel guilty about not being there when you're needed; and still another part may feel helpless.

Even when you're not physically there, you can help your loved one and the primary caregiver. You can participate in the planning stage, when you're evaluating care options or examining financial arrangements. You can attend important medical appointments, such as the initial medical evaluation, treatment planning, or annual follow-ups. You can help research local services to help. You can buy books on caregiving and inspirational texts to share with your loved one and the primary caregiver. If your loved one is moving in with one of your siblings or into a residential care facility, perhaps you can arrange your schedule so you can help with the move. Through phone calls, cards, emails, and texts, you can offer ongoing emotional support. You can contribute money for care, talk to doctors by phone, take a vacation week during a critical time to give the primary caregiver a break, and several other little things that show you care and want to help, even though you're far away.

This chapter reveals smart ways to contribute to the caregiving process, even from a distance, and points out some things you shouldn't do if you want to keep peace in your family. You find out how to recognize the Monday-morning-quarterback syndrome and ways to overcome your desire to second-guess everything the primary caregiver does. You also find tips to make your visits more productive and satisfying, even if you can visit only once a year.

Being hundreds of miles away when your loved one is facing a crisis like a memory disorder isn't the ideal situation, but with a little creative thinking, you can figure out ways to share your love, keep in touch, and offer a helping hand across the miles.

Understanding How Family Dynamics Affect Caregiving Decisions

Before you decide the best way to contribute to your loved one's care, think about your family dynamics. If your family members communicate well, get along, and treat each other with courtesy and respect, your family will obviously have an easier time caregiving than family members who don't speak because they're engaged in a 10-year feud. When a family is fighting, making satisfactory caregiving decisions is almost impossible.

The following sections explain how you can contribute to your loved one's care and support the primary caregiver when you can't be present on a regular basis.

Considering your proximity

When you live in a different town or state than the rest of your family, you may feel left out of the loop when it comes to caring for your loved one. Don't let those negative feelings create an even more difficult situation. Part of what you're feeling is a sense of conflict; you want to stay where you are and go on with your life, but you also want to be at your loved one's side 24 hours a day. You may feel like you have no control over the situation or that no one values your input, when in fact, they do. You have to work with your family members to find ways to help and stay informed about your loved one's condition.

If you live closest to the person with AD or dementia, other family members may automatically assume that you'll provide the bulk of the care, which can be a point of contention. Or if you're unmarried, divorced, or childless, you may be expected to step up to the plate even if you live far away and would have to give up your job and your current life to move home and provide care. Maybe you have small children or a tough job, or your other obligations are so demanding that you just don't see how you can help in the ways you're being asked to help. Good communication is the only way to get all of these unspoken assumptions and expectations out on the table and resolved fairly. Everyone involved needs to be heard, and everyone involved should be willing to compromise a bit to arrive at the best caretaking solutions.

Navigating family relationships

If you've always been the family leader and decision-maker or if you're the oldest child, your relatives may automatically look to you for guidance and direction, even if you're not the primary caregiver. If you're a middle child, you may be sensitive about your input being overlooked, whereas the youngest child may be either rebellious or resigned to someone else calling the shots in the family. Be careful that these old roles and feelings don't create new tensions in the family.

Even the nicest families may have a troublemaker — someone who thinks that Grandma's infirmity presents a swell opportunity to move in and drain the old girl's bank accounts. If this situation is possible in your family, you and your other family members must do everything you can to protect your loved one from fraud or intimidation.

You may also have family members who insist on characterizing your loved one's problem as just "old age," and they reject the diagnosis of dementia or AD altogether and express anger at family members who accept it. Don't expect much help from these naysayers until they can accept the true nature of the problem. In fact, they may actively work against what other family members are doing.

What you can do to help depends on your own situation, your strengths and talents, your resources, and your position within your family structure. No matter what your position is within the family, the primary caregiver may resent any suggestions anyone else makes, no matter how benign. Sit down with the primary caregiver and assure her that you appreciate her hard work and believe she's doing a great job. Tell her your suggestions are a way for you to stay connected to the situation and aren't an attempt to micromanage things from a distance. Open and honest discussion can be mutually reassuring and serves to forge a vital bond to help carry you through the difficult times ahead.

REMEMBER

Whatever role you played in the family growing up and whatever patterns of behavior dominated your family's interactions in the past are likely to re-emerge in full bloom under the stress of the situation, even if you thought those things were all in the past. Even if you're in your 50s, you may still be the baby of the family when it comes to family dynamics, unless you've planned ahead and are prepared to forge a new role for yourself. It's not easy to redefine your role within the family, but stay calm, stick to your agenda, and don't let anyone pull you back into an old argument. Stay focused on the present and redirect everyone's attention back to the problem at hand if they try to waste time and energy on old business.

If one of the reasons you moved far away from home was because your parent or grandparent who now has AD or dementia has a difficult personality or because your family is combative and you got tired of the fighting, then you probably dread coming back into the fold at this juncture in your life, even if you're just visiting for a week. Don't wreck your own life and sacrifice your serenity under the misguided belief that the only way you can help is to be physically present. Instead of getting caught in the middle of your family's drama again, think of other ways to be supportive that don't require your physical presence. (See "Discovering how to help" later in this chapter for some creative ideas.)

Staying in the loop

When you live in a different city or state than the rest of your family, you may feel left out of the loop when it comes to caring for your loved one. Although these feelings are natural, don't let your negative emotions fuel an already difficult situation. The primary caregiver already has her hands full and isn't necessarily leaving you out on purpose.

TIP

Take responsibility for keeping yourself in the loop. Set a time for a weekly phone meeting and keep the tone conversational and light. Make it clear that you're looking for information and feedback, not a fight. The primary caregiver may be sensitive to criticism, perceived or real, so try not to be the person who knows just how everything *should* be done, especially because you're not there dealing with the day-to-day reality. An I-know-it-all-from-afar attitude can be really maddening for the primary caregiver who is, after all, the real hero in the situation. Notice we didn't say the primary caregiver is the *only* hero — just the one who's most likely to get the Purple Caregiver's Heart for caring above and beyond the call of duty.

After you figure out how your family dynamics work and how those old roles may impact caregiving, you're ready for a family meeting to determine the new roles each person plays in the caretaking process.

Getting together

Whether family members agree or disagree about how to provide care for the patient, a family meeting is a good way to get thoughts out in the open and give everyone a chance to express his or her opinions. If emotions are really running high, you may want to consider scheduling your meeting with a counselor who can help you sort out your priorities and find workable compromises. Draw up guidelines for the meeting. Everyone can express his or her thoughts and feelings openly, without fear of being judged. Shouting and screaming aren't allowed; intense emotions don't accomplish anything and are very upsetting to everyone, especially your loved one. Be willing to accept compromise solutions.

TIP

Remember that caregiving is more than just changing sheets and preparing meals. Caregiving has a spiritual and emotional dimension as well, and this is an area where caregivers can often get overwhelmed, especially if they feel isolated and don't have anyone to talk to. Even though you're separated physically, you can help your family and the primary caregiver by regularly communicating and staying emotionally close.

After the care plan is chosen, assign jobs or responsibilities. Let each family member contribute in ways that suit his talents, finances, and availability. If no one can realistically take on the role of primary caregiver, you know that you must make other care arrangements.

Even if it's not physically possible for the whole family to meet for a planning session, you can arrange a telephone or Internet conference with all your family members who are directly involved. If that's not feasible, speak to everyone individually to discuss what needs to be done and how the work and responsibilities can be divided equally. Be sure to include your loved one in these meetings if at all possible; having input in the decisions that affect her care and quality of life is vitally important for the patient.

After the meeting, write out a care plan outlining the responsibilities of each family member who's involved. Send a copy to everyone for comment; this provides another opportunity for discussion and compromise. Pledge to keep each family member regularly informed about your loved one's condition, either by phone, letter, or email.

Discovering How to Help

When you first hear about your loved one's dementia or AD diagnosis, you feel a jumble of emotions. Your first instinct may be to pack a bag and fly to your loved one's side. Before using any vacation days you may need later, sit down and think about your options.

TIP

Trying to keep up with an AD or dementia patient from a distance? Put all correspondence, medical reports, legal documents, and anything else pertaining to your loved one's care in a portable file box. Keeping this information separate from your usual files helps you find it quickly when you need it.

Having young kids, financial or health issues of your own, or a demanding job constrains the amount of time and effort you can expend helping your loved one. Being in a structured situation, like college or the military, also limits what you can do to help and when you can do it. Take all of these factors into account when trying to determine how you can help.

You probably want to make at least one trip to visit your loved one, meet with your other family members, and assess the situation firsthand. If you return for a visit during your vacation, coordinate your schedule with the primary caregiver to make sure the timing is convenient. The caregiver may want to take a break during your visit or may want to stay and visit with you, enjoying your help and company. Let the caregiver decide how to spend her time and don't load her up with a lot of guilt.

Keeping in touch with each other is easier now than ever before. Cellphones and email have made staying in touch quick and inexpensive. How you choose to communicate with your family doesn't matter — just do it. Regular communication is one of the best ways to show you care and want to be part of the caregiving process, even from a distance.

Helping the primary caregiver

You can do a lot of things to make the primary caregiver's load lighter and strengthen your family bond at the same time. No one expects you to pull up stakes and move halfway across the country to provide care. That's just not realistic. But you can help in many other ways; the important thing is to make sure that whatever you're doing fulfills an actual need and doesn't add to the caregiving burden. You can express your love and support by offering to

- >> **Provide financial assistance.** Providing care for an AD or dementia patient is expensive. Having the means to offer financial assistance can ease the burden for the primary caregiver. Perhaps it allows a home health aide to be hired once a week to give the primary caregiver a break or maybe it pays for a daycare program or needed home modification or maintenance costs. Or you can offer to pay for medications not covered by insurance, co-pays for doctor visits, or even health insurance premiums to lessen the caregivers out of pocket expenses.

- >> **Offer telephone support.** Even though you're not physically present, taking five minutes a few times a week to call your loved one and the primary caregiver to let them know you love them and are thinking of them can go a long way toward relieving the isolation and loneliness that comes with being a caregiver.

- >> **Talk to your loved one's doctors.** When you have an opportunity to visit, be sure to accompany your loved one to the doctor and introduce yourself. You'll feel more comfortable and confident about the care being provided for your loved one after meeting her physicians.

- >> **Educate yourself.** Become knowledgeable about every aspect of dementia or AD, including its diagnosis, prognosis, and treatment. Utilize books and other resources at your local public library. Get online and do an Internet research. Share what you discover with the rest of your family. The Alzheimer's Association (www.alz.org) offers a wealth of information both on dementia in general and AD in particular. At the website you can sign up for the free weekly newsletter to stay informed with helpful tips and the latest research.

- >> **Help with recordkeeping.** Patients with a memory disorder have thick medical files and tons of paperwork to keep sorted. It's easy for caregivers to let paperwork slide, especially with all of the other tasks they must tend to. Offer to organize and file all of the paperwork during a visit. If you have a particular area of expertise such as accounting, law, or healthcare, offer to review documents relevant to your specialty on an ongoing basis.

- >> **Give emotional support.** Send regular letters or emails with support and encouragement and share funny stories, good news, your love, or anything to make your loved one smile.

- >> **Share visual memories.** Send old family photos or videos by email, reminding your loved one of good times in the past. Or share updated photos of your family to show how family events from afar or how the grandchildren are growing. Visual remembrances often can trigger memories even in moderate stages of dementia. Such reminiscence can be very therapeutic for both your loved one and the primary caregiver.

>> **Assist with gathering information.** When you're a primary caregiver, the last thing you have time to do is gather information. As a distant caregiver, you can help the primary caregiver by gathering information about care facilities and costs, clinical trials, memory research, medications, hired and substitute caregivers, and durable medical equipment.

>> **Be the family chronicler.** When a family faces a crisis like AD or dementia, communications not relating to AD and the patient tend to fall by the wayside. Maybe your niece is getting married, but all anyone talks about is the diagnosis. If you're good on the computer (or even if you're not), put together a family newsletter once a month and include all the positive news you can gather — births, engagements, weddings, graduations, birthdays, anniversaries, and job promotions. Also provide the latest update on your loved one's condition. Include photos, if possible, and send the newsletter via email or regular mail to all of your family members. Your newsletter will become very popular and help your family weather the difficult days of caregiving with hope and humor.

>> **Arrange a surprise.** You know how hard the primary caregiver works. To show your appreciation, arrange a surprise day or an evening out to recognize a special occasion like a birthday or anniversary. Enlist the help of other family members to hire a sitter and make reservations for a favorite restaurant. Depending on the caregiver's interests, throw in some movie or sporting event tickets, a few games of bowling, or a round of golf; make it something he really enjoys or doesn't get to do often because of his caregiving duties.

You can help from a distance in many other ways, in ways that are perhaps unique to your own family's situation. Be consistent, be persistent, and your family will feel your love and concern, even across the miles.

Offering financial assistance

Sometimes when you can't realistically do much else, you may feel better throwing money at the situation. Although providing financial support is fine if you can afford it, don't compromise your own financial wellbeing just to assuage your guilt for not being with your loved one all the time.

Money is tricky. Talking about finances is never easy, particularly if your family is close-mouthed about financial issues. But in order to make good decisions, you need all the facts, so ask whether a caregiving budget is in place. Don't make a big deal if there is no budget; simply offer to help draw one up. Compare resources against needs and determine whether there is a financial shortfall. (For complete information on how to assess the resources, see Chapter 13.) If the primary caregiver is sensitive about money issues, assure him that you only want to help, not take over.

Talk to the primary caregiver and your loved one about what is needed, what resources are available, and any anticipated shortage of funds. For example, if your loved one's adult daycare costs $600 a month and she can contribute just $200 a month, offer to split the remainder with the primary caregiver and any other siblings or relatives, if you're able.

If you're substantially better off than most of the members of your family, they may look to you to foot most of the bills. You need to figure out how you feel about this. If you're glad to help, that's one thing, but if you're going to act like a martyr, that's quite another. The help that you offer should be given freely with no emotional land mines attached. If you don't like the idea of shouldering the bulk of the financial burden, you'd better figure out another way to help.

If you're in worse financial shape than your other family members, they may try to get you to shoulder your portion of the burden by supplying services like sitting and transportation, which, of course, you can't do because you're so far away. Try some of the suggestions listed in the preceding section instead.

Dealing with Out-of-Towner's Guilt

No matter what you do, you may find yourself swamped with out-of-towner's guilt — the awful feeling that you could and should be doing more, if only you could figure out what. Feeling guilty is a normal part of the grieving process that accompanies a diagnosis of dementia or AD; you think you should do more, and the fact that you're physically distant only exaggerates your feelings. Deal with guilt in the same way you handle other negative, nonproductive emotions — head-on. Bring your feelings out in the open, try to figure out what's making you feel this way, talk it through, and then let it go. If you've tried and can't get out from under your guilt and keep thinking that you really need to be with your loved one, try a few counseling sessions to see if that helps. If it doesn't, consider the practicality of moving. If you're retired, moving may be a logical consideration, but if you have kids in school or a high-powered job, relocating may not make sense.

TIP

Look at your schedule and resources to determine how much time you really can spend with your loved one and make the most of your visits. Don't let guilt drag you down. Remember, you have a life of your own, and your loved one wouldn't want you to give up everything you've worked for to come sit and hold his hand. You can contribute to your loved one's care in other ways, so figure out what works for you and ditch the guilt complex.

5

The Part of Tens

IN THIS PART . . .

Look at some of the best advice for dealing with dementia if your loved one has been given the diagnosis, from discussing the condition with others to and planning financially for the future.

Find out how to be a good caregiver while ensuring that you have time to recharge your batteries.

Discover the truth about some of the most common and misleading myths about dementia.

Chapter 21

Ten Tips for Dealing with Dementia

However you look at it, being given the diagnosis of dementia or Alzheimer's disease (AD) is a difficult blow. And even though you or your close family may have had an inkling that the symptoms you were experiencing were due to this condition, the realization that you were right all along is still tough to take.

However, in the early days after your diagnosis, you still can do plenty to prepare for the challenges of your condition's later stages. Here are ten tips to consider putting into action as soon as you can.

Accept Changes

You may notice that some things aren't as easy as they used to be. You may be quite forgetful at times. Maybe you have missed appointments or forgotten to buy items on your shopping list. You may find calculations involving money trickier to manage. You may have gotten lost while driving even on familiar routes.

Trying to battle these new difficulties while simultaneously pretending they're not happening inevitably leads to frustration. If you accept your new limitations and work out ways around them with the help of family and friends, you'll feel more in control and cope better than if you bury your head in the sand.

You need to accept your new challenges and discover ways to adapt by maximizing your remaining functional abilities. Enlist memory aids. Consider displaying a wall calendar in an obvious place at home, listing all your activities so you don't miss important events. Establish a routine whereby you and the people you live with look at the calendar together at the same time every day. If you're still driving, use a GPS system in the car to prevent getting lost; if you're on foot, use a hand-held GPS app for walkers. Write lists instead of trying to remember everything. Make shopping lists and to do lists and keep them visible to help you stay on track. These small steps make it much easier to cope with the changes you are experiencing.

Keeping track of your prescription medications is essential, but it's commonly a challenge to remember to take your pills in the early stages of dementia. Use a weekly pillbox to help you remember to take your medications and to see whether you have already taken them, which is especially important because many medications can be toxic if taken a second time because you didn't remember that you took them earlier in the day. Forgetting to take pills can also be dangerous. If needed, consider an alarmed pill dispenser that rings when it's time for you to take your pills. Many options for such dispensers are available for purchase on the Internet.

Let People Know What's Happening

You must tell some people about your diagnosis as soon as possible, such as your boss if you're still working. Your boss may be able to organize workplace adaptations to make things easier for you to manage. Beyond that, it's up to you which of your friends, family, or colleagues to tell about your diagnosis. Health matters are obviously private, and you may not want every Tom, Diane, or Harry knowing your most intimate business.

However, telling relevant people has clear benefits:

>> You provide the information on your own terms and give people just the details you want them to know. If they hear it secondhand and in a gossipy fashion, they won't get the facts straight. Hence, they may assume what is wrong with you and come up with all sorts of weird theories that are untrue.

Better to be honest with those that you care about and ultimately want to be in the loop.

>> The more people who know what's going on and how your type of dementia usually progresses, the more people you have to support you as time goes on.

>> People that know what is going on with you will be able to make allowances for you when things don't go as they should as a direct result of your condition.

Be Realistic about Driving

When you're diagnosed with dementia, in certain states your doctor is required to tell the Department of Motor Vehicles (DMV). If you have an accident, it's possible there will be additional liability especially if your doctor has told you not to drive. Early in the disease, you may still be able to drive safely, but generally your ability to drive safely will erode with dementia progression. You'll face a time when you have to hang up your keys. (Check out Chapter 10 for more information about how to handle driving with an Alzheimer's or dementia patient.)

You won't necessarily need to surrender your driver's license especially early on, but you may be asked to take a driving test to assess whether you're still safe to be on the road. You may or may not be able to keep your license after the test depending on how you do. If you pass such a driving test, expect to be subject to regular review. This review may involve having your physician fill out a questionnaire for the DMV saying whether or not it's safe for you to drive based on your cognitive abilities.

TIP

If your loved one with the dementia diagnosis continues to drive, make sure that you personally experience his driving regularly. While driving with him, ask yourself whether you'd be happy if your children or grandchildren were in the car with him. If the answer is no or one of hesitation, then you need to think further. This litmus test for driving safety is important. Admitting that your loved one has reached this stage isn't easy, but you have to be honest about the reality of the disease and consider the safety of your loved one, his passengers, and those around him on the road.

People often say they only use a car to go in town to go shopping for groceries, to get their hair done, or to go to church services. But an accident can happen even when backing out of the driveway. Most people do most of their driving within a few miles of their homes, which is where most accidents occur. Just driving to get some groceries may be okay early in dementia, but as symptoms progress, any driving becomes more dangerous. Dementia affects a person's spatial perception and judgment especially in advanced stages.

It's better if your loved one chooses to stop driving for himself rather than you having to be the bad guy or having his license revoked by the DMV. If this issue is especially difficult for you to address with your loved one, then ask his doctor to address it. The doctor can be the bad guy and explain the medical reasons why it's necessary to quit driving. Unlike you, the doctor isn't living with your loved one and dealing with his daily frustrations. Hence, your loved one may accept this information more easily from a medical professional rather than from you. A driver's license is a powerful symbol of independence, so being told you can no longer have one can be a crushing blow.

Work Together with Your Partner

If you're in a long-term relationship, working together with your spouse or partner to manage your condition is important. Don't cut your partner off or, worse still, work against him. Now is the time when you need this partnership the most as you prepare to face the challenges of your dementia that will come down the road.

Your spouse or partner may well have thought that you had dementia for some time, but the diagnosis may still come as a shock, and she'll have to come to terms with the effects of your illness on your relationship. So be honest with her. Share your thoughts and feelings about your dementia or AD and allow her to share hers with you. Consider seeing a counselor together if you need help talking about this difficult subject. Continue doing activities together that you've always enjoyed. As your symptoms change, try new activities that are more manageable but allow you to continue to share the experience. Maybe you can go on a tour rather than traveling independently to lessen the stress of travel. You can still have a great trip. Flexibility at this time of change is essential.

Sometimes the psychological and emotional effects of the diagnosis affect your sexual relationship. But intimacy keeps you and your partner connected at this time of change. Again, talk together and seek counseling if needed to facilitate communication.

Keep Active

Dementia or AD isn't a prison sentence. You aren't confined within the four walls of your house for the rest of your life. Keeping fit and active is a great way to make sure your body and brain remain healthy for as long as possible.

If you normally play a sport or go to the gym, keep going for as long as you can (and want to). If you aren't sports oriented, then go for walks or bike rides. Perhaps you can join a bowling league. Any activity can help you keep connected to friends who can be supportive and understanding of your situation. Not only will remaining active keep you in shape, but it also helps you maintain relationships and meet new people.

Sort Out Your Finances

When you're newly diagnosed and still fully able to make rational decisions for yourself, spend some time with your family reviewing your financial situation. Consider hiring an independent financial advisor to help you better define where you stand financially. With his help, you can have a current picture of your income, expenses, and savings, and thus plan for whatever expenses the future may bring. This is especially important because you may need residential care in the future, and your family will need to know what financial resources you can bring to the table should that situation arise. As for paying bills, simple measures like making sure all your bills are paid automatically by direct debit from your checking account or savings can prevent late or missed payments.

You may be eligible for employee, retiree, veteran, or government-sponsored benefits. Enlist the help of family members or close friends to help you connect to potential resources.

Make a Will

You may think that making a will is a bit morbid, but everyone should have one. A *will* is the only way to ensure that your property, savings, and family heirlooms are passed on according to your wishes. Dying *intestate* — without a will — puts a huge burden on your family members that are left behind. In such situations, the government takes over and makes decisions for you. No one wants that.

Thus, while you still have the capacity to do so, consider who you want to benefit from your legacy. You'll want to provide for your spouse and maybe your children and grandchildren. It may be important for you to leave money to the animal shelter or the fund for the church roof. Maybe you want to leave instructions for your nearest and dearest to put a plaque honor you on your favorite park bench. It's your will — and at this point, you can still make the decisions, so get it done while you can.

You have many options for preparing a will. You can draw up a will yourself without legal help by simply downloading a form from the Internet and filling it in. However, make sure that the will you prepare meets any legal requirements in your state. Make sure your signature is appropriately witnessed to make your will valid. Alternatively, you can buy a ready-made will from a bookstore. If you have a lot of assets, you may want to hire an attorney to do a formal estate plan. Doing so can greatly decrease federal and state death tax implications for your family when you die. (For more information about wills and other legal issues, check out Chapter 12.)

Look After Your Physical Health

A diagnosis of dementia doesn't mean that your physical health automatically suffers. To remain in the best possible condition,

>> Eat a healthful, balanced diet that's low in carbohydrates, high in fiber, and includes at least five portions of fruit and vegetables per day. Cut out the sodas and sweets. Eat your greens.

>> Stay well hydrated by drinking lots of water each day. Watch your tea, coffee, and cola intake. Caffeine can make you anxious and irritable, so don't overindulge. Enjoy one cup, then switch to a noncaffeinated alternative like herbal tea.

>> Stick to the guidelines for safe alcohol intake; that's one drink per day for a woman and one to two for a man.

>> If you smoke, stop! Your physician, nurse practitioner, or pharmacist can provide advice about how to quit with the best chance of success.

>> Get a good night's sleep. Don't nap in the daytime. Keep a regular schedule to keep your circadian rhythms working appropriately. Day-night reversal can occur in dementia. Guard against this by keeping active during the day so you are tired when nighttime arrives.

Get Your Annual Checkups

Medicare offers an annual wellness visit for anyone over the age of 65 to review your health, arrange screenings, and obtain preventative care like vaccines. Take up the offer. If you already have ongoing chronic health problems, make sure you schedule and keep regular appointments with your primary care physician, nurse practitioner, or physician assistant. Other checks worth having include the following:

>> Six-month checkups at the dentist to ensure your teeth, mouth, and gums remain healthy and pain-free.

>> Annual eye exams at the optometrist (eyeglass doctor) to make sure your contacts or glasses maximize your vision. Or go to the ophthalmologist (medical eye doctor) if you have a diagnosed eye problem like glaucoma or cataracts.

>> Regular toenail/foot care from a podiatrist, especially if you have diabetes.

>> A medication review with your pharmacist. A pharmacist can advise you about side effects and interactions between your different medications. Pharmacists can also arrange for your pills to be supplied in a blister pack to help you remember what to take each day.

>> An annual flu shot from your local pharmacy because it no longer requires a doctor's order. Ask your physician about the shingles and pneumococcal pneumonia vaccinations because these shots often do require a doctor's order but are important preventative measures.

Continue Hobbies and Pastimes

In short, don't give up. Continue to do the things that you enjoy doing with your friends and family. Maintaining enjoyable activities as long as you can will do you a world of good. So continue to play golf or bridge with friends, make pottery, go bird watching, putter around in the garden, travel to interesting places, swim in the local pool, cycle up hills, windsurf, enter your dog in shows, go to your local library programs — get as much enjoyment out of life as possible. You can even take up something new to broaden your horizons and meet new people. In fact, any meaningful hobby can assist in keeping your brain active as possible.

Chapter 22

Ten Tips for Caregivers, Friends, and Families

Being the partner, friend, or relative of someone with dementia or Alzheimer's disease (AD) often throws you into the role of caregiver. And the closer you are to the person, the more likely you are to be involved.

People with dementia aren't always easy to care for, no matter how much you love them. Unfortunately, dementia not only affects people's intellectual functions like memory and planning, but it also invariably changes their mood and behavior. And what's more, you may not ever have considered yourself to be caregiver material in the first place. You may feel that your life is too busy, you don't have the patience, and you can't bear cleaning up after other people. But you may nevertheless be thrown, kicking and screaming, into that role.

Here are ten tips for the novice caregiver to help make life not only as easy as possible but also fulfilling.

Make Life as Normal as Possible for as Long as Possible

In the earlier stages of dementia, soon after someone has been given the diagnosis, she may well be able to continue doing all the things she's done up to this point. She may still be able to go to work, drive a car safely, indulge in her hobbies, and get out and about with friends. As long as this is the case, encourage her to continue. You may need to give a bit of extra help here and there because of the early effects of dementia, but by and large, things will likely carry on for some time as they were. No one goes from diagnosis to total disability in the way that a sports car accelerates from 0 to 60.

Going about her usual life also helps keep your loved one's spirits up after the diagnosis of dementia, which can be a crushing blow. So keep encouraging her to carry on normally as much as possible. Meanwhile, involve her in making decisions about the future for when her dementia progresses. Get her input while she can give it.

Encourage Her to Plan for the Future

Although you don't want the person you're caring for to think the future is inevitably bleak, it's a good idea to help her sort out the financial and legal issues that will ultimately affect her future while she still has the capacity to express her desires.

The most important issues are as follows:

>> **Sorting out finances:** The person with dementia should see a financial advisor to review her income, expenses, and savings to estimate her resources if she retires. In addition, figure out what personal expenses there will be if she needs residential or nursing home care in the future. Make a plan about how to cover these expenses if they're needed. (See Chapter 13 for more about financial issues.)

>> **Making a will:** Most people have an idea about whom they want to benefit from their estate when they die and whom they want to be the executor(s) of the will. Sorting out these details while she can participate takes a weight off her mind and yours.

Dying *intestate* (without a will) can create huge — and potentially expensive — problems for those left behind. Refer to Chapter 12 for more details about wills.

>> **Setting up direct debits for auto-pay of bills:** The memory problems that affect people with dementia or AD can make it impossible to remember when to pay important bills on time. And missing payments may result in having utilities cut off or having creditors calling for payment. Paying bills automatically by direct debit from a checking or savings account significantly reduces this risk from happening (as long as the account has sufficient funds to cover expenses). This is one less worry for both of you.

>> **Applying for benefits:** Some benefits may be available to assist your loved one. Employees (including family), veterans, and Medicaid-recipients may have specific resources available that aren't available to the general population. Apply for these benefits as early as possible to receive the maximum advantage.

>> **Establishing durable power of attorney:** *This point is of critical importance.* People with a memory disorder *must* have someone to manage their affairs when they're no longer able to do so. Two types of durable power of attorney exist:

- Healthcare decisions

- Finance management

You don't need a lawyer to set up durable power of attorney; just download the forms from the Internet. Remember that these documents must be notarized in order to be valid. If it makes you more comfortable that all everything is legal, then you may choose to hire a lawyer to assist in the preparation of these documents.

One website that provides durable power of attorney forms is http:// powerofattorrney.com/durable/. Note that this website requires you to select forms based on your state of residence. Although the forms may be specific to your state, these documents are valid across state lines. If you move to another state, a signed durable power of attorney document from the prior state remains functional, which is especially important when a move occurs when the individual with dementia no longer has capacity to make changes to these legal documents. (Chapter 12 has more information about these legal documents.)

Ensure That She Remains Healthy

People with dementia require attention to personal care (bathing and clean clothes), nutrition, and general health maintenance just like anyone else. However, as dementia progresses, you may need to prompt and assist the person whom you're caring for to do these basics of daily life.

Encourage a healthful diet including five servings of fruit and vegetables daily and limit carbohydrates. Remind your loved one to drink eight cups of water daily. Avoid or at least limit alcohol use to one drink for women and one to two drinks for men per day. If your loved one smokes, help him to quit. (As dementia progresses, smoking can become increasingly hazardous due to a person lighting a cigarette and not remembering to handle it properly or not snuffing it out fully causing fire risk.) You may have your hands full if drinking and/or smoking are important to your loved one. Be pragmatic and just do your best.

Encourage exercise. If your loved one has always exercised, then encourage her to continue. If exercise has never been a priority, then encourage her to start. Of course, exercise is good for heart health, but it also improves mood, provides social opportunities, and makes people naturally tired so they sleep better at night. You may find that you can both exercise by taking a walk together. Then you can both benefit. Exercise is a win-win activity.

In time, you may need to remind the person you're caring for about basic hygiene. She may need prompting to wash her hands after using the toilet and before preparing food. Reminders may be needed to bathe, change soiled clothes regularly, and do laundry. Don't forget oral hygiene. Brushing teeth remains important, but many people often forgot to do it.

Attention to personal hygiene fades as all forms of dementia progress. Hence these basics of personal care will likely require more of your caregiving attention as time goes on.

Take Her for Health Checks

Medicare provides for a free annual wellness visit. When someone you care for has dementia, you need to utilize this benefit for all it's worth. After all, you don't get much free these days, especially in healthcare.

REMEMBER

Assist your loved one in scheduling regular visits to her primary care physician. Stick to the same doctor as much as possible to ensure continuity of care. If your loved one appears to have rapidly progressing confusion, agitated behavior, or lethargy, then get an appointment promptly to evaluate for an underlying medical problem. If her usual doctor isn't available for such an urgent or unexpected visit, then get an appointment with a doctor or nurse practitioner in the same group so your loved one's medical records are available for reference. Doing so helps to ensure appropriate and thoughtful medical care.

Other professionals who should be involved in monitoring your loved one's health are the dentist, optometrist, podiatrist, and pharmacist. Finally, ensure the person is up-to-date with recommended vaccinations and screening checks such as mammograms. (See Chapter 12 for more about helping your loved one maintain her health.)

Consider Underlying Reasons for Changes in Behavior

As dementia progresses, you'll be presented with a variety of new challenges as your loved one loses cognitive function. However, if you notice a rapid change, such as new onset or escalating agitated behavior, don't assume it simply results from a worsening of the memory disorder. A variety of reasons may explain the change, from constipation to urinary tract infections. As your loved one loses her ability to communicate effectively, new agitation or lethargy may be the only way she can express her symptoms or tells you she's in pain.

WARNING

When communication becomes difficult, people with memory loss may express fear or irritability, or react to pain by becoming withdrawn and refusing to interact, eat, or participate in bathing. Alternatively, they may become aggressive when they're normally placid. If your loved one behaves differently for no obvious reason, bring her to see her primary care physician to check for underlying physical causes.

Accept Professional Help

As a friend or relative, you may think that all caring responsibilities for your loved one should fall on your shoulders. Many people feel guilty when they have to enlist outside help or place someone in an assisted living facility or nursing home, but that's what professional caregivers are for. Think of it like this: Getting extra help relieves you of some pressure. It frees you to do more things with the person you're caring for that you both enjoy. So consider getting help with housecleaning rather than always doing the cleaning yourself. Order Meals on Wheels, rather than preparing food three times a day. Hire a handyman to do home adaptations rather than getting out your tools and trying to put up handrails in your spare time.

Continue to Be Involved When She Enters Residential Care

You obviously don't have to stay with your loved one for 24 hours a day at the assisted living facility or nursing home because that would defeat the entire purpose of her being cared for by someone else. Of course, helping your loved one become acclimated to her new surroundings by introducing her to the staff is important so the staff members get to know her quickly. Bring in some knick-knacks from home to decorate her room to make it a more familiar setting. (See Chapter 15 for more about these topics.)

REMEMBER

You don't have to visit daily but do visit regularly so the staff also gets to know you. Participate in social activities provided by the facility. Don't forget to bring grandchildren to visit whenever possible. The presence of children in the facility cheers up everyone — residents and staff alike. Bulletin boards with family photos provide material for reminiscence as well as giving the staff a window into her family life. It's important that the staff understands who your loved one is as a person, where she worked, and what she enjoys doing. These strategies help the facility staff to see her as a person, not just as a patient.

Think about End-of-Life Care

Experiencing a good death is as important as having a good life. With planning, your loved one's passing is more likely to be peaceful. If she still has the capacity to make decisions, discuss her end-of-life wishes with her. If not, discuss these decisions with other family members, her doctor and the staff at the facility if that's where she's living.

A key issue that you need to consider is whether your loved one should be resuscitated if her heart stops or she stops breathing. Her primary care physician will be happy to discuss these matters with you and formalize them by defining her *code status* in the medical record.

In the advanced stages of dementia, hospice may be an option. To approve hospice services for your loved one, her physician must certify that her life expectancy is less than six months, based on her current medical status. (See Chapter 11 for details on end-of-life care issues, including hospice.)

Look After Yourself

Being a caregiver isn't a 9-to-5 job; it is more like 24/7. Such responsibility can be physically, mentally, and emotionally stressful. Obviously, if you become ill or burnt out, you will be of no use whatsoever to your loved one. Like your loved one, you too should eat a healthful diet, get a good night's sleep, exercise, drink sensibly if at all, and avoid smoking.

You need to schedule regular visits and preventive care with your family physician to maintain your own health. If you have ongoing medical problems such as diabetes or asthma, make sure you take your medication.

TIP

To cope with the emotional and psychological effects of caregiving, stay in touch with other family members and friends. Maintain open lines of communication so you have a support system when you need someone to talk because things are tough.

Consider joining a caregiver support group. The Alzheimer's Association can assist you to find a local group. Support groups can be incredibly helpful by providing a forum to share practical knowledge and experience between caregivers. Such meetings help you to realize that you are not alone in the daily challenges you are facing. Likely what you are struggling with today, another group member struggled with in the past. The solutions they previously discovered can be a lifesaver for you. Shared wisdom by those individuals who are in the same boat provides practical tips to help you care for your loved one with less stress. The Alzheimer's Association has a great website (www.alz.org) with a wealth of information, practical advice, and suggestions for dealing with the strain of caregiving.

If you feel as though you're collapsing under the strain and don't know where to turn, talk to your physician. He can advise extra support available. He can also point you in the direction of professional counseling if that's what he thinks you need. Chapter 17 includes other support networks we suggest you investigate.

Take a Break

Everyone needs a break sometimes, even caregivers. To cope with the demands of caring, make sure that you take time for you, such as regular evenings out relaxing with friends, weekend breaks, and holidays. If no one in your family or friends can take over from time to time, you can hire a paid caregiver to be with your loved one while you take a break for a few hours or days.

If you can't find a paid caregiver to come to your home, you may have to arrange a respite care admission at your local assisted living facility or nursing home if you need an extended absence. Don't feel guilty about taking time for yourself. Time out is essential to your physical and mental wellbeing and can help you to be a better caregiver in the long run.

Chapter 23

Busting Ten Myths about Dementia and Alzheimer's Disease

There are many myths about dementia in general and Alzheimer's disease (AD) in particular. These false and misleading beliefs have led many people to try the wrong treatments and avoid seeking appropriate help. Such myths need busting! But what is actually true? This chapter looks at ten common myths and why they're wrong.

Dementia Is a Natural Part of Aging

Dementia *isn't* a part of normal aging. Most people know seniors who remain mentally sharp despite advanced years, which clearly busts this myth, although it's true that dementia (and AD) is more common in older people. Most people who are diagnosed with dementia including AD are in their senior years.

But advancing age isn't the only risk factor for dementia. Lifestyle issues such as smoking, lack of exercise, and poor diet and medical issues like high blood pressure and high cholesterol play a part. Genetics and family history are involved as well. However, just because your Great Aunt Martha had dementia doesn't mean that you'll be afflicted.

Thus even though older people may be a bit forgetful at times and appear confused about what day it is or forget where they put their keys, having a few such "senior moments" doesn't amount to dementia. Dementia is a clearly defined medical diagnosis that thankfully doesn't apply to everyone as they age.

Dementia Is the Same as Alzheimer's Disease

This myth is like saying beer is the same as alcohol. Beer is a type of alcoholic drink, but it certainly isn't the only one. Wine, gin, whiskey, scotch, vodka, tequila, rum, hard cider, champagne, and port, are also alcoholic drinks. In the same way, dementia is the big category.

Alzheimer's disease is the most common and well-known cause of dementia, with its own society to boot (www.alz.org) and makes up more than 60 percent of all dementias. The other main types of dementia are vascular dementia, frontotemporal dementia, and Lewy body disease, which together make up about 30 percent. The remaining 10 percent are comprised of the more rare forms of dementia including Parkinson's dementia, normal pressure hydrocephalus, Creutzfeldt-Jakob disease, Huntington's disease, and Wernicke-Korsakoff syndrome among others.

Everyone with Dementia Becomes Aggressive

Thankfully, they don't. Anger and aggression can be behavioral symptoms of dementia, but they're by no means universal.

Everyone is capable of being annoyed, losing their tempers, and getting cantankerous. However, some people are naturally hot headed and can blow their lid at the drop of a hat, whereas others have the patience of a saint and only lose control when they're pushed to the limit. People maintain elements of their own personality even in severe dementia. However, that's not to say that dementia-triggered disinhibition can't make warlords out of pacifists sometimes. Yet those who were grumpy pre-dementia will often stay grumpy, shouting, cussing, and moaning their way through the illness. However, there is the chance that they will become more serene. Likewise, if people were calm, cool, and collected pre-dementia, they may remain so or become more irritable.

REMEMBER

After language skills have declined in more advanced dementia, these individuals may show agitation, anger, or aggression because they can't otherwise communicate their discomfort or pain. Although what is bothering these folks can be difficult to sort out, changing something in their surroundings or treating the underlying physical problem often will resolve these behaviors.

Alzheimer's Disease Only Affects Old People

Although AD is more common in older people, it isn't only a disease of old age. Younger people in their 40s or 50s may develop early onset AD, although it's much less common. Up to 5 percent of all Americans with AD fall into this category. Although the age of onset is younger, early onset AD follows the same progression of cognitive and functional losses as AD affecting older people. Doctors don't understand the cause of early onset AD, although some cases of rare familial AD that develop in this age group do exist. These individuals have inherited specific genes that cause early onset AD in multiple family members over multiple generations.

Aluminium Gives You Dementia

The myth describing a link between dementia and aluminum in cooking pots, pop cans, and antiperspirants began in the 1960s. That is when some scientists took it upon themselves to inject aluminum into the brains of live rabbits to see what happened. Not surprisingly, the rabbits fared poorly: they developed protein tangles in their brains, similar to those found in people diagnosed with AD. Consequently, these researchers linked AD to aluminum exposure, and a conspiracy theory was born. Since then, further research hasn't corroborated any link, so the Alzheimer's Association is very keen to dismiss this myth.

Alzheimer's Disease Can Be Cured

At present, no cure for AD (as well as most other forms of dementia) is available. The FDA approved drugs used in AD may slow progression for 6 to 12 months in half the people who take them, but this effect is temporary. These drugs don't cure AD, although they can be beneficial. Much research is currently underway to understand the causes of AD and search for a cure. Refer to Chapter 8 for an in-depth discussion on these medications.

Alzheimer's Disease Is Progressive and Debilitating but Not Fatal

Actually, AD can kill you. Although other disease processes like heart attack can kill you before AD does the job, in 2015 about 700,000 Americans older than 65 died from AD. In fact, AD is the only condition in the top ten causes of death in the United States that isn't preventable or curable. Between 2000 and 2013, deaths from AD increased by more than 70 percent, whereas deaths from the number one killer, heart disease, declined almost 15 percent.

Women Are More Likely to Develop Alzheimer's Disease than Men

It's true that more women than men develop dementia; in fact, two-thirds of Americans with AD are women. Among AD sufferers, the proportion of women to men increases with age. However, women aren't necessarily more susceptible to the causes of dementia than men. Rather, they tend to live longer (a woman's life expectancy in the United States is 81.2 years compared to 76.4 for a man), thus increasing their likelihood of developing dementia, which is more common with advancing age.

If You're Forgetting Things, You're Definitely Developing Dementia

Memory loss is one of the most common symptoms of all types of dementia, but it's by no means the only symptom. To be diagnosed with dementia, people need to have symptoms affecting not only their cognitive functions (like memory and thinking), but also their ability to carry out the normal activities of daily life.

A forgetful person may never develop these other problems and so steer clear of full-on dementia. However, if a person has noticeable cognitive impairment that isn't severe enough to interfere with daily life, he may be suffering from Mild Cognitive Impairment (MCI). MCI may affect up to 10 to 20 percent of people older than 65. Although MCI increases the risk of developing dementia, it doesn't always lead to dementia.

Red Wine Can Reverse Alzheimer's Disease

You may think this is purely wishful thinking, but scientific research is finding that a compound in red wine may be beneficial in preventing or even treating AD. But the idea that drinking a glass of merlot nightly will reverse AD is definitely false. Researchers have identified that red wine contains polyphenols including resveratrol that have been shown to decrease memory deterioration in mice by decreasing the development of amyloid plaques in their brains.

This study led to the idea that red wine may help prevent and treat AD. In 2015, the Alzheimer's Association funded a clinical trial to study the effect of these red grape-derived polyphenols in people experiencing the early stages of AD. Hopefully, this study will identify a new approach to AD treatment. But remember, no one is suggesting that drinking a lot of red wine will protect your brain from AD. It's clear that too much alcohol can negatively affect the brain. Although the jury is still out, having *one* glass of cabernet sauvignon nightly may be beneficial.

Appendix

Resources for Caregivers

I solation is a common problem among those caring for dementia and Alzheimer's patients because the demands of their caregiving responsibilities on top of the day-to-day demands of their lives leave very little time to socialize. That's where the Internet can help. It not only gives you the opportunity to meet other caregivers and discuss problems and concerns with them but also gives you an invaluable tool to research information about dementia and Alzheimer's disease (AD). (*Note:* Even though many of the websites listed here have "Alzheimer's" in their title, they generally have a good amount of information on dementia too.)

In this appendix, we introduce you to several invaluable Internet resources for caregivers. We provide the web address as well as a brief description of what type of information is available on the site. If none of the resources we've listed address your questions or concerns, simply pull up your favorite search engine and type in a couple of keywords related to your concern. You're bound to find something helpful; if not, contact someone at the Alzheimer's Association for help. We also include one book that has endured for more than 30 years and is recommended by the *Journal of the American Medical Association* and the *New York Times.*

AARP Caregiving

The AARP is one of the best sources in the country for information about aging (whether your own or a loved one's). At www.aarp.org/home-family/caregiving, you can get information about caregiving issues, find a local caregiver if you need a break, find out how to be a caregiver across the miles, and connect with experts.

ADEAR (Alzheimer's Disease Education and Referral)

The National Institute on Aging maintains an excellent website (www.nia.nih.gov/alzheimers) with a vast store of information about every aspect of Alzheimer's disease, from symptoms and causes to diagnosis and treatment. You can sign up for its emails and download a PDF of a terrific full-color book, *Alzheimer's Disease: Unraveling the Mystery.* The site also has information about current clinical trials and AD research centers. You can reach ADEAR experts by email (listed on the home page of the website) or its toll-free number (800-438-4380) from 8:30 a.m. until 5 p.m., Eastern Standard Time, Monday through Friday.

Alzheimer's Association

The Alzheimer's Association maintains a vast and comprehensive website (www.alz.org) for Alzheimer's patients and their families. It has up-to-date information about research, clinical trials, diagnosis, treatments, caregiving, and advocacy. Enter your zip code, and you get contact information for your local chapter. The site also offers resources in Spanish, French, Japanese, Korean, Vietnamese, and Chinese.

Alzheimer's Caregiver Support Online

Sponsored by the University of Florida, this site (www.alzonline.net) offers a lot of information of interest to caregivers. The site also includes a message board, a classroom with helpful videos, and a reading room with a variety of excellent articles for caregivers.

The Alzheimer's Foundation of America

The Alzheimer's Foundation of America is dedicated to improving the quality of life for AD patients and their families. Visit its website at www.alzfdn.org for a wealth of information about the disease, its diagnosis and treatment, and current research. The foundation also provides links to education, social services resources, and professional development for individuals who have dedicated their careers to AD research, treatment, and caregiving.

Benefitscheckup.org

The National Council on Aging maintains a website at www.benefitscheckup.org to help people age 55 and older find programs that may pay part or all of their cost for prescription drugs, healthcare, utilities, and other services. Just fill out a short questionnaire and the site will let you know what programs are available in your area and if you qualify.

Caregiver.com

This website offers information about a variety of topics that caregivers face when taking care of their loved one, including mental health, nutrition, and how to handle a patient's incontinence. The Alzheimer's Channel at www.caregiver.com/channels/alz/index.htm offers articles on a host of topics that caregivers face.

Caregiver Action Network

Caregivers created the Caregiver Action Network (http://caregiveraction.org; formerly the National Family Caregivers Association) for caregivers to share information, promote education and self-care for caregivers, and offer mutual support. The group hosts an active online forum and has posted videos about what it's like to be a caregiver.

Family Caregiver Alliance

The Family Caregiver Alliance maintains one of the very best sites for caregivers on the Web (www.caregiver.org). It has loads of statistics regarding caregivers and excellent, in-depth fact sheets for a variety of conditions that require a caregiver, including dementia and AD. Its monthly newsletters, available online, contain information and advice about a variety of topics of interest to caregivers. You can access Caregiver Connect, a place for caregivers to find and offer support. It also offers webinars for caregivers, plus an archive of past webinars.

Leeza's Care Connection

Leeza Gibbons has been an advocate of families affected by dementia and Alzheimer's disease ever since her mother was diagnosed with AD and her family became caregivers. Her foundation, the Leeza Gibbons Memory Foundation, operates www.leezascareconnection.org, which offers resources for caregivers that Gibbons wishes she'd had when access to caring for her mother. In addition to information about the disease and caregiving, you can find helpful articles on everything from legal and financial matters to mantras to get you through each day.

Medlineplus.gov

The National Institutes of Health and the United States National Library of Medicine maintain this comprehensive site (www.medlineplus.gov) with information on more than 600 health topics, including the latest information about dementia and AD. You can also find information about prescription and over-the-counter drugs and a medical encyclopedia and dictionary to help you understand some of the jargon your healthcare providers may throw at you. There's also a directory to help you find a healthcare provider near you and a breaking news section to help you keep up with the latest information.

Needymeds.com

Many older Americans live on limited budgets and have trouble finding the money to pay for the medicines they need. This site (www.needymeds.com) is an information source that links people who need help paying for medication to scholarship and charitable programs that pay part or all of the cost of their prescription drugs. Programs are available for all three widely used AD medications, including brand name Aricept, Exelon, and Reminyl. The site is easy to use and very informative.

One Book to Add to Your Shelf

If you're looking for a comprehensive guide to dementia and Alzheimer's disease that isn't a website (and in addition to this book), we recommend *The 36 Hour Day: A Family Guide to Caring for People with Alzheimer's Disease, related Dementias, and Memory Loss* by Nancy L. Mace, MA, and Peter V. Rabins, MD, MPH (published by Grand Central Life & Style). Originally published in 1981 and now in its fifth edition, this book remains the go-to reference for lay people on the subject of memory loss.

Index

endorphins, 333

end-stage dementia, in Clinical Dementia Rating (CDR) Scale, 121–122

energy, using up, 27

entertaining activities, offering, 190–191

environmental triggers, 59

estazolam (Prosom), as sleeping pills, 136

eszopiclone (Lunesta), as sleeping pills, 136

evaluating

capacity, 221

choices of evaluators, 77

communication skills, 99

competency, 221

coordination, 104–105

determining need for, 36–38

eye movements, 104–105

eye-hand coordination skills, 103

finding evaluators, 74–79

insurance coverage, 257–262

judgment, 102

memory, 101

motor skills, 103

orientation, 102–103

reasoning skills, 102

self-care skills, 99

simple math skills, 99

stages via cognitive and functional impairment, 116–122

exaggerated language, 161

examinations, for diagnosis, 85–89

executive functioning, 62

Exelon (Rivastigmine), 126, 129

exercise

for caregivers, 326

importance of, 390

providing, 189–190

as a risk factor for dementia, 54

extrapyramidal signs, identifying, 35

eye movements, evaluating, 104–105

eye specialists, 207–208

eye-hand coordination skills, evaluating, 103

F

failure to recognize, 316–317

Failure to Thrive, in Global Deterioration Scale (GDS), 115

falls, as symptom of dementia, 122

familiar objects, 353

family

balancing for caregivers, 362–365

caregiving and dynamics of, 368–371

getting help from, 264

navigating relationships, 369–370

prioritizing time with, 365–366

providing information on, 296–299

support from, 343–344

tips for, 387–394

Family and Medical Leave Act (FMLA) (1993), 357–358

Family Caregiver Alliance, 276, 310, 341, 360, 366, 404

family chronicler, 374

family doctor, for evaluations, 74–75

family history

dementia and, 50–51

for evaluation, 85

as a risk factor for Alzheimer's disease, 55

role of, 48–51

fatigue, fighting, 327

fats, 181

fear, 172, 315

fee based financial advisers, 254

fee only financial advisers, 254

feeding problems, as symptom of dementia, 121

fence, 194

fiber, 181

fight-or-flight hormone, 312

financial advisers

about, 251

cost issues, 253–255

types of, 252–253

what to look for with, 251–252

financial durable POA, 225

financial issues

  about, 243–244

  of caregivers, 337–338

  changes in tax status, 250

  evaluating insurance coverage, 257–262

  financial advisers, 251–255

  getting advice, 338

  managing, 383–389

  providing financial assistance, 373–375, 374–375

  quitting work, 255–257

  reviewing needs and resources, 244–247

  running out of resources, 263–264

  taking over, 247–250

flavonoids, 143

flexible working, changing to, 337–338

flu shot, for caregivers, 327

fluids, ingesting, 182

folic acid, 148

follow-up, 89–94

Folstein test, 98

foods, medical, 149–150

Forgetfulness Stage, in Global Deterioration Scale (GDS), 114

forgetting things, 22–26

formal support, 340–343

Foundation for Health in Aging (website), 291

fraud, 249

free radicals, 56, 142

fresh air, providing, 189–190

friends

  importance of, 336–337

  meeting, 330

  support from, 344

  tips for, 387–394

frontal lobe, 41, 43

frontotemporal dementia, 14, 47, 51

fruits, 180–181

frustration, as a negative emotion of caregivers, 319–320

Full code, 211

function, brain, 40–44

Functional Assessment Staging Tool (FAST), 113, 115–116

functional impairment, assessing stages via, 116–122

functional problems, 32–34

functional skills, measured by Clinical Dementia Rating (CDR) Scale, 117

funeral planning, 215

future costs, projecting, 245–246

future planning, encouraging, 388–389

G

galantamine (Razadyne), 127, 130, 134

gardening, 329, 333

gates, for stairs, 195

gender, Alzheimer's disease (AD) and, 398

general durable POA, 225

genes, role of, 48–51

genetic theories, 56–57

geriatricians, 76

Gibbons, Leeza (TV personality), 404

gingko biloba, 141–144

glabellar reflex, 104

Global Deterioration Scale (GDS), 15–16, 113

glutamate, 127

golf, 332

"good enough," 318

government agencies, 340–342

Grannie-cams, 195

grantor, 235

gray matter, 43

grief, as a negative emotion of caregivers, 321–322

grooming, simplifying, 174–175

Guanine (G), 49

guardianships

  about, 231–232

  awarding of, 232–233

  choosing, 233–234

  compared with durable POA, 234

  duties of guardians, 232

guilt, of caregivers, 313–315

H

habit, continuing with a, 27

habit training, 178

Halidol (haloperidol), 35

hallucinations, as a symptom, 30, 108, 121

haloperidol (Halidol), 35

handicap placards, 200

Harper, David (research psychologist), 192

Hartford Insurance Company (website), 199

head trauma theory, 59

health checks, importance of, 390–391

Health in Aging (website), 327

healthcare durable POA, 225

healthcare issues, 200–202

healthcare providers, 342

Heimlich maneuver, 188

Helicobacter pylori, 58

help and helping
  for abusive tendencies, 345–346
  for anger, 320
  from a distance, 372–375
  with eating, 185–188, 354
  from employers, 358–359
  for primary caregiver, 372–375
  sufficiency of existing, 268
  when to ask for, 344–346

hemispheres, 41

high blood pressure, as a risk factor for Alzheimer's disease, 55

high cholesterol, as a risk factor for Alzheimer's disease, 55

hippocampus, 44

hobbies, 330–331, 3857

home
  cost of adaptations, 273
  patient proofing your, 194–195

home and hobbies, measured by Clinical Dementia Rating (CDR) Scale, 116

home care, providing, 270–282

home health agencies, finding, 278–279

home health aides, finding, 275–277

home health-care aide, 269

home safety, 193–196

homocysteine, 148

Honor Guard, 176

hormonal causes, of dementia and Alzheimer's disease, 66–67

hospice programs, 245–246

hospitalizations
  admission process, 350–352
  emergency room process, 350–352
  helping at mealtimes, 354
  staff and doctors, 352–353
  visiting regularly, 353–354

household chores, paid in-home care for, 274

humor, as a coping mechanism, 333–334

Huntington's disease, as a cause of dementia and Alzheimer's disease, 66

huperzine A, 14–147

hydrocodone (Vicodin, Norco, Lortab), as a cause of dementia and Alzheimer's disease, 68

hyperparathyroidism, as a cause of dementia and Alzheimer's disease, 66–67

hypnotics, 136

I

icons, explained, 3

illness, fighting, 327

immune system theory, 59

impaired motor ability, 36

'in the loop,' 370–371

incontinence
  bowel, 178
  as symptom of dementia, 122
  urinary, 176–178

independence, ensuring, 169–170

infections, as symptom of dementia, 122

infectious causes, of dementia and Alzheimer's disease, 67–68

influenza, as a cause of dementia and Alzheimer's disease, 68

informal support, 340, 343–344

paid in-home care, hiring, 273–274

pain, relieving, 27

palliative care, 213–214

pampering, 328–329, 332–333

paperwork, managing, 247

paranoia, as a symptom, 29, 31–32, 121

parathyroid glands, 66–67

parent, becoming to your parent, 323

parietal lobe, 41, 44

Parkinson's disease, as a cause of dementia and Alzheimer's disease, 64–65

Part A coverage (Medicare), 258

Part B coverage (Medicare), 258

Part D coverage (Medicare), 258–259

partner, working with your, 382

pastimes, 385

patient, letting them know, 90

patient emotions, 202–204

patient proofing your home, 194–195

people, memory of, 25

percentage fee financial advisers, 254

permanent assets, 263

personal care
  importance of, 390–391
  measured by Clinical Dementia Rating (CDR) Scale, 117
  paid in-home care for, 274

personal care home, 270

personality, changes in, 21–22

pets, 191

Phantom Boarder syndrome, 31

phenytoin (Dilantin), as a cause of dementia and Alzheimer's disease, 68

photos, 191

physical aggression, 29–30

physical exams, 105–107

physical frailty, as symptom of dementia, 120

physical health
  of caregivers, 324–327
  managing, 384

physical restraints, 192

physical symptoms, 34–36, 312

physical therapists, 208

Physician Orders for Life Sustaining Treatment (POLST), 238

Physician Orders for Scope of Treatment (POST), 238

pill boxes, 202

places
  confusion over, 20
  memory of, 25

plan for care, ongoing, 89–94

planning, difficulty with, 19–20

Plavix (clopidogrel), 145

pneumonia, as a cause of dementia and Alzheimer's disease, 68

podiatrists, 201, 208

polyphenols, 399

portfolio managers, 253

positron emission tomography (PET) scan, 88, 107

Possible Mild Cognitive Impairment, in Global Deterioration Scale (GDS), 114

power of attorney (POA), 81, 212. See also durable power of attorney (POA)

practical issues, addressing, 94

Pradaxa, 145

prednisone, as a cause of dementia and Alzheimer's disease, 68

prescriptions
  as cause of dementia and Alzheimer's disease, 68
  providing information on, 300–301

prevalence, of Alzheimer's disease (AD), 60

primary auditory cortex, 44

primary care physicians (PCP), 206–207

primary caregiver, helping, 372–375

primitive reflexes, 104

principal, 224, 228

private companies, for meals, 183

private insurance, 261

probate, 235

problem solving
  difficulty with, 19–20
  measured by Clinical Dementia Rating (CDR) Scale, 117

S

Safe Return program, 195, 341

safety
  in the home, 193–196
  paid in-home care for, 274

salary financial advisers, 254

Savaysa, 145

scams, 161–162

Scharre, Douglas (Director of Cognitive Neurology), 160

scheduled toileting, 178

scheduling, 363–364

screening
  for Alzheimer's disease (AD), 98–103
  for dementia, 98–103

second opinions, 90

Securities and Exchange Commission (SEC), 253

self, memory of, 26

self-administered Gerocognitive Exam (SAGE), 160

self-administered tests, 160–161

self-care, lack of, as symptom of dementia, 120

self-care skills, assessing, 99–100

self-interest, 326

self-referred, 160

senior moments, compared with dementia, 18

sensory abilities, checking, 105

serenity, finding, 323–324

Severe Dementia
  in Functional Assessment Staging Tool (FAST), 116
  in Global Deterioration Scale (GDS), 115

Severe Impairment, in Clinical Dementia Rating (CDR) Scale, 120–121

sexual disinhibition, 31

short breaks, 3313

short-term memory, 23, 25, 45

side effects
  of antidepressant drugs, 135
  of antipsychotic drugs, 138
  of gingko biloba, 143–144
  of huperzine A, 147
  of medical treatments, 131–133
  of sleeping pills, 137
  of VITACOG, 148
  of vitamin E, 145

sight, reminiscence therapy and, 152

simple math skills, assessing, 99

single-photon emission computed tomography (SPECT) scan, 87–88

sitting service, paid in-home care for, 274

sleep aids, 136–137, 326–327

smell, reminiscence therapy and, 153

smoke alarms, 195

smoking, as a risk factor for dementia, 53

social aggression, 30

social history, 85

social opportunities, offering, 190–191

social problems, 30

Social Security (website), 277

social services, paid in-home care for, 274

social supports, managing, 93–94

Sonata (zaleplon), as sleeping pills, 136

sound, reminiscence therapy and, 152

Source for Senior Living (website), 276

Souvenaid (Nutricia), 1493

specialists
  bringing in, 207–209
  choosing, 75–77
  ear, teeth, and eye, 207–208
  mobility, 208
  referrals to, 88–89

Specialized Early Care for Alzheimer's (SPECAL), 157

speech
  checking, 105
  as symptom of dementia, 121

spiritual health, 324

sporting events, 332

spouse, working with your, 382

springing durable POA, 228, 234

staff, hospital, 352–353

T

take-out food, 332

tardive dyskinesia, 138

taste, reminiscence therapy and, 153

tax deductions, applying for, 338

tax status, changes in, 250

tea, 330

teams, building, 206–209

Technical Stuff icon, 3

teeth specialists, 207–208

Tegretol (carbamazepine), as a cause of dementia and Alzheimer's disease, 68

telephone support, providing, 373

temazepam (Restoril), as sleeping pills, 136

temporal lobe, 41, 44

terminal dementia, in Clinical Dementia Rating (CDR) Scale, 121–122

terpenoids, 143

testator, 239

testimonials, undocumented, 162

tests
  for diagnosing Alzheimer's disease, 95–109
  for diagnosis, 85–89
  driving, 197–198
  not recommended, 157–161

theories, on causes of Alzheimer's disease, 56–60

"They Can't Hang Up" document, 249

The 36 Hour Day: A Family Guide to Caring for People with Alzheimer's Disease, related Dementias, and Memory Loss (Mace and Rabins), 405

thought-processing problems, recognizing, 22–28

Thymine (T), 49

thyroid disease, as a cause of dementia and Alzheimer's disease, 66

thyroxine, 66

times
  confusion over, 20
  memory for, 24–25

Tip icon, 3

toileting, 178

touch, reminiscence therapy and, 152

tramadol (Ultram), as a cause of dementia and Alzheimer's disease, 68

transitions
  about, 295–296
  acting as an advocate, 304–306
  informing staff members about loved one, 296–299
  involvement in, 392
  to residential care, 283–285
  taking part in care/activities in the home, 303–304
  visiting regularly, 302–303

Transportable Physician Orders for Patient Preferences (TPOPP), 238

transportation providers, 199

treatments, not recommended, 157–161

triage, 350

trustee, 235

U

Ultram (tramadol), as a cause of dementia and Alzheimer's disease, 68

undocumented testimonials, 162

University of Florida (website), 342, 402

urinary incontinence, 176–178

urinary tract infection (UTI), 68, 178

US Department of Health and Human Services, 340

V

vacations, 331–332

validation therapy, 156

Valium (diazepam), 68, 136

vapories, aromatherapy and, 151

vascular dementia
  about, 13
  features of, 47
  genetics and, 50
  prevalence of, 64

vegetables, 180–181

ventricles, functions of, 44

Notes

Notes

About the American Geriatrics Society

Founded in 1942, the American Geriatrics Society (AGS) is a nationwide, nonprofit society of geriatrics healthcare professionals dedicated to improving the health, independence, and quality of life of older people. Its nearly 6,000 members include geriatricians, geriatric nurses, social workers, family practitioners, physician assistants, pharmacists, and internists. The Society provides leadership to healthcare professionals, policymakers, and the public by implementing and advocating for programs in patient care, research, professional and public education, and public policy. For more information, visit www.americangeriatrics.org.

About The Health in Aging Foundation

The Health in Aging Foundation is a national nonprofit organization established in 1999 by the American Geriatrics Society to bring the knowledge and expertise of geriatrics healthcare professionals to the public. The Foundation is committed to ensuring that the public is empowered to advocate for high quality care for themselves or their loved ones, by providing them with trustworthy information and resources. For more information, visit www.healthinagingfoundation.org.

About the Authors

Michael Wasserman, MD, completed his medical degree at the University of Texas, Medical Branch before completing his internal medicine residency at Cedars-Sinai Medical Center and Geriatric Fellowship at UCLA. He co-founded Senior Care of Colorado, which became one of the largest privately owned primary care geriatric practices in the country over a period of ten years. A Certified Medical Director, he is presently Director, Nursing Home QIN-QIO, for Health Services Advisory Group in California, where he is focused on bringing person-centered care to residents of nursing facilities.

Wasserman previously was president and chief medical officer for GeriMed of America, a geriatric medical management company in Denver, Colorado. He is past chair of the American Geriatric Society's Managed Care Task Force and presently serves on the Public Policy Committee. He was formerly a public commissioner for the Continuing Care Accreditation Commission. Wasserman serves on the Boards of The Wish of a Lifetime Foundation and The Foundation for Health In Aging. He has spoken extensively and been published on a variety of topics, involving geriatrics, Alzheimer's disease, practice management, and managed care.

Simon Atkins, MD, qualified as a doctor in 1995 and has been a full-time GP partner in Bristol since 2000. He holds degrees in physiology with psychology from Southampton University and medicine from Bristol University, and has a master's degree in science communication from the University of the West of England.

Mark Edwin Kunik, MD, MPH, is a leading expert on dementia. He is a practicing geropsychiatrist who has conducted extensive clinical and health services research on dementia. Kunik has done a lot to improve the quality of life for people with dementia, both as a caring physician to his patients and as a researcher who has published more than 40 papers on dementia-related issues alone.

Mary Kenan, PhD, is a faculty member with the Department of Neurology at Baylor College of Medicine and is a licensed clinical psychologist. She received her B.A. from the University of Oklahoma and her doctorate in clinical psychology from Indiana State University. She completed her clinical internship and a postdoctoral fellowship in geriatric psychology at the Houston Veterans Affairs Medical Center, where she then served as a staff psychologist. In 1999, Kenan assumed her current position as the Director of Education and patient/family counselor for Baylor College of Medicine's Alzheimer's Disease Center.

Patricia Burkhart Smith is an award-winning health and medical writer. She wrote for *People* magazine for six years. She co-reported a 1998 cover story on breast cancer that won the Society of Professional Journalists' Peter Lisagor Award for Excellence in Journalism. She also co-reported a 1999 cover story on anorexia that won a second place Time Inc. Luce Award. In 1984, Ms. Smith lost her mother to Alzheimer's and in 1995, her favorite aunt lost her battle with the disease. The two deaths fueled Ms. Smith's desire to learn as much as she could about Alzheimer's and share that information with people dealing with the same problems and decisions her own family faced.

Publisher's Acknowledgments

Compiler: Victoria M. Adang

Senior Acquisitions Editor: Tracy Boggier

Project Manager: Chad R. Sievers

Development Editor/Copy Editor: Chad R. Sievers

Technical Editor: Allison J. Batchelor, MD, CMD

Production Editor: Siddique Shaik

Cover Image: goa novi/Shutterstock

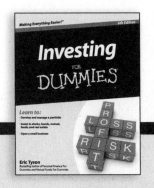
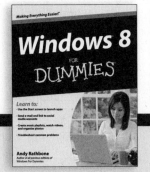
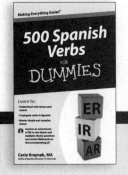
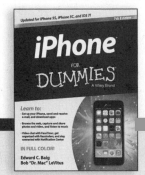

Math & Science

Algebra I For Dummies,
2nd Edition
978-0-470-55964-2

Anatomy and Physiology
For Dummies, 2nd Edition
978-0-470-92326-9

Astronomy For Dummies,
3rd Edition
978-1-118-37697-3

Biology For Dummies,
2nd Edition
978-0-470-59875-7

Chemistry For Dummies,
2nd Edition
978-1-118-00730-3

1001 Algebra II Practice
Problems For Dummies
978-1-118-44662-1

Microsoft Office

Excel 2013 For Dummies
978-1-118-51012-4

Office 2013 All-in-One
For Dummies
978-1-118-51636-2

PowerPoint 2013
For Dummies
978-1-118-50253-2

Word 2013 For Dummies
978-1-118-49123-2

Music

Blues Harmonica
For Dummies
978-1-118-25269-7

Guitar For Dummies,
3rd Edition
978-1-118-11554-1

iPod & iTunes
For Dummies, 10th Edition
978-1-118-50864-0

Programming

Beginning Programming
with C For Dummies
978-1-118-73763-7

Excel VBA Programming
For Dummies, 3rd Edition
978-1-118-49037-2

Java For Dummies,
6th Edition
978-1-118-40780-6

Religion & Inspiration

The Bible For Dummies
978-0-7645-5296-0

Buddhism For Dummies,
2nd Edition
978-1-118-02379-2

Catholicism For Dummies,
2nd Edition
978-1-118-07778-8

Self-Help & Relationships

Beating Sugar Addiction
For Dummies
978-1-118-54645-1

Meditation For Dummies,
3rd Edition
978-1-118-29144-3

Seniors

Laptops For Seniors
For Dummies, 3rd Edition
978-1-118-71105-7

Computers For Seniors
For Dummies, 3rd Edition
978-1-118-11553-4

iPad For Seniors
For Dummies, 6th Edition
978-1-118-72826-0

Social Security
For Dummies
978-1-118-20573-0

Smartphones & Tablets

Android Phones
For Dummies, 2nd Edition
978-1-118-72030-1

Nexus Tablets
For Dummies
978-1-118-77243-0

Samsung Galaxy S 4
For Dummies
978-1-118-64222-1

Samsung Galaxy Tabs
For Dummies
978-1-118-77294-2

Test Prep

ACT For Dummies,
5th Edition
978-1-118-01259-8

ASVAB For Dummies,
3rd Edition
978-0-470-63760-9

GRE For Dummies,
7th Edition
978-0-470-88921-3

Officer Candidate Tests
For Dummies
978-0-470-59876-4

Physician's Assistant Exam
For Dummies
978-1-118-11556-5

Series 7 Exam For Dummie
978-0-470-09932-2

Windows 8

Windows 8.1 All-in-One
For Dummies
978-1-118-82087-2

Windows 8.1 For Dummies
978-1-118-82121-3

Windows 8.1 For Dummies
Book + DVD Bundle
978-1-118-82107-7

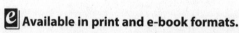 **Available in print and e-book formats.**

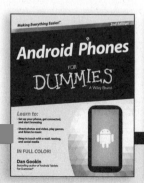

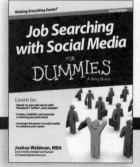

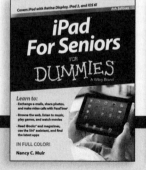

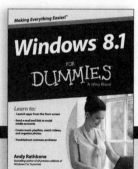

Available wherever books are sold. **For more information or to order direct visit www.dummies.com**

Take Dummies with you everywhere you go!

Whether you are excited about e-books, want more from the web, must have your mobile apps, or are swept up in social media, Dummies makes everything easier.

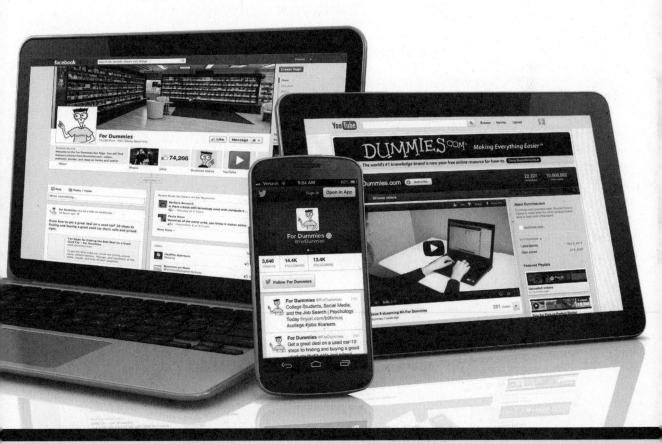

 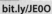

For Dummies is the global leader in the reference category and one of the most trusted and highly regarded brands in the world. No longer just focused on books, customers now have access to the For Dummies content they need in the format they want. Let us help you develop a solution that will fit your brand and help you connect with your customers.

Advertising & Sponsorships

Connect with an engaged audience on a powerful multimedia site, and position your message alongside expert how-to content.

Targeted ads • Video • Email marketing • Microsites • Sweepstakes sponsorship

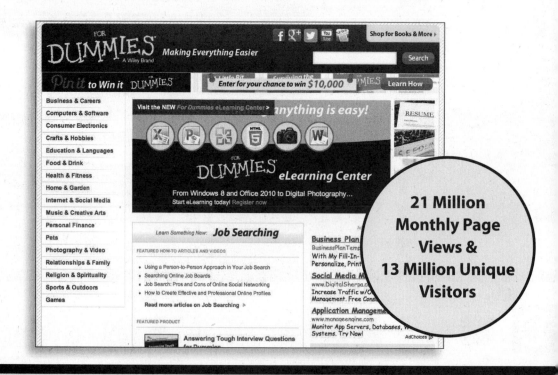

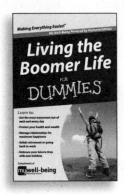
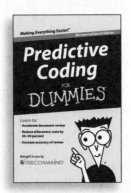
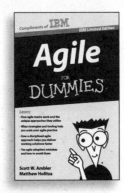
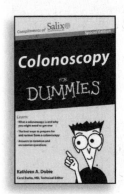
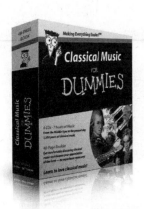
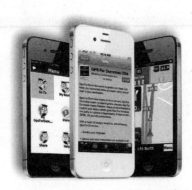
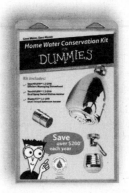
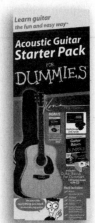
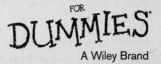

Dummies products make life easier!

- DIY
- Consumer Electronics
- Crafts

- Software
- Cookware
- Hobbies

- Videos
- Music
- Games
- and More!

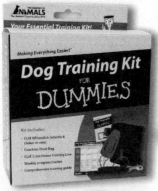

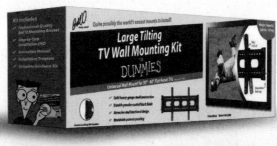
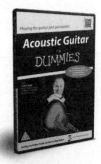

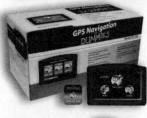
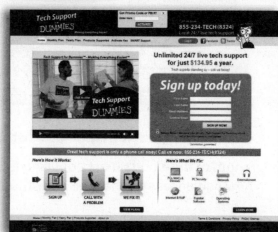
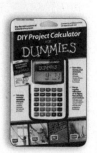

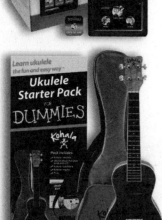
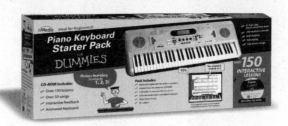
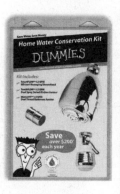

For more information, go to **Dummies.com** and search the store by category.

FOR
DUMMIES

A Wiley Brand